Nutrition, Diet Quality, Aging and Frailty

Nutrition, Diet Quality, Aging and Frailty

Editors

Cristiano Capurso
Catherine Féart

MDPI • Basel • Beijing • Wuhan • Barcelona • Belgrade • Manchester • Tokyo • Cluj • Tianjin

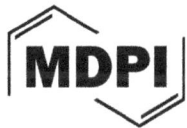

Editors
Cristiano Capurso
University of Foggia
Italy

Catherine Féart
University of Bordeaux
France

Editorial Office
MDPI
St. Alban-Anlage 66
4052 Basel, Switzerland

This is a reprint of articles from the Special Issue published online in the open access journal *Nutrients* (ISSN 2072-6643) (available at: https://www.mdpi.com/journal/nutrients/special_issues/Nutrition_Frailty).

For citation purposes, cite each article independently as indicated on the article page online and as indicated below:

LastName, A.A.; LastName, B.B.; LastName, C.C. Article Title. *Journal Name* **Year**, *Volume Number*, Page Range.

ISBN 978-3-0365-6065-6 (Hbk)
ISBN 978-3-0365-6066-3 (PDF)

© 2022 by the authors. Articles in this book are Open Access and distributed under the Creative Commons Attribution (CC BY) license, which allows users to download, copy and build upon published articles, as long as the author and publisher are properly credited, which ensures maximum dissemination and a wider impact of our publications.

The book as a whole is distributed by MDPI under the terms and conditions of the Creative Commons license CC BY-NC-ND.

Contents

About the Editors vii

Preface to "Nutrition, Diet Quality, Aging and Frailty" ix

Austin M. Reilly, Andy P. Tsai, Peter B. Lin, Aaron C. Ericsson, Adrian L. Oblak and Hongxia Ren
Metabolic Defects Caused by High-Fat Diet Modify Disease Risk through Inflammatory and Amyloidogenic Pathways in a Mouse Model of Alzheimer's Disease
Reprinted from: *Nutrients* **2020**, *12*, 2977, doi:10.3390/nu12102977 1

Daljeet Singh Dhanjal, Sonali Bhardwaj, Ruchi Sharma, Kanchan Bhardwaj, Dinesh Kumar, Chirag Chopra, Eugenie Nepovimova, Reena Singh and Kamil Kuca
Plant Fortification of the Diet for Anti-Ageing Effects: A Review
Reprinted from: *Nutrients* **2020**, *12*, 3008, doi:10.3390/nu12103008 19

Alejandro Gaytán-González, María de Jesús Ocampo-Alfaro, Francisco Torres-Naranjo, Roberto Gabriel González-Mendoza, Martha Gil-Barreiro, Maritza Arroniz-Rivera and Juan R. López-Taylor
Dietary Protein Intake Patterns and Inadequate Protein Intake in Older Adults from Four Countries
Reprinted from: *Nutrients* **2020**, *12*, 3156, doi:10.3390/nu12103156 43

Hendrik Nieraad, Natasja de Bruin, Olga Arne, Martine C. J. Hofmann, Mike Schmidt, Takashi Saito, Takaomi C. Saido, Robert Gurke, Dominik Schmidt, Uwe Till, Michael J. Parnham and Gerd Geisslinger
Impact of Hyperhomocysteinemia and Different Dietary Interventions on Cognitive Performance in a Knock-in Mouse Model for Alzheimer's Disease
Reprinted from: *Nutrients* **2020**, *12*, 3248, doi:10.3390/nu12113248 61

Jian Zhang, Ai Zhao, Wei Wu, Zhongxia Ren, Chenlu Yang, Peiyu Wang and Yumei Zhang
Beneficial Effect of Dietary Diversity on the Risk of Disability in Activities of Daily Living in Adults: A Prospective Cohort Study
Reprinted from: *Nutrients* **2020**, *12*, 3263, doi:10.3390/nu12113263 89

Yoshiaki Nomura, Erika Kakuta, Ayako Okada, Ryoko Otsuka, Mieko Shimada, Yasuko Tomizawa, Chieko Taguchi, Kazumune Arikawa, Hideki Daikoku, Tamotsu Sato and Nobuhiro Hanada
Impact of the Serum Level of Albumin and Self-Assessed Chewing Ability on Mortality, QOL, and ADLs for Community-Dwelling Older Adults at the Age of 85: A 15 Year Follow up Study
Reprinted from: *Nutrients* **2020**, *12*, 3315, doi:10.3390/nu12113315 101

Adriana Caldo-Silva, Guilherme Eustáquio Furtado, Matheus Uba Chupel, André L. L. Bachi, Marcelo P. de Barros, Rafael Neves, Emanuele Marzetti, Alain Massart and Ana Maria Teixeira
Effect of Training-Detraining Phases of Multicomponent Exercises and BCAA Supplementation on Inflammatory Markers and Albumin Levels in Frail Older Persons
Reprinted from: *Nutrients* **2021**, *13*, 1106, doi:10.3390/nu13041106 117

Marlene Gojanovic, Kara L. Holloway-Kew, Natalie K. Hyde, Mohammadreza Mohebbi, Nitin Shivappa, James R. Hebert, Adrienne O'Neil and Julie A. Pasco
The Dietary Inflammatory Index Is Associated with Low Muscle Mass and Low Muscle Function in Older Australians
Reprinted from: *Nutrients* **2020**, *13*, 1166, doi:10.3390/nu13041166 135

Zi Chen, Wei-Ying Li, Mandy Ho and Pui-Hing Chau
The Prevalence of Sarcopenia in Chinese Older Adults: Meta-Analysis and Meta-Regression
Reprinted from: *Nutrients* **2021**, *13*, 1441, doi:10.3390/nu13051441 147

Berna Rahi, Hermine Pellay, Virginie Chuy, Catherine Helmer, Cecilia Samieri and Catherine Féart
Dairy Product Intake and Long-Term Risk for Frailty among French Elderly Community Dwellers
Reprinted from: *Nutrients* **2021**, *13*, 2151, doi:10.3390/nu13072151 163

Nathalie Yaghi, Cesar Yaghi, Marianne Abifadel, Christa Boulos and Catherine Feart
Dietary Patterns and Risk Factors of Frailty in Lebanese Older Adults
Reprinted from: *Nutrients* **2021**, *13*, 2188, doi:10.3390/nu13072188 177

Cristiano Capurso
Whole-Grain Intake in the Mediterranean Diet and a Low Protein to Carbohydrates Ratio Can Help to Reduce Mortality from Cardiovascular Disease, Slow Down the Progression of Aging, and to Improve Lifespan: A Review
Reprinted from: *Nutrients* **2021**, *13*, 2540, doi:10.3390/nu13082540 193

About the Editors

Cristiano Capurso

Cristiano Capurso is currently working as Associate Professor at the Department of Surgical and Medical Sciences of the University of Foggia, Italy. He holds a medical degree and a specialization in Geriatric Medicine from the University of Bari, Italy. She also holds a PhD in Carcinogenesis, Aging and Immunoregulation from the University of Bari, Italy. His research interests include cognitive decline, hyperlipidaemia, atherosclerosis, diet pattern, i.e., the Mediterranean Diet, and markers for human longevity. He has more two decades of experience in these fields. He has published approximately 129 papers in peer-reviewed journals. He has also collaborated with other researchers to publish a scientific book in English with Springer and a chapter of the volume "Principles of Nutrigenetics and Nutrigenomics" with Elsevier. He is a member of the Italian Society of Gerontology and Geriatrics, of the Italian Society for the Study of Atherosclerosis, and of Italian Society of Internal Medicine.

Catherine Féart

Catherine Féart is currently working as tenured researcher at the Bordeaux Population Health research center of the INSERM, University of Bordeaux, France. She holds a PhD in Nutrition and Food Sciences, and a Qualification to Direct Researches (HDR) in Public Health and Epidemiology. Her research focuses on the relationship between nutrition and food intake and the onset of geriatric syndromes, using the tools of the nutritional epidemiology field. She is mainly interested in the potential benefit of specific nutrients, foods and dietary patterns on the risk of developing mental disorders, including dementia and depression, and physical frailty and by the underlying mechanisms, including the role of gut microbiota and inflammation on these relationships. She has published around 120 papers (original articles and reviews) in peer-reviewed journals. She is a member of the steering committees of the French Society of Nutrition (SFN) and of the Group Lipids and Nutrition (GLN) and is the leader of the University Diploma (DU) Nutritional epidemiology via the internet at the University of Bordeaux.

Preface to "Nutrition, Diet Quality, Aging and Frailty"

In the last century, the average life expectancy at birth increased from roughly 45 years in the early 1900s to more than 80 years of age at present. However, living longer is often related to different levels of frailty. There is no curative treatment for frailty—the interventions that have been described as effective to slow or delay the onset of frailty are physical activity and nutritional interventions. Maintaining adequate nutrition status is important to reduce the risk of chronic diseases, many of which are age-related. On the other hand, frailty itself may have a negative effect on eating and, thus, on the nutritional status.

The main goal of this Special Issue is to address existing knowledge on nutrition regarding the causative factors of frailty and disease due to aging, i.e., strategies for delaying the pathological effects of aging.

Published articles cover original research, protocol development, methodological studies, narrative or systematic reviews, and meta-analyses regarding the role of dietary patterns and the different aspects of frailty, from reduced muscle mass and strength to cognitive function, to impaired autonomy, or the slowing of aging. In addition, the articles published are concerned with the role of specific elements, such as albumin, homocysteine, fatty acids, and dairy products, in the different aspects of frailty and aging in cohort studies and animal models.

Beyond this Special Issue, of course, there remains a need for further research to address the multiple factors that determine longevity and aging, which naturally also involve nutrition.

Finally, we would like to express our most profound appreciation to the MDPI Book staff, the editorial team of Nutrients journal, the Assistant Editor of this Special Issue Ms. Stella Duo, the Managing Editor Ms. Chloe Wang, and all authors and the hardworking and professional reviewers.

Cristiano Capurso and Catherine Féart
Editors

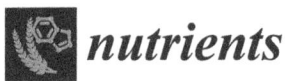

Article

Metabolic Defects Caused by High-Fat Diet Modify Disease Risk through Inflammatory and Amyloidogenic Pathways in a Mouse Model of Alzheimer's Disease

Austin M. Reilly [1], Andy P. Tsai [1], Peter B. Lin [1], Aaron C. Ericsson [2], Adrian L. Oblak [1] and Hongxia Ren [1,3,4,5,6,7,*,†]

1. Stark Neurosciences Research Institute, Medical Neuroscience Graduate Program, Indiana University School of Medicine, Indianapolis, IN 46202, USA; aureilly@iu.edu (A.M.R.); tandy@iu.edu (A.P.T.); pblin@iu.edu (P.B.L.); aoblak@iupui.edu (A.L.O.)
2. Metagenomics Center, University of Missouri, Columbia, MO 65201, USA; EricssonA@missouri.edu
3. Herman B. Wells Center for Pediatric Research, Department of Pediatrics, Indiana University School of Medicine, Indianapolis, IN 46202, USA
4. Center for Diabetes and Metabolic Diseases, Indiana University School of Medicine, Indianapolis, IN 46202, USA
5. Department of Biochemistry & Molecular Biology, Indiana University School of Medicine, Indianapolis, IN 46202, USA
6. Department of Pharmacology & Toxicology, Indiana University School of Medicine, Indianapolis, IN 46202, USA
7. Department of Anatomy and Cell Biology, Indiana University School of Medicine, Indianapolis, IN 46202, USA
* Correspondence: renh@iu.edu; Tel.: +1-317-274-1567
† Postal address: Indiana University School of Medicine, 635 Barnhill Dr., MS2031, Indianapolis, IN 46202, USA.

Received: 31 August 2020; Accepted: 25 September 2020; Published: 29 September 2020

Abstract: High-fat diet (HFD) has been shown to accelerate Alzheimer's disease (AD) pathology, but the exact molecular and cellular mechanisms remain incompletely understood. Moreover, it is unknown whether AD mice are more susceptible to HFD-induced metabolic dysfunctions. To address these questions, we used 5xFAD mice as an Alzheimer's disease model to study the physiological and molecular underpinning between HFD-induced metabolic defects and AD pathology. We systematically profiled the metabolic parameters, the gut microbiome composition, and hippocampal gene expression in 5xFAD and wild type (WT) mice fed normal chow diet and HFD. HFD feeding impaired energy metabolism in male 5xFAD mice, leading to increased locomotor activity, energy expenditure, and food intake. 5xFAD mice on HFD had elevated circulating lipids and worsened glucose intolerance. HFD caused profound changes in gut microbiome compositions, though no difference between genotype was detected. We measured hippocampal mRNAs related to AD neuropathology and neuroinflammation and showed that HFD elevated the expression of apoptotic, microglial, and amyloidogenic genes in 5xFAD mice. Pathway analysis revealed that differentially regulated genes were involved in insulin signaling, cytokine signaling, cellular stress, and neurotransmission. Collectively, our results showed that 5xFAD mice were more susceptible to HFD-induced metabolic dysregulation and suggest that targeting metabolic dysfunctions can ameliorate AD symptoms via effects on insulin signaling and neuroinflammation in the hippocampus.

Keywords: diet; metabolism; nutrient; glucose; lipid; insulin; neuroinflammation; Alzheimer's disease

1. Introduction

Alzheimer's disease (AD) is the most prevalent cause of dementia in the elderly. AD is a progressive and devastating neurological disease, which begins with mild memory loss and eventually can seriously compromise a person's ability to carry out daily activities. With its increasing prevalence in today's aging society, AD has become a pressing global health concern [1]. The most characteristic neuropathological hallmarks of AD are the accumulation of extracellular Aβ plaques and intracellular neurofibrillary Tau tangles in the brain [2]. Additional AD biomarkers may lead to earlier diagnosis and interventions targeting the preclinical, asymptomatic stages of the disease [3]. Key molecular pathways have been implicated in the initiation and progression of the neuropathological cascade, which could provide potential targets for developing biomarkers and therapeutic strategies. A growing body of recent studies shows that increased neuroinflammation and impaired cellular metabolism may be the underlying cause of AD pathology [4–7]. Compelling epidemiological evidence points to a mechanistic connection between impaired metabolic homeostasis, age-associated cognitive impairment, and neurodegenerative diseases characterized by cognitive disorders [8,9]. Patients with diabetes develop more cognitive dysfunction and have a greater incidence of AD than non-diabetics [8]. In a meta-analysis of prospective studies, diabetes increased the relative risk of AD by 56% [10]. Glycated hemoglobin (HbA1c), a biomarker of diabetes severity and duration, is a top correlate of brain atrophy [11]. Aberrant glucose metabolism has been linked to amyloid deposition and brain cognitive dysfunction [12–14]. Brain insulin resistance causes metabolic and bioenergetic defects, which is a potential contributing factor to cognitive impairment and AD pathogenesis [9,15–17]. With the prevalence of both AD and diabetes on the rise, studies of potential mechanisms that underlie common predisposing factors are paramount.

Studies have suggested that diet and nutrition may play a role in the development of AD [18]. The Mediterranean diet (MeDi) is associated with a lower incidence of chronic diseases and shows protective effects against cognitive decline in aging individuals [19–22]. Conversely, the overconsumption of high-sugar and high-fat diets coupled with sedentary lifestyle predisposes individuals to metabolic diseases and neurocognitive defects during the aging process. High-fat diet (HFD) causes nutritional excess and promotes obesity and other key components of metabolic syndrome, such as systemic inflammation, dyslipidemia, insulin resistance, and elevated blood glucose [23] thereby contributing to AD pathogenesis. Indeed, previous studies showed that HFD feeding in a transgenic mouse model harboring five familial AD mutations (5xFAD) had increased amyloid deposition and impaired performance in memory and learning tasks [24,25]. 5xFAD is an early onset mouse model of Alzheimer's disease harboring five AD-associated mutations in human *APP* and *PS1* which causes rapid progression of amyloid pathology due to the increased generation of insoluble Aβ isoforms [26]. However, the mechanisms linking high-fat diet to AD progression are still under investigation, and it remains unknown whether transgenic AD mouse models are more susceptible to HFD-induced metabolic derangements. Moreover, the exact molecular mechanisms of how nutrient excess caused by HFD feeding exacerbates AD pathophysiology remain largely undefined. In the present study, we set out to address these questions by studying the metabolic phenotype in the 5xFAD mouse model on normal chow diet (NCD) and high-fat diet (HFD). Our results demonstrated that HFD more severely impacted the metabolic homeostasis of transgenic AD mice compared to control mice. Furthermore, we characterized the changes in the gut microbiome and profiled hippocampal gene transcription of transgenic AD mice on NCD versus HFD. We revealed the specific effects of HFD on the hippocampi of the transgenic AD mice in terms of individual gene transcription and the collective changes in the neuropathology and neuroinflammatory pathways, thereby providing potential targets for AD therapy.

2. Experimental Procedures

2.1. Experimental Animals

All mice were maintained in the Indiana University School of Medicine Lab animal resource center (LARC) facility on a 12:12 h light: dark cycle. All animal protocols were approved by Indiana University IACUC (IACUC#11121, 11258, 19013, 20007, PI's Ren and Oblak).). 5xFAD (mouse line Tg6799) heterozygous mice [26] are available from The Jackson Laboratory (https://www.jax.org/strain/008730) and a colony is maintained at Indiana University. Age-matched littermates lacking 5xFAD, hereafter called wild type (WT) mice, were used as controls. For gene expression studies, NCD mice were anesthetized with Avertin and transcardially perfused with ice-cold PBS. Frozen brain tissue was homogenized in T-PER buffer, RNase-free water, and stored in an equal volume of STAT-60 (tel-test inc, CS502) at −80 °C. HFD mice were euthanized with CO_2 and tissues were stored at −80 °C.

2.2. Dietary Treatment

For metabolic profiling studies presented in Figures 1–4 and Supplemental Figures S2 and S4, mice were raised on 62.1% of calories from carbohydrates, 24.6% from protein, and 13.2% from fat (LabDiet, catalog #5053, Richmond, IN, USA) prior to starting HFD (Supplemental Figure S1A). At 3 months old, mice were switched to HFD containing 60% calories from lard-based fat, 20% from protein, 20% from carbohydrate (Research Diets, catalog #D12492, New Brunswick, NJ, USA). Mice had ad libitum access to food except for fasting/refeeding experiments as indicated in the figures and legends. Lean mass and fat mass were determined by MRI scan (EchoMRI-100, EchoMRI Houston, TX, USA). For microbiome and gene expression profiling studies presented in Figures 5 and 6 and (Supplemental Figures S3 and S5), age-matched NCD-fed WT and 5xFAD mice were fed 19.3% protein, 16.6% fat, 61.3% carbohydrates (LabDiet, catalog #5K52, Richmond, IN, USA) (Supplemental Figure S1B).

2.3. Glucose Measurements

Tail blood glucose was measured with AlphaTRAK 2 (Zoetis Inc., catalog #71681-01 and 71676-01, Kalamazoo, MO, USA) during ad libitum feeding, after 5 h of daytime fasting, or after 16 h overnight fasting. Oral glucose tolerance test (oGTT, 2 g/kg) in NCD-fed mice was performed after 16-h fasting. HFD-fed mice were given oGTT (3 g/kg) after 5-h fasting.

2.4. Serum Biochemistries

Serum was collected by tail vein bleeding or cardiac puncture during ad libitum feeding, daytime short fasting (5 h), overnight fasting (~16 h), and refeeding (4–5 h of feeding after overnight fast). Serum insulin was measured by ELISA (EMD Millipore, catalog #EZRMI-13K, Bellerica, MA, USA). Colorimetric assays were used to detect serum triglycerides (Thermo Fisher, catalog #TR22421, Middletown, VA, USA), free cholesterol E (Wako, catalog #990-02511, Chuo-Ku Osaka, Japan), glycerol (Sigma, catalog #F6428-40mL, St. Louis, MO, USA), and non-esterified fatty acids (NEFA) (Wako, catalog #999-34691, 995-34791, 991-34891, 993-35191, Chuo-Ku Osaka, Japan). All reactions were performed according to manufacturer protocols.

2.5. Indirect Calorimetry

Indirect calorimetry measurements were collected using a TSE PhenoMaster Platform (TSE Systems, Chesterfield, MO, USA) as described previously [27]. Briefly, mice were individually housed for a 48 h acclimation period before recording data used for analysis. Metabolic parameters (locomotor activity, food intake, energy expenditure, oxygen consumption, respiratory exchange ratio) were measured at 36 min intervals during a normal 12-h light/dark cycle. Total body weight and lean mass were determined beforehand by MRI scan (EchoMRI-100, EchoMRI Houston, TX, USA) for calculations.

2.6. Hippocampal mRNA Quantitation

For each mouse, RNA was extracted from one hippocampus. HFD samples (left or right hippocampi) were extracted using Trizol reagent (Invitrogen, catalog #15596018, Carlsbad, CA, USA). NCD samples (left hippocampus) were extracted using STAT-60 reagent (Tel-Test, catalog #CS-502, Friendswood, TX, USA) and purified by using the Purelink RNA Mini Kit (Life Technologies, catalog #12183025, Carlsbad, CA, USA). The mRNA transcripts were detected using sequence-specific fluorescently barcoded probes (Nanostring Technologies, nCounter Neuropathology and nCounter Neuroinflammation; catalog numbers XT-CSO-MNROP1-12 and XT-CSO-MNROI1-12, respectively, Seattle, WA, USA). 200 ng of RNA was loaded for all samples and hybridized with probes for 16 h at 65 degrees Celsius. Results obtained from nCounter MAX Analysis System (NanoString Technologies, catalog #NCT-SYST-LS, Seattle WA) were imported to nSolver Analysis Software (v4.0; NanoString Technologies) for QC verification, normalization, and data statistics using Advanced Analysis (v2.0.115; NanoString Technologies). Probes were only included if the read count was more than 3 standard deviations above background, and probes that had <100 reads for 6 or more samples were removed from analysis. For comparisons between genes of interest, expression data were normalized to WT mice on the same diet. All assays were performed according to manufacturer protocols.

2.7. 16S rRNA Library Preparation and Sequencing

Library preparation and sequencing were performed at the University of Missouri DNA Core Facility. Bacterial 16S rRNA amplicon libraries were generated via amplification of the 16S rRNA gene with primers (U515F/806R) previously developed against the V4 region, flanked by Illumina standard adapter sequences [28,29]. Dual-indexed F and R primers were used in all reactions. Amplification was performed in 50 µL reactions containing 100 ng fecal DNA, F and R primers (0.2 µM each), dNTPs (200 µM each), and Phusion high-fidelity DNA polymerase (1U). PCR parameters were as follows: $98\,°C^{(3min)} + [98\,°C^{(15sec)} + 50\,°C^{(30sec)} + 72\,°C^{(30sec)}] \times 25$ cycles $+ 72\,°C^{(7min)}$. Following PCR, amplicon pools (5 µL/reaction) were combined, mixed, and purified using Axygen™ Axyprep MagPCR clean-up beads at an equal volume of 50 µL of amplicons and incubation at room temperature (RT) for 15 min. Following clean-up, products were washed multiple times with 80% ethanol, resuspended in 32.5 µL EB buffer, incubated for two minutes at RT, and then placed on a magnetic stand for five minutes. Final amplicon pools were evaluated using an Advanced Analytical Fragment Analyzer automated electrophoresis system, quantified using a Qubit 2.0 fluorometer and quant-iT HS dsDNA kits, and diluted according to Illumina's standard protocol for sequencing on the MiSeq instrument using V2 chemistry kits.

2.8. Informatics Analysis of 16S rRNA Sequences

Sequenced DNA was assembled and annotated at the University of Missouri Informatics Research Core. Primers were designed to match the 5′ ends of forward and reverse reads. Using Cutadapt (version 2.6; https://github.com/marcelm/cutadapt; [30]) software, the primer sequence and its reverse complement were removed from the 5′ end of the forward read, along with all bases downstream of the latter. The same approach was applied to the reverse read, with primers in the opposite roles. The 16S rRNA libraries were generated at 25 cycles. Read pairs were rejected if either read failed to match a 5′ primer, using an allowed error-rate of 0.1. The Qiime2 dada2 plugin (version 1.10.0; [31]) was used to denoise, de-replicate, and count amplicon sequence variants (ASVs), based on the following parameters: (1) forward and reverse reads were trimmed to 150 bases, (2) forward and reverse reads with >2 expected errors were discarded, and 3) chimera detection and removal were performed using the "consensus" method. R version 3.5.1 and Biom version 2.1.7 were used in Qiime2. Taxonomies were assigned to trimmed sequences using the Silva.v132 database [32], using the classify-sklearn procedure.

2.9. Statistics

Statistical methods and number of mice per group can be found in the corresponding figure legends, with the exception of microbiome analyses, which can be found in 'Methods'.

2.10. Statistical Analysis of Annotated Sequences

Statistical analysis of β-diversity between groups was performed using $\frac{1}{4}$ root transformed relative amplicon sequence variant (ASV) abundances. Experimental groups were compared with one-way permutational multivariate analysis of variance (PERMANOVA) of Bray-Curtis and Jaccard distances using Past 3.26b. The corrected p-values for pairwise statistical comparisons were calculated using Bonferroni's method. Heatmaps and hierarchical clustering dendrograms were generated in Metaboanalyst 4.0 (https://www.metaboanalyst.ca/). Data were cube-root transformed and clustered using Ward's method based on Euclidean distances. The top 50 most statistically significant ASV's were determined by ANOVA.

3. Results

3.1. Young Male 5xFAD Mice Exhibited Normal Overall Energy Homeostasis When Fed Normal Chow Diet (NCD)

In order to evaluate baseline energy homeostasis in 5xFAD mice compared to WT mice, we used indirect calorimetry for metabolic profiling and measured locomotor activity, energy expenditure, oxygen consumption, nutrient utilization, and food intake in WT and 5xFAD animals fed NCD. In order to minimize the confounding effect of advanced neurodegeneration on energy homeostasis, we used male 5xFAD and control animals at 2 months of age. We determined that WT and 5xFAD mice had comparable body weight and body composition (Figure 1A–C). Then, mice were housed individually in a home cage environment and acclimated for 48 h before recording. 5xFAD mice had a normal diurnal rhythm of locomotor activity during ad libitum feeding (Figure 1D,E). Energy expenditure (EE) and oxygen consumption (VO_2) were also similar between 5xFAD and WT control mice (Figure 1F–I). Energy partitioning measured by respiratory exchange ratio (RER) was used to gauge carbohydrate and lipid utilization as metabolic fuel. An RER of 1.0 indicates carbohydrate being the predominant fuel source, while a value of 0.7 indicates the combustion of fatty acids as the predominant fuel source. We found no significant differences of RER in WT and 5xFAD mice during ad libitum feeding (Figure 1J,K). WT and 5xFAD mice also had comparable food intake during ad libitum feeding (Figure 1L,M). In order to further evaluate the potential impact on neuroendocrine system for energy balance regulation in the 5xFAD mice, we applied the fasting-refeeding experimental paradigm in the indirect calorimetry experiment. Consistent with the results from ad libitum feeding, we found that the metabolic parameters were virtually indistinguishable between WT and 5xFAD mice during fasting-refeeding challenge (Supplemental Figure S2). Collectively, our results showed that 5xFAD mice on normal chow diet were able to maintain energy homeostasis with normal food intake, energy expenditure, and nutrient utilization.

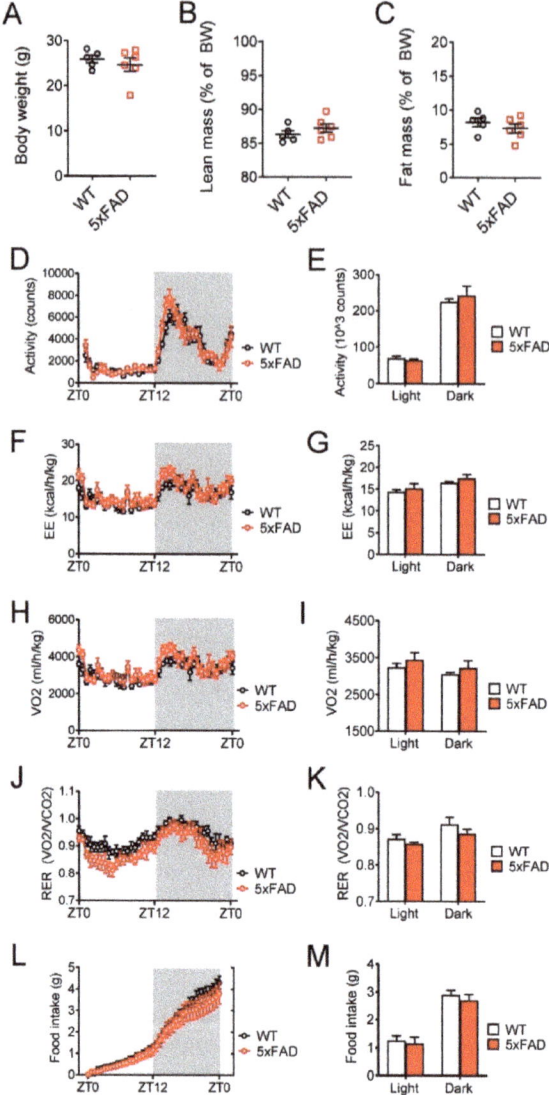

Figure 1. Young male 5xFAD mice fed normal chow diet (NCD) had normal energy homeostasis. Male 5xFAD and wild type (WT) mice were 2 months old and fed normal chow diet (NCD). Metabolic profiling was performed during ad libitum feeding. (**A**) Body weight. (**B**) Lean mass as a percentage of body weight (BW). (**C**) Fat mass as a percentage of body weight. (**D**) Lateral locomotor activity and (**E**) total locomotor activity. (**F**) Energy expenditure (EE) normalized to total body weight and (**G**) average EE normalized to total body weight. (**H**) Oxygen consumption (VO_2) and (**I**) average VO_2. (**J**) Respiratory exchange ratio (RER) and (**K**) average RER. (**L**) Cumulative food intake and (**M**) total food intake during each light/dark phase. Data are displayed as means ± standard error of the mean. Statistical comparisons for time-course data were calculated with Fisher's least squared difference method. Statistical comparisons for light/dark averages were calculated with student's t-test. $n = 5$ for WT mice and $n = 6$ for 5xFAD mice.

3.2. 5xFAD Mice Fed Normal Chow Diet Exhibited Age-Dependent Sexual Dimorphic Effects on Body Weight Maintenance

Though younger 5xFAD mice were able to maintain energy balance, advanced neuropathology in older 5xFAD mice could impair the maintenance of whole-body energy homeostasis due to defects in feeding-related locomotion and neurocognitive function. We analyzed 7.5-month-old male and female WT and 5xFAD mice fed on normal chow diet to measure body weight and adiposity. Female 5xFAD mice had lower body weight, whereas male 5xFAD mice were comparable to WT mice (Supplemental Figure S3A). We collected the liver, epididymal white adipose tissue (EWAT), and pancreas from both male and female mice and measured the organ masses and found that female 5xFAD had lower masses of liver, EWAT, and pancreas (Supplemental Figure S3B–D). When tissue weights were normalized to total body weight, female 5xFAD mice had significantly lower relative EWAT mass (Supplemental Figure S3F). Our results suggested that mechanisms governing energy homeostasis in 5xFAD mice were impaired in an age-dependent sexually dimorphic manner and that female 5xFAD mice on chow diet were more prone to have lower body weight due to adiposity loss.

3.3. 5xFAD Mice Displayed Metabolic Defects after High-Fat Diet (HFD) Feeding

In order to evaluate the effect of HFD on energy homeostasis in 5xFAD mice, we switched the diet from NCD comprised of 13.2% calories from fat to HFD comprised of 60% calories from fat for two months and then repeated metabolic profiling. 5xFAD mice exposed to HFD feeding had similar body weight (Figure 2A), lean mass (Figure 2B), and fat mass (Figure 2C) as WT mice. However, 5xFAD mice had greater nocturnal locomotor activity during ad libitum feeding, particularly towards the end of the dark phase when mice typically exhibit declined activity (Figure 2D,E). The increases in locomotor activity were accompanied by increases in energy expenditure and oxygen consumption (VO_2) in 5xFAD mice during ad libitum feeding (Figure 2F–I). However, we did not observe differences in respiratory exchange ratio (RER), suggesting that energy partitioning was not different between 5xFAD and WT mice (Figure 2J,K). During ad libitum feeding, 5xFAD mice consumed more HFD than WT mice especially during the dark phase (Figure 2L,M, significant after 31.7 h).

As we observed changes in feeding and energy expenditure during ad libitum feeding in HFD-fed 5xFAD mice, we further examined the satiety and energy balance regulation using the fasting-refeeding challenge. In response to food deprivation, 5xFAD mice had significantly increased locomotor activity, indicating increased hunger and food foraging behavior (Supplemental Figure S4A,B). After refeeding, 5xFAD mice had significantly increased locomotor activity, energy expenditure, and oxygen consumption, indicating increased feeding behavior (Supplemental Figure S4A–F). Consistent with foraging behaviors, 5xFAD mice consumed more HFD during the 24-h refeeding phase (Supplemental Figure S4I,J, significant after 20.9 h). Taken together, we concluded that 5xFAD mice on HFD had reduced satiety and increased caloric intake but increased energy expenditure.

3.4. 5xFAD Mice on High-Fat Diet (HFD) Have Altered Glycemia and Blood Lipid Profile Compared with WT Mice

We investigated whether increased ad libitum HFD food intake in 5xFAD mice would alter serum metabolites that are involved in metabolic syndrome and also implicated as AD risk factors [33–35]. Male 5xFAD mice on HFD had decreased blood glucose concentration during ad libitum feeding but not during fasting or refeeding (Figure 3A). WT and 5xFAD mice had similar concentrations of serum insulin and cholesterol throughout the changes to physiological status (Figure 3B,C). We observed higher serum non-esterified fatty acids (NEFA) during fasting and higher glycerol during refeeding (Figure 3D,E), suggesting 5xFAD mice had increased lipolysis during the fasting-refeeding challenge. During refeeding, we also observed significantly increased serum triglycerides (TG) in 5xFAD mice (Figure 3F). Taken together, we concluded that 5xFAD mice on HFD have increased serum lipid metabolites (e.g., increased NEFA and TG) compared to WT mice, which is consistent with their metabolic defects on HFD (e.g., food intake) (Figure 2).

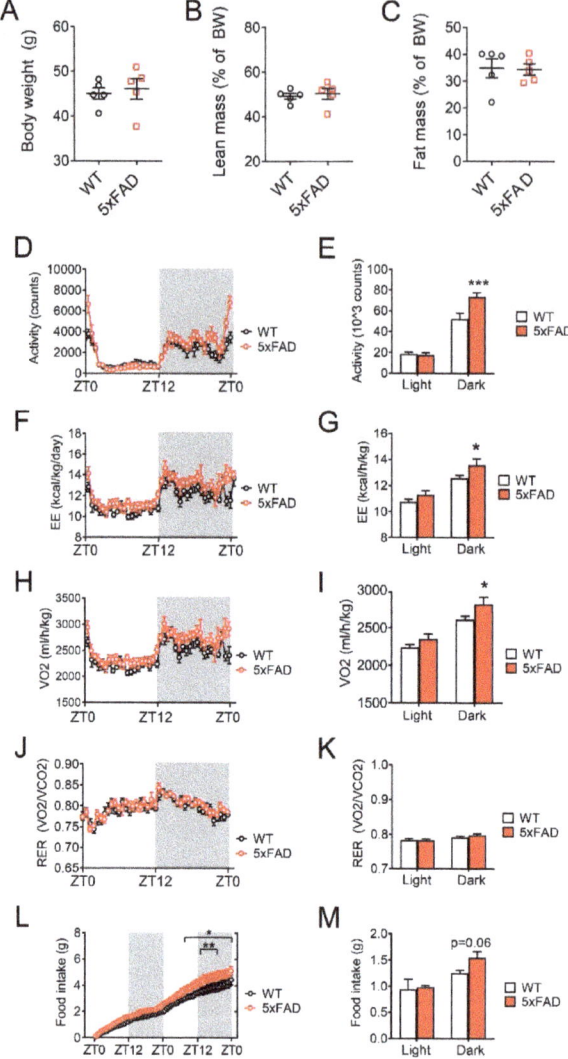

Figure 2. 5xFAD male mice displayed metabolic defects after high-fat diet (HFD) feeding. Male 5xFAD and wild type (WT) mice were fed HFD for 2 months. Metabolic profiling was performed during ad libitum feeding on HFD. (**A**) Body weight. (**B**) Lean mass as a percentage of body weight (BW). (**C**) Fat mass as a percentage of body weight (BW). (**D**) Lateral locomotor activity and (**E**) total locomotor activity. (**F**) Energy expenditure (EE) normalized to total body weight and (**G**) average EE normalized to total body weight. (**H**) Oxygen consumption (VO_2) and (**I**) average VO_2. (**J**) Respiratory exchange ratio (RER) and (**K**) average RER. (**L**) Cumulative food intake and (**M**) total food intake during each light/dark phase. Data are displayed as means ± standard error of the mean. Statistical comparisons for time-course data were calculated with Fisher's least squared difference method. Statistical comparisons for light/dark averages were calculated with student's *t*-test. Statistical comparisons for bar graphs were calculated with student's *t*-test. (*) indicates $p < 0.05$; (**) indicates $p < 0.01$; (***) indicates $p < 0.001$. $n = 5$ for each group.

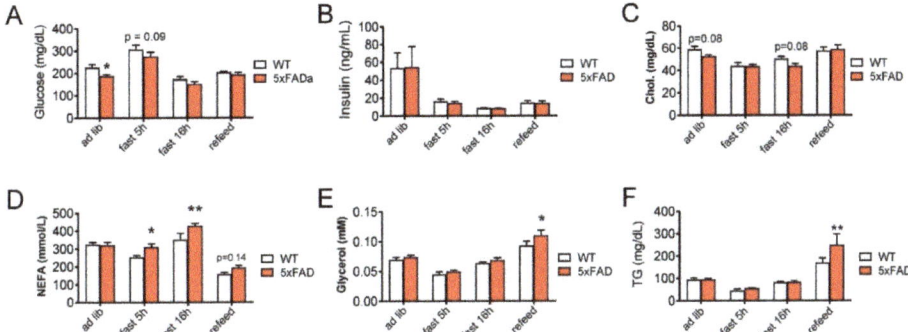

Figure 3. 5xFAD male mice on high-fat diet (HFD) had altered blood glucose and lipid metabolites compared with wild type (WT) mice. Serum metabolites were measured in 6-month-old mice fed HFD for 3 months. (**A**) blood glucose, (**B**) serum insulin, (**C**) serum free cholesterol, (**D**) serum non-esterified fatty acids (NEFA), (**E**) serum glycerol, (**F**) serum triglycerides (TG). Data are displayed as means ± standard error of the mean. $n = 5$ for WT mice and $n = 6$ for 5xFAD mice. Statistical comparisons were calculated with student's *t*-test, * $p < 0.05$, ** $p < 0.01$; additional *p*-values were noted in the panels for clarity.

3.5. High-Fat Diet (HFD) Exacerbated the Glucose Intolerance Phenotype in Male 5xFAD Mice

Impaired glucose metabolism and cellular bioenergetics in the brain have been associated with AD pathology [4,5,12]. HFD feeding causes nutritional excess and impairs hypothalamic regulation of energy balance and glucose homeostasis [36,37]. In order to investigate the dietary effect on glucose metabolism in 5xFAD mice, we evaluated the glucose tolerance phenotype using male 5xFAD and control mice fed with NCD and HFD. We first performed an oral glucose tolerance test (oGTT) using young male 5xFAD and WT mice fed NCD with comparable weight and adiposity. 5xFAD mice had a modest but significantly higher peak glucose concentration at 30 min (Figure 4A). After 2 months of HFD feeding, we performed a glucose tolerance test again and found that 5xFAD mice showed decreased glucose clearance during oGTT (Figure 4B). In addition, we measured the body weight throughout the time course of HFD feeding and found that 5xFAD and WT mice fed HFD had similar weight gain (Figure 4C), suggesting that glucose intolerance was not confounded by differences in body weight adiposity gain. Therefore, we concluded that male 5xFAD mice were more susceptible to HFD-induced glucose intolerance.

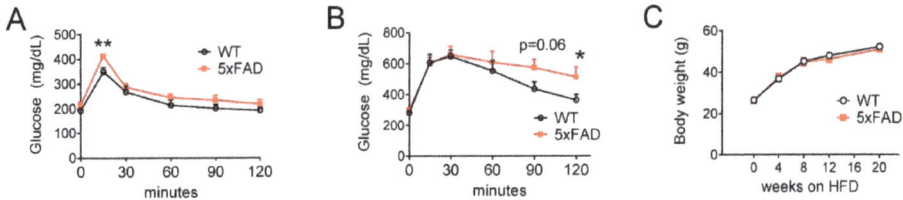

Figure 4. High-fat diet (HFD) exacerbated the glucose intolerance phenotype in male 5xFAD mice. (**A**) Glucose excursion of 2-month-old male mice fed NCD during oral glucose tolerance test (oGTT) (2 g/kg). (**B**) Glucose excursion during oGTT (3 g/kg) in wild type (WT) and 5xFAD male mice fed HFD for 2 months. (**C**) Body weight of WT and 5xFAD mice on HFD. Data are displayed as means ± standard error of the mean. $n = 5$ per group. Statistical comparisons for each timepoint were calculated with student's *t*-test, (*) indicates $p < 0.05$, (**) indicates $p < 0.01$.

3.6. High-Fat Diet (HFD) Altered the Gut Microbiome Composition in Both WT and 5xFAD Mice

As dietary change causes rapid and profound change in the gut microbiome composition, we investigated the relative contribution of the 5xFAD genetic background and HFD to alterations in the microbiome composition and the possibility of specific interactions between HFD and the 5xFAD background. We measured the relative abundance of bacterial taxa in feces of WT and 5xFAD mice on NCD or HFD by 16S rRNA gene sequencing. In 28 samples, 1404 amplicon sequence variants (ASV's) were identified with an average read count of 7.3×10^4 per sample. The results were then rarefied to 258 ASV's that were used for downstream analyses to characterize the microbiome composition (Figure 5). We determined that HFD changed the relative abundance in the phyla *Firmicutesi*, *Bacteroidetes* and *Actinobacteria*, with no discernable differences between WT and 5xFAD mice of the same diet (Figure 5A,B).

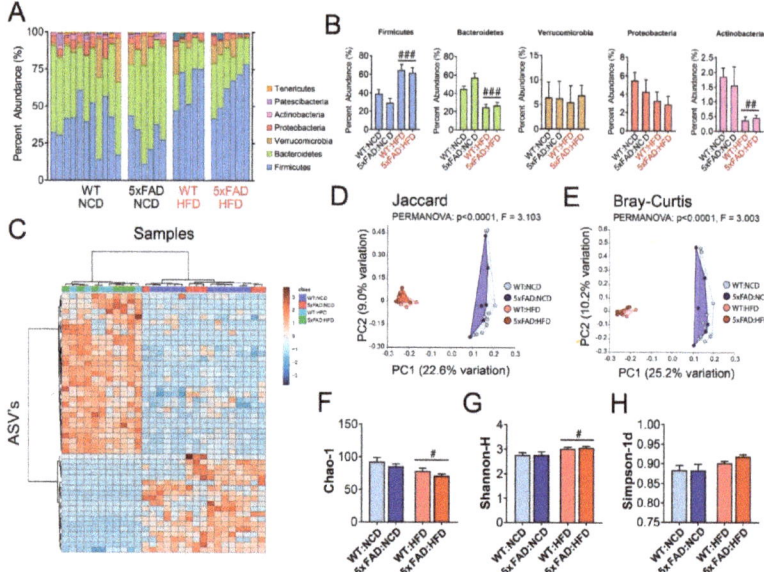

Figure 5. High-fat diet (HFD) altered the gut microbiome composition in both WT and 5xFAD mice. The microbiome compositions and diversity in fecal samples from 6-month-old wild type (WT) and 5xFAD mice fed normal chow diet (NCD) or high-fat diet (HFD) were determined by 16S rRNA sequencing. (**A**) Stacked bar chart of the relative abundance of detected bacterial phyla. Each stacked bar represents an individual mouse with genotypes indicated on the x-axis. Low abundance phyla <1% were omitted from the legend. (**B**) Average relative abundance of detected bacterial phyla: *Firmicutes*, *Bacteroidetes*, *Verrucomicrobia*, *Proteobacteria*, and *Actinobacteria*. (**C**) Hierarchical clustering heatmap of the top 50 significant amplicon sequence variants (ASV's). Columns represent individual mice with respective genotypes indicated by the legend. (**D**) Principle coordinate analysis (PCoA) of Jaccard distances. (**E**) Principle coordinate analysis (PCoA) of Bray-Curtis distances. (**F**) Richness measurement using Chao-1 index. (**G**) α-diversity measurement using Shannon-H index. (**H**) α-diversity measurement using Simpson-1d index. Statistical comparisons in PCoA were made using one-way permutational multivariate analysis of variance (PERMANOVA). Bonferroni-corrected pairwise comparisons between genotypes on the same diet were not statistically significant. Statistical comparisons in B, F-H were made using two-way ANOVA, where (#) indicates $p < 0.05$ between different diets, (##) indicates $p < 0.01$, and (###) indicates $p < 0.001$ between different diets. Tukey-corrected pairwise comparisons between genotypes on the same diet were not statistically significant. $n = 11, 6, 5, 6$ mice per group for WT:NCD, 5xFAD:NCD, WT:HFD, and 5xFAD:HFD, respectively.

We also selected the top 50 of the most statistically significant ASV's and performed hierarchical clustering (HC) based on Euclidean distances. HC showed that the differences in microbial compositions were mainly attributed to the diet, and that dissimilarities between WT and 5xFAD mice were relatively small compared to the dissimilarities between diets (Figure 5C). We further confirmed this result using principle coordinate analysis (PCoA) based on Jaccard and Bray-Curtis distances (Figure 5D,E). In both analyses, the only significant comparisons were between the different diets, which shows that the dissimilarities between samples were mainly driven by diet and not genotype (Figure 5D,E).

Finally, we determined the α-diversity and richness of the gut microbiome in 5xFAD and WT mice fed either NCD or HFD. The richness of the gut microbiome was decreased in HFD samples compared to NCD samples, but no effect of genotype was observed (Figure 5F). We measured α-diversity, which considers the evenness and richness of the microbiome compositions, using the Shannon-H and Simpson-1d indices. Diet caused a significant change in the Shannon-H index and a nearly significant change in the Simpson-1d index, but no genotype effects were observed (Figure 5G,H). Taken together, we concluded that changes in gut microbiome composition were mainly driven by HFD and that 5xFAD and WT mice on the same diet have similar gut microbiome compositions.

3.7. Amyloidogenic and Inflammatory Pathways in the Hippocampus of 5xFAD Mice Are Exacerbated by High-Fat Diet (HFD)

We examined the transcripts of genes with known functions in metabolism and AD pathology. First, the mRNA of genes involved in the insulin signaling pathway, such as *Insr*, *Akt3*, and *Pik3r2*, were downregulated in NCD-fed 5xFAD mice but upregulated in HFD-fed 5xFAD mice compared to WT mice (Figure 6A). Of note, *Mtor*, which mediates nutrient sensing and interacts with the insulin signaling pathway, was increased in 5xFAD mice on HFD. Therefore, our data demonstrated increased transcription for key regulators of cellular energy metabolism in 5xFAD mice on HFD, which suggests compensatory response to diet-induced nutrient excess at the transcription level. Secondly, genes genetically associated with AD risk, including *Apoe*, *Lrp1*, *Clu*, *App*, and *Psen2*, had further increased mRNA levels in 5xFAD mice on HFD (Figure 6B). Thirdly, in order to determine whether HFD could exacerbate the neurotoxicity of plaques in 5xFAD mice, we assessed the expression of apoptosis and pro-apoptosis pathway genes in HFD-fed 5xFAD mice and found that many were further upregulated by HFD feeding (Figure 6C). *Casp8*, *Casp6*, *Nfkb1*, and *Atm* showed increased transcription in 5xFAD mice fed on HFD compared to NCD. Lastly, many of the genes with the highest fold change in 5xFAD mice were microglial markers (Figure 6D). Of note, *Cx3cr1* and *Tmem119* were further upregulated in HFD-fed 5xFAD mice, suggesting that HFD feeding increased the expression of microglia-specific marker genes. Taken together, our results demonstrated that HFD feeding promoted pathological progression of AD in 5xFAD hippocampi, possibly due to increased plaque burden, neuronal death, and microglial mediated neuroinflammatory response. In addition to the individual genes with well-established roles in metabolism and AD pathology, we unbiasedly analyzed the differentially expressed genes in 5xFAD mice fed NCD versus HFD based on fold change and statistical significance (Figure 6E). The top hits were plotted in Figure 6F, which provides a list of potential targets to mitigate the effects of HFD in 5xFAD mice.

In order to understand the overall physiological impact of HFD on cellular pathways in the hippocampus of 5xFAD mice, we performed Nanostring pathway analyses for 5xFAD mice on NCD versus HFD (Figure 6G and Supplemental Figure S5). Consistent with our findings based on analyses of individual gene expression (Figure 6A–D), many of the top differentially regulated pathways were related to insulin signaling, cellular stress, neurotransmission, cytokine signaling, microglial function, and immune response. Furthermore, we performed gene set enrichment analysis (GSEA) with DAVID 6.8 (https://david.ncifcrf.gov/) to identify and rank the pathways that are altered in HFD-fed 5xFAD mice (Figure 6H). The 10 most significant pathways from Kyoto Encyclopedia of Genes and Genomes (KEGG) Pathway and Gene Ontology (GO) terms were selected and ranked by fold-enrichment. Our GSEA results revealed that the top HFD-induced changes to pathways in 5xFAD mice were related to the regulation of neurological function (e.g., synaptic plasticity, neurotransmission, and neuronal death) and metabolic function (e.g., epigenetic and rhythmic regulation, protein phosphorylation, and cAMP signaling).

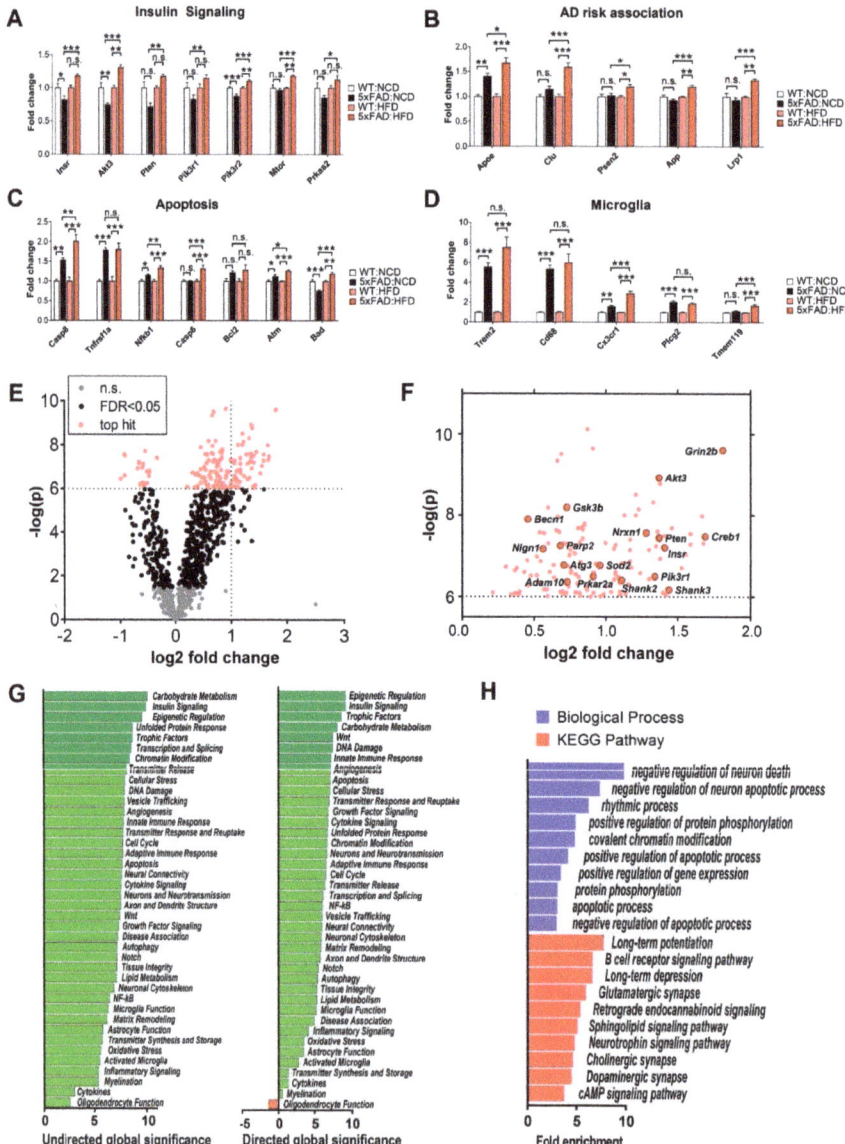

Figure 6. Amyloidogenic and inflammatory pathways in the hippocampus of 5xFAD mice were exacerbated by high-fat diet (HFD). RNA profiling was performed using samples isolated from the hippocampi of wild type (WT) and 5xFAD mice fed NCD and HFD. (**A**) NanoString gene expression analysis of insulin signaling genes, (**B**) AD risk-associated genes, (**C**) apoptosis-related genes, (**D**) microglia

associated genes. (**E**) Volcano plot of hippocampal transcripts from 5xFAD mice fed HFD versus NCD. Top hits are genes with −log10(*p*) > 6. Out of a total 979 gene probes, 302 were non-significant and 677 gene probes were significant at Benjamini-Hochberg false-discovery rate (FDR) < 0.05. (**F**) Labeled genes of interest that were top hits identified in Figure 6E (**G**) Nanostring undirected global significance (left) and directed global significance (right). Undirected global significance is a measure of differential expression of genes belonging to each pathway, calculated as the square root of the mean squared t-statistics. Similarly, directed global significance measures the tendency to have up or down regulated genes, calculated as the square root of the mean of signed (positive/negative) squared t-statistics. (**H**) Gene set enrichment analysis (GSEA) of significant hippocampal mRNAs (FDR < 0.05) from 5xFAD mice fed NCD versus HFD. The top 10 KEGG pathways and Gene Ontology (GO) term biological processes were identified based on *p*-value, then sorted by highest fold-enrichment. Data are displayed as means ± standard error of the mean. n = 6,6,5,6 for WT:NCD, 5xFAD:NCD, WT:HFD, and 5xFAD:HFD, respectively. Statistical comparisons between groups in A-D were performed using two-way ANOVA and Tukey post-hoc tests. (*) indicates $p < 0.05$, (**) indicates $p < 0.01$. (***) indicates $p < 0.001$. Comparisons that were non-significant (n.s.) are also indicated for clarity.

4. Discussion

Epidemiological and clinical studies have highlighted the role of diet and nutrition in the development of AD [18,21]. Given the ethical and technical barriers to conduct mechanistic studies in human subjects, the emerging Alzheimer's disease animal models present as excellent alternative preclinical models for identifying biomarkers and developing therapeutics in basic and translational research [38]. In the current study, we used 5xFAD mice as an Alzheimer's disease model to study the physiological and molecular underpinning between diet-induced metabolic defects and AD pathology. Specifically, we set to address two questions–(1) whether 5xFAD mice were more susceptible to high-fat diet (HFD)-induced metabolic disorders; (2) whether HFD could increase stress on AD-related neurological pathways. The dietary fat in HFD was rendered from lard and comprised 60% of the calories. First, we systematically characterized the metabolic parameters of 5xFAD and control mice on normal chow diet (NCD) versus high-fat diet (HFD) using indirect calorimetry. We found that HFD feeding disrupted energy balance in male 5xFAD mice, leading to increased locomotor activity, energy expenditure, and food intake. We further measured the glucose tolerance and circulating lipid metabolites under different feeding statuses. Our results demonstrated that 5xFAD mice had glucose intolerance, which was worsened by HFD feeding. Moreover, high dietary fat intake led to elevated circulating lipids (i.e., TG and NEFA) in 5xFAD mice. We also characterized the gut microbiome composition of the WT and 5xFAD mice fed NCD and HFD. Though we found no taxonomical differences associated with genotype, HFD caused profound changes in the microbiome composition, which could cause altered microbial products and host immune response. Finally, we isolated and quantified hippocampal mRNAs related to AD neuropathology and neuroinflammation and showed that HFD elevated the expression of apoptotic, microglial, and amyloidogenic genes in 5xFAD mice. We performed comprehensive analysis of the cellular pathways in 5xFAD mice fed NCD vs. HFD. Our gene ontology (GO) analysis showed that the differentially expressed genes were enriched in GO terms which included long-term synaptic plasticity, insulin signaling, and neuron death.

In our current studies, 5xFAD mice on HFD displayed increased energy intake and expenditure compared to WT animals (Figure 2). Moreover, 5xFAD mice on HFD displayed more glucose and lipid metabolism defects compared to WT animals (Figures 3 and 4). Therefore, our studies demonstrate that 5xFAD mice were more susceptible to HFD-induced metabolic defects, which could create a vicious cycle of impaired metabolic fitness and cognitive decline. Several mechanisms may contribute to this phenotype and connect metabolic disorders with AD. HFD compromises brain glucose and insulin sensing, which are required for maintaining metabolic homeostasis [39,40]. Increased triglycerides were reported to cross the blood-brain barrier, leading to inhibition of neuronal insulin receptor signaling [41]. HFD causes inflammation in the hypothalamus and impairs energy balance regulation by reducing hypothalamic proopiomelanocortin (POMC) neurons and increasing gliosis [37,42]. Our previous studies have shown that increasing the hormonal sensitivity in POMC neurons ameliorates the metabolic derangements caused by long-term HFD feeding in aged mice [27]. Future study is warranted to understand whether the neuroendocrine system is more severely impacted in 5xFAD fed HFD. Alternatively, HFD could precipitate Aβ deposition and inhibit Aβ degradation. For example, HFD feeding in another AD mouse model (APP23 mice) caused cognitive deficits and increased hippocampal and cortical Aβ deposition [43] and insulin resistance was reported to increase hyperphosphorylation of Tau via GSK-3β activity [44].

We performed the hippocampal gene transcript profiling using NanoString nCounter assays, which enables accurate and higher-throughput transcriptional analysis of gene panels related to AD neuropathology and neuroinflammation. Our key finding was that the transcription of insulin signaling genes, AD risk genes and microglial markers were among the most significantly upregulated genes in HFD-fed 5xFAD hippocampi (Figure 6). (I) We found Insulin signaling pathway genes, including *InsR*, *Akt3*, *Mtor*, and *Prkaa2*, were upregulated in HFD-fed 5xFAD mice compared NCD-fed 5xFAD mice (Figure 6A). mTOR and AMPK are important cellular sensors for energy status and were implicated in AD-related pathologies [6,45,46]. Since HFD increases insulin resistance in the hippocampus, resulting in impaired cognitive performance [47–50], our findings suggest that these genes were upregulated in order to compensate for insulin resistance. (II) We discovered that the expression of several AD risk-associated genes was further increased in 5xFAD mice fed HFD (Figure 6B). *Apoe* and its receptor, *Lrp1*, were further upregulated in HFD-fed 5xFAD mice, suggesting that HFD caused disturbances of brain cholesterol metabolism. 5xFAD is an amyloid pathology model that expresses human *APP* and *PSEN1* transgenes with a total of five AD-linked mutations. The amyloid plaque burden is mainly driven by the human transgene expression. In our study, we detected mouse *App* and *Psen2* were also upregulated in 5xFAD mice fed HFD, suggesting that HFD may have increased endogenous App generation and App processing. *Clu*, which interacts with extracellular Aβ plaques, was also increased. Therefore, our data suggest that HFD modifies the expression of AD risk-associated genes which are likely to increase amyloid generation in 5xFAD mice. (III) We discovered that HFD further increased transcripts encoding *Casp8* and *Casp6* in 5xFAD mice suggesting that increased apoptosis (Figure 6C). *Nfkb1*, which is a pro-apoptotic gene, was also upregulated. Therefore, we concluded that HFD increased neurotoxicity in 5xFAD hippocampi which may lead to greater apoptosis and neurodegeneration. (IV) Microglial markers, including *Trem2*, *Cd68*, *Cx3cr1*, *Plcg2*, and *Tmem119*, were selectively upregulated with the highest fold changes in 5xFAD mice compared with WT mice (Figure 6D). Interestingly, the expression of *Cx3cr1* and *Tmem119* was further upregulated on HFD, indicating the dietary effects were significantly associated with expression levels of microglia-specific marker genes. (V) We performed differential expression analysis by comparing HFD-fed with NCD-fed 5xFAD mice (Figure 6E,F). The top hits with the most statistical significance are genes involved in insulin signaling and cellular energetics, such as *Insr*, *Akt3*, *Pten*, *Creb1*, *Prkar2a*, *Becn1*, *Atg3*, and *Gsk3b*. (VI) In addition to identifying the differential expression of individual genes, we performed pathway analysis to pinpoint altered molecular and cellular pathways in HFD-fed versus NCD-fed 5xFAD mice (Figure 6G,H and Supplementary Figure S5). Of note, innate and adaptive immune response, cytokine signaling, microglia function, activated microglia, and inflammatory signaling pathways had high undirected global significance (>5), suggesting that HFD feeding caused greater inflammatory response and microglial activation in the hippocampi of 5xFAD mice (Figure 6G). Our findings in HFD-fed 5xFAD mice were consistent with previous reports that HFD increases microglial activation in the hippocampus [51–53] which may promote synapse loss [51]. Collectively, our data showed that HFD combined with amyloid pathology is likely to increase stress on multiple pathways and cause detrimental effects on long-term synaptic plasticity, neuronal apoptosis, and neuroinflammation.

Multiple experimental and clinical studies have pointed out that changes in gut microbiome composition contribute to the progression of metabolic and neurodegeneration diseases via altered microbial metabolites, immune activation, and bacterial amyloids [54–57]. The role of the gut microbiome in neurodegenerative diseases is beginning to be elucidated. The gut microbiome is a source of bacterial amyloids (which can cross-seed with Aβ), endotoxins (i.e., lipopolysaccharides), and inflammatory cytokines which can prime immune cells in the brain [54–57]. Treating APP/PS1 mice with antibiotics reduced plaque formation, suggesting that the microbiome secretes factors which accelerate disease pathogenesis [58]. Studies in human patients found correlations between Aβ and phospho-Tau peptides in the cerebrospinal fluid and specific genera of microbes [57]. Interestingly, transplantation of HFD-associated microbiomes increased anxiety behaviors and impaired auditory-cued fear learning compared to NCD-transplanted microbiomes [59]. However, it is unclear whether the different microbiome compositions in AD patients are directly causal to impaired cognitive function. In our study, the effects of 5xFAD on the microbiome were negligible compared to the effect of HFD feeding (Figure 5), suggesting that diet-induced changes to the gut microbiome are more rapid and of greater magnitude than changes induced by AD pathology.

A previous study reported that HFD enhances cerebral amyloid angiopathy and cognitive impairment in 5xFAD mice independently of metabolic disorders [24]. The major difference between that study and ours was the age difference when 5xFAD mice were used for metabolic analyses. When 13 month-old 5xFAD mice were switched to HFD for another 10 weeks, they gained less weight and glucose tolerance was not affected compared to WT mice [24]. 5xFAD mice demonstrate age-dependent rapid progression to neurodegeneration [26]. Therefore, the reduced body mass and weight gain of older 5xFAD mice could be caused by the advanced state of neurodegeneration. Moreover, lower body weight of aged 5xFAD mice could be a confounding factor for the glucose tolerance tests. In order to minimize these confounding factors associated with the older 5xFAD mice, we used younger mice for metabolic profiling. Male 5xFAD mice on either NCD or HFD had similar body weight and body composition as the WT mice and were used in our studies. Meanwhile, another group used younger 5xFAD mice to start HFD feeding and found increased amyloid deposition and defects in glucose metabolism [25], which was consistent with our findings in the current study. We found NCD-fed female (but not male) 5xFAD mice at 7.5 months of age had reduced body weight and adiposity (Supplemental Figure S3), indicating an association between cognitive decline and frailty [60]. Differences in body composition would be a confounding factor for characterizing the glucose and energy metabolic phenotype in female mice, therefore we focused the current study on male mice. How female 5xFAD mice would respond to dietary changes in terms of metabolism and neuropathology is an interesting question and will be investigated in future studies.

5. Conclusions

In conclusion, our studies demonstrated that 5xFAD mice were more susceptible to HFD-induced metabolic disorders and that HFD could exacerbate stress on AD-related neuropathological and neuroinflammatory pathways. Altogether, our data suggest that targeting metabolic dysfunctions caused by high dietary fat intake can ameliorate AD symptoms via effects on insulin signaling, neuroinflammation, Aβ deposition, and microglia activation in the hippocampus.

Supplementary Materials: The following are available online at http://www.mdpi.com/2072-6643/12/10/2977/s1, Figure S1: Study Design, Figure S2: Indirect calorimetry during fasting/refeeding challenge in male 5xFAD and WT mice fed NCD, Figure S3: 5xFAD mice fed normal chow diet exhibited age-dependent sexually dimorphic effects on body weight maintenance., Figure S4: Indirect calorimetry during fasting/refeeding challenge in male 5xFAD and WT mice fed high-fat diet (HFD), Figure S5: Heatmap of Nanostring pathway scores of 5xFAD mice on NCD versus HFD.

Author Contributions: Conceptualization, A.M.R., H.R., A.L.O.; methodology, A.M.R., H.R., A.L.O., A.C.E., P.B.L., A.P.T.; data curation, A.M.R., A.P.T., P.B.L., A.C.E.; formal analysis, A.M.R., A.P.T.; visualization, A.M.R.; investigation, A.M.R.; resources, H.R., A.L.O., A.C.E.; writing—original draft preparation, A.M.R. and H.R.; writing—review and editing, A.M.R. and H.R. All authors have read and agreed to the published version of the manuscript.

Funding: This work was supported by Indiana University Multi-Center Collaborative Award (H. Ren, A. Oblak), NIH R00DK098294, NIH R01DK120772, P&F grant from P30DK097512 and UL1TR002529, and Showalter Scholarship (H. Ren); Paul and Carole Stark Fellowship award, and Diabetes and Obesity Research Training award T32DK064466 (A. Reilly).

Acknowledgments: We would like to thank Indira Medina-Rodriguez (senior technical applications scientist from NanoString) for excellent technical support, Gary Landreth for critically reviewing the manuscript, Cynthia Ingraham, Christopher Lloyd, Deborah Baker, Shijun Yan, and Jason Conley for their help in collecting samples, Shijun Yan for assisting with GTT, Natalie Stull for assisting with indirect calorimetry measurements, Giedre Turner for 16S rRNA sequencing, Kara Orr for assisting with echoMRI scans, and Courtney Jewett for manuscript editing.

Conflicts of Interest: The authors declare no conflict of interest.

References

1. Ballard, C.; Gauthier, S.; Corbett, A.; Brayne, C.; Aarsland, D.; Jones, E. Alzheimer's disease. *Lancet* **2011**, *377*, 1019–1031. [CrossRef]
2. Lane, C.A.; Hardy, J.; Schott, J.M. Alzheimer's disease. *Eur. J. Neurol.* **2018**, *25*, 59–70. [CrossRef] [PubMed]
3. Scheltens, P.; Blennow, K.; Breteler, M.M.B.; de Strooper, B.; Frisoni, G.B.; Salloway, S.; Van der Flier, W.M. Alzheimer's disease. *Lancet* **2016**, *388*, 505–517. [CrossRef]
4. Johnson, E.C.B.; Dammer, E.B.; Duong, D.M.; Ping, L.; Zhou, M.; Yin, L.; Higginbotham, L.A.; Guajardo, A.; White, B.; Troncoso, J.C.; et al. Large-scale proteomic analysis of Alzheimer's disease brain and cerebrospinal fluid reveals early changes in energy metabolism associated with microglia and astrocyte activation. *Nat. Med.* **2020**, *26*, 769–780. [CrossRef] [PubMed]
5. Baik, S.H.; Kang, S.; Lee, W.; Choi, H.; Chung, S.; Kim, J.-I.; Mook-Jung, I. A Breakdown in Metabolic Reprogramming Causes Microglia Dysfunction in Alzheimer's Disease. *Cell Metab.* **2019**, *30*, 493–507.e6. [CrossRef]

6. Ulland, T.K.; Song, W.M.; Huang, S.C.-C.; Ulrich, J.D.; Sergushichev, A.; Beatty, W.L.; Loboda, A.A.; Zhou, Y.; Cairns, N.J.; Kambal, A.; et al. TREM2 Maintains Microglial Metabolic Fitness in Alzheimer's Disease. *Cell* **2017**, *170*, 649–663.e13. [CrossRef]
7. Calsolaro, V.; Edison, P. Neuroinflammation in Alzheimer's disease: Current evidence and future directions. *Alzheimers Dement* **2016**, *12*, 719–732. [CrossRef]
8. McCrimmon, R.J.; Ryan, C.M.; Frier, B.M. Diabetes and cognitive dysfunction. *Lancet* **2012**, *379*, 2291–2299. [CrossRef]
9. Strachan, M.W.J.; Reynolds, R.M.; Marioni, R.E.; Price, J.F. Cognitive function, dementia and type 2 diabetes mellitus in the elderly. *Nat. Rev. Endocrinol.* **2011**, *7*, 108–114. [CrossRef]
10. Gudala, K.; Bansal, D.; Schifano, F.; Bhansali, A. Diabetes mellitus and risk of dementia: A meta-analysis of prospective observational studies. *J. Diabetes Investig.* **2013**, *4*, 640–650. [CrossRef]
11. Enzinger, C.; Fazekas, F.; Matthews, P.M.; Ropele, S.; Schmidt, H.; Smith, S.; Schmidt, R. Risk factors for progression of brain atrophy in aging: Six-year follow-up of normal subjects. *Neurology* **2005**, *64*, 1704–1711. [CrossRef] [PubMed]
12. Macauley, S.L.; Stanley, M.; Caesar, E.E.; Yamada, S.A.; Raichle, M.E.; Perez, R.; Mahan, T.E.; Sutphen, C.L.; Holtzman, D.M. Hyperglycemia modulates extracellular amyloid-β concentrations and neuronal activity in vivo. *J. Clin. Investig.* **2015**, *125*, 2463–2467. [CrossRef] [PubMed]
13. Winkler, E.A.; Nishida, Y.; Sagare, A.P.; Rege, S.V.; Bell, R.D.; Perlmutter, D.; Sengillo, J.D.; Hillman, S.; Kong, P.; Nelson, A.R.; et al. GLUT1 reductions exacerbate Alzheimer's disease vasculo-neuronal dysfunction and degeneration. *Nat. Neurosci.* **2015**, *18*, 521–530. [CrossRef] [PubMed]
14. Jais, A.; Solas, M.; Backes, H.; Chaurasia, B.; Kleinridders, A.; Theurich, S.; Mauer, J.; Steculorum, S.M.; Hampel, B.; Goldau, J.; et al. Myeloid-Cell-Derived VEGF Maintains Brain Glucose Uptake and Limits Cognitive Impairment in Obesity. *Cell* **2016**, *165*, 882–895. [CrossRef]
15. Cholerton, B.; Baker, L.D.; Craft, S. Insulin resistance and pathological brain ageing. *Diabet. Med.* **2011**, *28*, 1463–1475. [CrossRef]
16. Talbot, K.; Wang, H.-Y.; Kazi, H.; Han, L.-Y.; Bakshi, K.P.; Stucky, A.; Fuino, R.L.; Kawaguchi, K.R.; Samoyedny, A.J.; Wilson, R.S.; et al. Demonstrated brain insulin resistance in Alzheimer's disease patients is associated with IGF-1 resistance, IRS-1 dysregulation, and cognitive decline. *J. Clin. Investig.* **2012**, *122*, 1316–1338. [CrossRef]
17. Neth, B.J.; Craft, S. Insulin Resistance and Alzheimer's Disease: Bioenergetic Linkages. *Front. Aging Neurosci.* **2017**, *9*, 345. [CrossRef]
18. Yusufov, M.; Weyandt, L.L.; Piryatinsky, I. Alzheimer's disease and diet: A systematic review. *Int. J. Neurosci.* **2017**, *127*, 161–175. [CrossRef]
19. Capurso, C.; Bellanti, F.; Lo Buglio, A.; Vendemiale, G. The Mediterranean Diet Slows Down the Progression of Aging and Helps to Prevent the Onset of Frailty: A Narrative Review. *Nutrients* **2019**, *12*, 35. [CrossRef]
20. Feart, C.; Samieri, C.; Barberger-Gateau, P. Mediterranean diet and cognitive health: An update of available knowledge. *Curr. Opin. Clin. Nutr. Metab. Care* **2015**, *18*, 51–62. [CrossRef]
21. McGrattan, A.M.; McGuinness, B.; McKinley, M.C.; Kee, F.; Passmore, P.; Woodside, J.V.; McEvoy, C.T. Diet and Inflammation in Cognitive Ageing and Alzheimer's Disease. *Curr. Nutr. Rep.* **2019**, *8*, 53–65. [CrossRef] [PubMed]
22. Féart, C.; Samieri, C.; Rondeau, V.; Amieva, H.; Portet, F.; Dartigues, J.-F.; Scarmeas, N.; Barberger-Gateau, P. Adherence to a Mediterranean diet, cognitive decline, and risk of dementia. *JAMA* **2009**, *302*, 638–648. [CrossRef] [PubMed]
23. Czech, M.P. Insulin action and resistance in obesity and type 2 diabetes. *Nat. Med.* **2017**, *23*, 804–814. [CrossRef]
24. Lin, B.; Hasegawa, Y.; Takane, K.; Koibuchi, N.; Cao, C.; Kim-Mitsuyama, S. High-Fat-Diet Intake Enhances Cerebral Amyloid Angiopathy and Cognitive Impairment in a Mouse Model of Alzheimer's Disease, Independently of Metabolic Disorders. *JAHA* **2016**, *5*. [CrossRef] [PubMed]
25. Medrano-Jiménez, E.; Jiménez-Ferrer Carrillo, I.; Pedraza-Escalona, M.; Ramírez-Serrano, C.E.; Álvarez-Arellano, L.; Cortés-Mendoza, J.; Herrera-Ruiz, M.; Jiménez-Ferrer, E.; Zamilpa, A.; Tortoriello, J.; et al. Malva parviflora extract ameliorates the deleterious effects of a high fat diet on the cognitive deficit in a mouse model of Alzheimer's disease by restoring microglial function via a PPAR-γ-dependent mechanism. *J. Neuroinflamm.* **2019**, *16*, 143. [CrossRef]

26. Oakley, H.; Cole, S.L.; Logan, S.; Maus, E.; Shao, P.; Craft, J.; Guillozet-Bongaarts, A.; Ohno, M.; Disterhoft, J.; Van Eldik, L.; et al. Intraneuronal beta-amyloid aggregates, neurodegeneration, and neuron loss in transgenic mice with five familial Alzheimer's disease mutations: Potential factors in amyloid plaque formation. *J. Neurosci.* **2006**, *26*, 10129–10140. [CrossRef]
27. Reilly, A.M.; Zhou, S.; Panigrahi, S.K.; Yan, S.; Conley, J.M.; Sheets, P.L.; Wardlaw, S.L.; Ren, H. Gpr17 deficiency in POMC neurons ameliorates the metabolic derangements caused by long-term high-fat diet feeding. *Nutr. Diabetes* **2019**, *9*, 29. [CrossRef]
28. Walters, W.A.; Caporaso, J.G.; Lauber, C.L.; Berg-Lyons, D.; Fierer, N.; Knight, R. PrimerProspector: De novo design and taxonomic analysis of barcoded polymerase chain reaction primers. *Bioinformatics* **2011**, *27*, 1159–1161. [CrossRef]
29. Caporaso, J.G.; Lauber, C.L.; Walters, W.A.; Berg-Lyons, D.; Lozupone, C.A.; Turnbaugh, P.J.; Fierer, N.; Knight, R. Global patterns of 16S rRNA diversity at a depth of millions of sequences per sample. *Proc. Natl. Acad. Sci. USA* **2011**, *108*, 4516–4522. [CrossRef]
30. Martin, M. Cutadapt removes adapter sequences from high-throughput sequencing reads. *EMBnet.journal* **2011**, *17*, 10–12. [CrossRef]
31. Kuczynski, J.; Stombaugh, J.; Walters, W.A.; González, A.; Caporaso, J.G.; Knight, R. Using QIIME to analyze 16S rRNA gene sequences from microbial communities. *Curr. Protoc. Bioinform.* **2011**. [CrossRef] [PubMed]
32. Pruesse, E.; Quast, C.; Knittel, K.; Fuchs, B.M.; Ludwig, W.; Peplies, J.; Glöckner, F.O. SILVA: A comprehensive online resource for quality checked and aligned ribosomal RNA sequence data compatible with ARB. *Nucleic Acids Res.* **2007**, *35*, 7188–7196. [CrossRef] [PubMed]
33. Bernath, M.M.; Bhattacharyya, S.; Nho, K.; Barupal, D.K.; Fiehn, O.; Baillie, R.; Risacher, S.; Arnold, M.; Jacobson, T.; Trojanowski, J.Q.; et al. Serum triglycerides in Alzheimer's disease: Relation to neuroimaging and CSF biomarkers. *Neuroscience* **2018**, *94*, e2088–e2098.
34. Choi, H.J.; Byun, M.S.; Yi, D.; Choe, Y.M.; Sohn, B.K.; Baek, H.W.; Lee, J.H.; Kim, H.J.; Han, J.Y.; Yoon, E.J.; et al. Association Between Serum Triglycerides and Cerebral Amyloidosis in Cognitively Normal Elderly. *Am. J. Geriatr. Psychiatry* **2016**, *24*, 604–612. [CrossRef]
35. Raffaitin, C.; Gin, H.; Empana, J.-P.; Helmer, C.; Berr, C.; Tzourio, C.; Portet, F.; Dartigues, J.-F.; Alperovitch, A.; Barberger-Gateau, P. Metabolic Syndrome and Risk for Incident Alzheimer's Disease or Vascular Dementia: The Three-City Study. *Diabetes Care* **2009**, *32*, 169–174. [CrossRef] [PubMed]
36. Jais, A.; Brüning, J.C. Hypothalamic inflammation in obesity and metabolic disease. *J. Clin. Investig.* **2017**, *127*, 24–32. [CrossRef] [PubMed]
37. Valdearcos, M.; Douglass, J.D.; Robblee, M.M.; Dorfman, M.D.; Stifler, D.R.; Bennett, M.L.; Gerritse, I.; Fasnacht, R.; Barres, B.A.; Thaler, J.P.; et al. Microglial Inflammatory Signaling Orchestrates the Hypothalamic Immune Response to Dietary Excess and Mediates Obesity Susceptibility. *Cell Metab.* **2017**, *26*, 185–197.e3. [CrossRef]
38. Scearce-Levie, K.; Sanchez, P.E.; Lewcock, J.W. Leveraging preclinical models for the development of Alzheimer disease therapeutics. *Nat. Rev. Drug Discov.* **2020**, *19*, 447–462. [CrossRef]
39. Schwartz, M.W.; Seeley, R.J.; Tschöp, M.H.; Woods, S.C.; Morton, G.J.; Myers, M.G.; D'Alessio, D. Cooperation between brain and islet in glucose homeostasis and diabetes. *Nature* **2013**, *503*, 59–66. [CrossRef]
40. Bentsen, M.A.; Mirzadeh, Z.; Schwartz, M.W. Revisiting How the Brain Senses Glucose-And Why. *Cell Metab.* **2019**, *29*, 11–17. [CrossRef]
41. Banks, W.A.; Farr, S.A.; Salameh, T.S.; Niehoff, M.L.; Rhea, E.M.; Morley, J.E.; Hanson, A.J.; Hansen, K.M.; Craft, S. Triglycerides cross the blood–brain barrier and induce central leptin and insulin receptor resistance. *Int. J. Obes.* **2018**, *42*, 391–397. [CrossRef] [PubMed]
42. Thaler, J.P.; Yi, C.-X.; Schur, E.A.; Guyenet, S.J.; Hwang, B.H.; Dietrich, M.O.; Zhao, X.; Sarruf, D.A.; Izgur, V.; Maravilla, K.R.; et al. Obesity is associated with hypothalamic injury in rodents and humans. *J. Clin. Investig.* **2012**, *122*, 153–162. [CrossRef] [PubMed]
43. Fitz, N.F.; Cronican, A.; Pham, T.; Fogg, A.; Fauq, A.H.; Chapman, R.; Lefterov, I.; Koldamova, R. Liver X Receptor Agonist Treatment Ameliorates Amyloid Pathology and Memory Deficits Caused by High-Fat Diet in APP23 Mice. *J. Neurosci.* **2010**, *30*, 6862–6872. [CrossRef]
44. Hooper, C.; Killick, R.; Lovestone, S. The GSK3 hypothesis of Alzheimer's disease. *J. Neurochem.* **2008**, *104*, 1433–1439. [CrossRef] [PubMed]

45. Kim, B.; Figueroa-Romero, C.; Pacut, C.; Backus, C.; Feldman, E.L. Insulin Resistance Prevents AMPK-induced Tau Dephosphorylation through Akt-mediated Increase in AMPK $^{Ser-485}$ Phosphorylation. *J. Biol. Chem.* **2015**, *290*, 19146–19157. [CrossRef] [PubMed]
46. Vingtdeux, V.; Davies, P.; Dickson, D.W.; Marambaud, P. AMPK is abnormally activated in tangle- and pre-tangle-bearing neurons in Alzheimer's disease and other tauopathies. *Acta Neuropathol.* **2011**, *121*, 337–349. [CrossRef]
47. Arnold, S.E.; Lucki, I.; Brookshire, B.R.; Carlson, G.C.; Browne, C.A.; Kazi, H.; Bang, S.; Choi, B.-R.; Chen, Y.; McMullen, M.F.; et al. High fat diet produces brain insulin resistance, synaptodendritic abnormalities and altered behavior in mice. *Neurobiol. Dis.* **2014**, *67*, 79–87. [CrossRef]
48. Park, H.-S.; Park, S.-S.; Kim, C.-J.; Shin, M.-S.; Kim, T.-W. Exercise Alleviates Cognitive Functions by Enhancing Hippocampal Insulin Signaling and Neuroplasticity in High-Fat Diet-Induced Obesity. *Nutrients* **2019**, *11*, 1603. [CrossRef]
49. McNay, E.C.; Ong, C.T.; McCrimmon, R.J.; Cresswell, J.; Bogan, J.S.; Sherwin, R.S. Hippocampal memory processes are modulated by insulin and high-fat-induced insulin resistance. *Neurobiol. Learn. Mem.* **2010**, *93*, 546–553. [CrossRef]
50. Stranahan, A.M.; Norman, E.D.; Lee, K.; Cutler, R.G.; Telljohann, R.S.; Egan, J.M.; Mattson, M.P. Diet-induced insulin resistance impairs hippocampal synaptic plasticity and cognition in middle-aged rats. *Hippocampus* **2008**, *18*, 1085–1088. [CrossRef]
51. Hao, S.; Dey, A.; Yu, X.; Stranahan, A.M. Dietary obesity reversibly induces synaptic stripping by microglia and impairs hippocampal plasticity. *Brain Behav. Immun.* **2016**, *51*, 230–239. [CrossRef] [PubMed]
52. Tucsek, Z.; Toth, P.; Sosnowska, D.; Gautam, T.; Mitschelen, M.; Koller, A.; Szalai, G.; Sonntag, W.E.; Ungvari, Z.; Csiszar, A. Obesity in Aging Exacerbates Blood-Brain Barrier Disruption, Neuroinflammation, and Oxidative Stress in the Mouse Hippocampus: Effects on Expression of Genes Involved in Beta-Amyloid Generation and Alzheimer's Disease. *J. Gerontol. Ser. A Biol. Sci. Med. Sci.* **2014**, *69*, 1212–1226. [CrossRef] [PubMed]
53. Vinuesa, A.; Bentivegna, M.; Calfa, G.; Filipello, F.; Pomilio, C.; Bonaventura, M.M.; Lux-Lantos, V.; Matzkin, M.E.; Gregosa, A.; Presa, J.; et al. Early Exposure to a High-Fat Diet Impacts on Hippocampal Plasticity: Implication of Microglia-Derived Exosome-like Extracellular Vesicles. *Mol. Neurobiol.* **2019**, *56*, 5075–5094. [CrossRef] [PubMed]
54. Beli, E.; Prabakaran, S.; Krishnan, P.; Evans-Molina, C.; Grant, M.B. Loss of Diurnal Oscillatory Rhythms in Gut Microbiota Correlates with Changes in Circulating Metabolites in Type 2 Diabetic db/db Mice. *Nutrients* **2019**, *11*, 2310. [CrossRef]
55. Kowalski, K.; Mulak, A. Brain-Gut-Microbiota Axis in Alzheimer's Disease. *J. Neurogastroenterol. Motil.* **2019**, *25*, 48–60. [CrossRef]
56. Qin, J.; Li, Y.; Cai, Z.; Li, S.; Zhu, J.; Zhang, F.; Liang, S.; Zhang, W.; Guan, Y.; Shen, D.; et al. A metagenome-wide association study of gut microbiota in type 2 diabetes. *Nature* **2012**, *490*, 55–60. [CrossRef]
57. Vogt, N.M.; Kerby, R.L.; Dill-McFarland, K.A.; Harding, S.J.; Merluzzi, A.P.; Johnson, S.C.; Carlsson, C.M.; Asthana, S.; Zetterberg, H.; Blennow, K.; et al. Gut microbiome alterations in Alzheimer's disease. *Sci. Rep.* **2017**, *7*. [CrossRef]
58. Harach, T.; Marungruang, N.; Duthilleul, N.; Cheatham, V.; Mc Coy, K.D.; Frisoni, G.; Neher, J.J.; Fåk, F.; Jucker, M.; Lasser, T.; et al. Reduction of Abeta amyloid pathology in APPPS1 transgenic mice in the absence of gut microbiota. *Sci. Rep.* **2017**, *7*, 41802. [CrossRef]
59. Bruce-Keller, A.J.; Salbaum, J.M.; Luo, M.; Blanchard, E.; Taylor, C.M.; Welsh, D.A.; Berthoud, H.-R. Obese-type Gut Microbiota Induce Neurobehavioral Changes in the Absence of Obesity. *Biol. Psychiatry* **2015**, *77*, 607–615. [CrossRef]
60. De Morais Fabrício, D.; Chagas, M.H.N.; Diniz, B.S. Frailty and cognitive decline. *Transl. Res.* **2020**, *221*, 58–64. [CrossRef]

© 2020 by the authors. Licensee MDPI, Basel, Switzerland. This article is an open access article distributed under the terms and conditions of the Creative Commons Attribution (CC BY) license (http://creativecommons.org/licenses/by/4.0/).

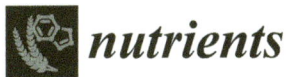

Review

Plant Fortification of the Diet for Anti-Ageing Effects: A Review

Daljeet Singh Dhanjal [1,†], Sonali Bhardwaj [1,†], Ruchi Sharma [2], Kanchan Bhardwaj [3], Dinesh Kumar [2], Chirag Chopra [1], Eugenie Nepovimova [4], Reena Singh [1,*] and Kamil Kuca [4,*]

[1] School of Bioengineering and Biosciences, Lovely Professional University, Phagwara 144411, Punjab, India; daljeetdhanjal92@gmail.com (D.S.D.); sonali.bhardwaj1414@gmail.com (S.B.); chirag.18298@lpu.co.in (C.C.)

[2] School of Bioengineering and Food Technology, Shoolini University of Biotechnology and Management Sciences, Solan 173229, Himachal Pradesh, India; mails4sharmaruchi@gmail.com (R.S.); dineshkumar@shooliniuniversity.com (D.K.)

[3] School of Biological and Environmental Sciences, Shoolini University of Biotechnology and Management Sciences, Solan 173229, Himachal Pradesh, India; kanchankannu1992@gmail.com

[4] Department of Chemistry, Faculty of Science, University of Hradec Kralove, 50003 Hradec Kralove, Czech Republic; eugenie.nepovimova@uhk.cz

* Correspondence: reena.19408@lpu.co.in (R.S.); kamil.kuca@uhk.cz (K.K.); Tel.: +420-603-289-166 (K.K.)

† These authors contributed equally to this work.

Received: 31 August 2020; Accepted: 29 September 2020; Published: 30 September 2020

Abstract: Ageing is an enigmatic and progressive biological process which undermines the normal functions of living organisms with time. Ageing has been conspicuously linked to dietary habits, whereby dietary restrictions and antioxidants play a substantial role in slowing the ageing process. Oxygen is an essential molecule that sustains human life on earth and is involved in the synthesis of reactive oxygen species (ROS) that pose certain health complications. The ROS are believed to be a significant factor in the progression of ageing. A robust lifestyle and healthy food, containing dietary antioxidants, are essential for improving the overall livelihood and decelerating the ageing process. Dietary antioxidants such as adaptogens, anthocyanins, vitamins A/D/C/E and isoflavones slow the ageing phenomena by reducing ROS production in the cells, thereby improving the life span of living organisms. This review highlights the manifestations of ageing, theories associated with ageing and the importance of diet management in ageing. It also discusses the available functional foods as well as nutraceuticals with anti-ageing potential.

Keywords: anti-ageing; diet; eating habits; functional foods; skin ageing

1. Introduction

Ageing is a progressive biological process which affects the normal functions of cells and tissue, thereby imperiling the person towards diseases and mortality [1]. For a layman, it is the process of maturing and growing old. Both internal and external factors play an integral role in ageing [2]. Internal factors comprise the usual biological processes of the cell, whereas the external factors involve chronic sun-exposure, hormonal imbalance, nutritional deficiencies, ultraviolet (UV) irradiation and other factors such as pollution and smoking [3]. The hallmarks associated with ageing have been illustrated in Figure 1. Skin ageing, characterized by wrinkling, can be reduced via suitable preventive measures involving the consumption of antioxidant-rich supplements, a balanced diet and undertaking skincare [4]. By opting for these measures, the harmful effects induced by free radicals can be restrained [5].

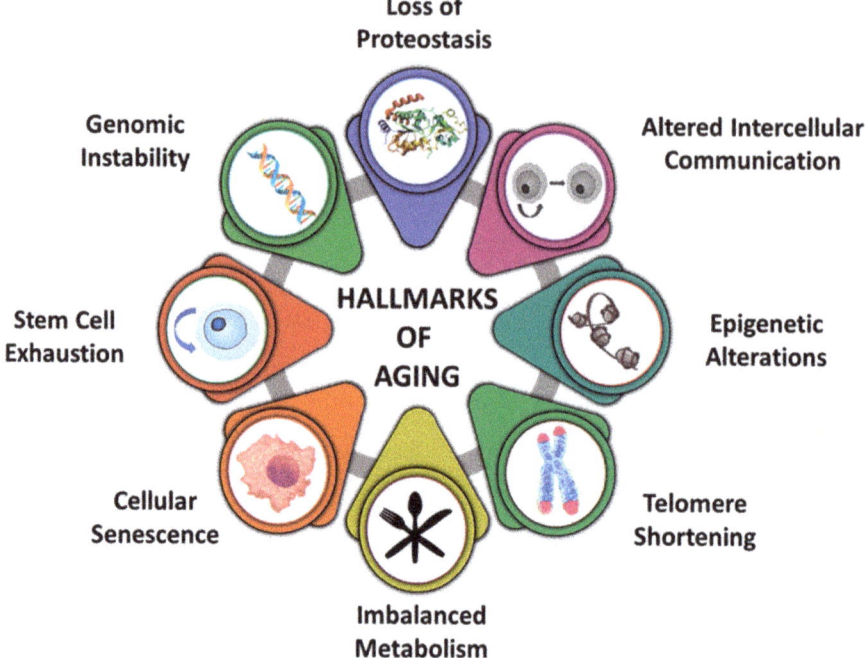

Figure 1. Hallmarks contributing to ageing.

Over the past few decades, the relationship between nutrition and ageing has been extensively studied in both animals and humans [6]. Nutraceuticals are nutritional elements with medicinal characteristics; hence the name, where "Nutra" stands for food and "ceutical" means therapeutic properties [7]. As per the definition of Foundation for Innovation in Medicine (FIM), nutraceuticals are the "food and food products" that have medicinal value and provide health benefits, especially in preventing and treating age-related diseases [8]. These products include functional foods, dietary supplements and herbal extracts, which provide health benefits in the long-run when consumed as supplements in the diet [9]. Even researchers have suggested that antioxidants have propitious effects on both chronic as well as age-related diseases, especially neurodegenerative diseases and cancer [10]. Various food supplements that exhibit an antioxidant potential, such as carotenoids, flavonoids and vitamins, prevent and treat ROS-associated chronic conditions, which results in healthier and longer lifespans [10]. Food supplements produce antagonistic effects against the degenerative and inflammatory processes in the body, and have beneficial effects on the immune and digestive system, hence improving the quality of life [11].

The current review focusses on highlighting the manifestations of ageing and theories associated with ageing. Additionally, it also discusses the importance of diet management in ageing and functional food, as well as nutraceuticals with anti-ageing potential.

2. Manifestation of Ageing

Clinical manifestations of intrinsic ageing can be determined by assessing the regenerative ability of the damaged tissues or organs [12]. All dividing and differentiating cells are vulnerable to insults causing intrinsic ageing [13]. The visual traits of ageing start appearing in the early 40s. Most cells, tissues and organs steadily undergo ageing and become incompetent [14]. A significant effect can be observed on the skin, which turns loose, thin wrinkled and inelastic [15]. The face fat also reduces, leading to hollowed eye sockets and cheeks.

Furthermore, the hair starts thinning from the armpits, pubic area and scalp [16]. As melanin content decreases, the hair strands become thinner grey, and the nails become thinner as well [17]. At over 80 years old, more noticeable visual changes can be observed, such as the compression of spinal disks, vertebrae and joints. The hearing abilities also diminish depending on the severity of the ageing phenomenon [18].

Other than this, the elderly population gets presbyopia and may require reading glasses [19]. In comparison to healthy adults, they lack deep sleep and are unable to take sufficient rest as required by the body at this stage [20]. The bone density decreases and becomes weaker, increasing the risk of fracture [21]. Due to slow metabolism and hormonal changes, there is a reduction in muscle mass and an increase in body fat [22]. Besides this, older adults also suffer from lapses of memory and vagueness, preventing them from recalling names and memories [23]. The heart and lungs become less efficient with time, and kidney functions are abated [24]. The accumulated harmful metabolic waste later appears as dangerous diseases and allergies, causing significant discomfort to older people [25]. Moreover, females at menopause produce reduced amounts of estrogen, due to which they experience various changes, such as vaginal dryness, hot flashes, chills, night sweats, sleeping problems, mood swings, weight gain and slowed metabolism [26]. Besides this, an unhealthy diet and indolent lifestyle further increase the risk of occurrence of chronic diseases in elderly people, such as cancer, osteoarthritis, type 2 diabetes, obesity, coronary artery disease osteoporosis and high blood pressure [27].

3. Theories of Ageing

Several theories have been formulated to define the ageing phenomenon. These theories have been postulated based on certain assumptions, but none of them provide a satisfactory explanation [28]. There are three major theories for ageing, i.e., genetic theories, dysfunction of interlinked organs and physiological approaches [29]. Of these, three physiological theories have been extensively studied, which comprise the cross-linking theory, the waste material accumulation theory and the free radical theory [30].

In 1950, Denham Harman stated that ageing is the result of the massive production of free radicals [31]. In general, free radicals are those atoms or molecules that have unpaired electrons and possess the ability to form electronic couples [32]. This explains the short life and high reactiveness of these molecules. These free radicals are usually formed during the metabolic reactions under normal conditions [33]. Moreover, the generation of these free radicals also takes place during exposure to cigarette smoke, UV rays and toxic substances, as well as during emotional stress [34]. Even though free radicals are involved in normal metabolic processes, but they do not generally infiltrate the cells. Still, when they do, they have harmful and deleterious effects on various organs [35].

Free radicals released from food are essential for energy production within the cell [36]. Additionally, their production also protects the body from opportunistic infections and elicits the synthesis of hormones involved in effective communication within the body [37]. However, the excessive production of free radicals has detrimental effects on DNA, collagen, elastin and blood vessels [38]. Oxidative damage to different biomolecules, such as DNA, macromolecules and proteins, takes place over time [39]. It is considered a significant factor, but is not the only factor responsible for ageing [40]. Fundamentally, oxygen has a dual role in our body, i.e., it is necessary for life and is one of the chief components of harmful compounds like free radicals [41]. Free radicals are generated by the aerobic metabolism. They liberate different types of reactive oxygen species, such as singlet oxygen ($^1[O_2]$), superoxide anion radicals (O_2^-), hydroxyl radicals (OH^-), hydroperoxyl radicals (HO_2), peroxide radicals (R = lipid) (ROO^-) and hydrogen peroxide (H_2O_2) [42]. The various sources involved in the generation of free radicals are illustrated in Figure 2.

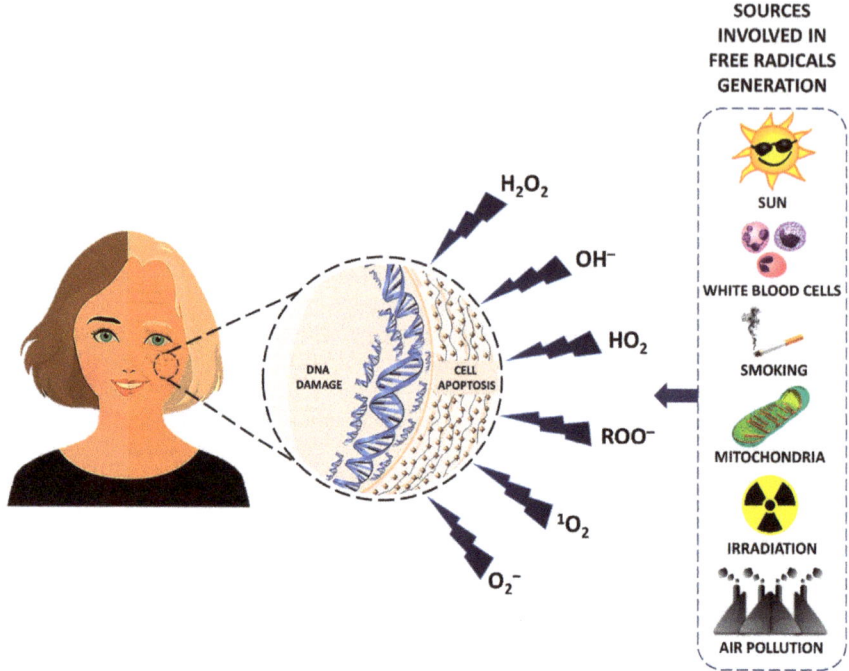

Figure 2. Schematic representation of sources involved in the formation of free radicals and their association with the ageing process.

For example, if the free-radical-mediated DNA mutations are left uncorrected via repair mechanisms, this defect persists even after successive replication cycles, transcription and translation [43]. It is well-known that free radicals are formed by the aerobic metabolism for the synthesis of energy-rich molecules like ATP, which are synthesized in mitochondria (also known as cell factories) [44]. As humans start ageing, the efficacy of mitochondria in synthesizing ATP substantially decreases, thereby allowing the accumulation of free radicals in mitochondria as well as permitting the passage of free radicals through the mitochondrial membrane, thereby damaging other parts of the cell [45]. These alterations have helped to determine the key factors which favor ageing, i.e., increases in oxidative stress and a decrease in energy production [46]. Even the published literature has stated that a high degree of mutation is observed in mitochondrial DNA in contrast to nuclear DNA due to oxidative stress [47]. Therefore, calorie restriction (CR) impedes the process of ageing and increases the lifespans of flies, fish, spiders and mammals (mice and rats) [48]. This happens because CR decreases the oxidative load, which reduces the free radical formation in mitochondria [49]. The reduction in the free radical formation substantially reduces the number of oxidized proteins, lipids and mutated mitochondrial DNA [50]. Extensive studies have been conducted on rodent models to assess the effects of a diet enriched with minerals and vitamins in ageing [44]. As such, it is believed that calorie restriction and the consumption of food rich in antioxidants can considerably prolong the life span of individuals [51].

An important theory that explains the process of ageing is the shortening of the telomeres. Due to the end-replication problem, the telomeres are shortened in every generation of the cell till they reach a critical length in the crisis stage of ageing [52]. At this stage, the cell division slows down considerably, causing the cell to slowly die. This may be referred to as "replicative mortality". Cells involved in growth, development and reproduction express high levels of the enzyme telomerase, which maintains the length of the telomeric DNA [53]. These cells include the stem cells and reproductive cells (eggs and sperms). However, most adult cells have low expressions or no expression of telomerase, which causes these cells to age and eventually die [54].

4. Plant-Based Supplements with Anti-Ageing Potential

Plants and their inherent components are well known to exhibit antioxidant potentials, sch as carotenoids, flavonoids and vitamins, that aid in the prevention and treatment of ROS-associated chronic conditions [55]. These supplements have antagonistic effects against the degenerative and inflammatory processes in the body and show beneficial effects on the immune and digestive system, hence improving the quality of life [56]. Some of the predominantly used plant-based supplements have been discussed below.

4.1. Adaptogens

Adaptogens are compounds obtained from herbal plants for maintaining homeostasis and stabilizing the physiological processes in humans [57]. These compounds reduce cellular sensitivity to stress and improve the ability of the body to resist the damage from other risk factors [58]. Moreover, they also help in restoring and promoting normal physiological function [59]. A few of the highly known adaptogens have been discussed below.

4.2. Bacopa monnieri

Bacopa monnieri, also known as Brahmi, is a perennial herb with small oblong leaves and purple flowers [60]. Highly valuable nootropic phytochemicals, such as bacosides, are found in this medicinal herb [61]. Brahmine and Herpestine are the two essential phytochemicals that are predominantly extracted from this herb [62]. The phytochemicals obtained from Brahmi aid in protecting the brain from the attack of free radicals and stimulating cognitive functioning and learning [63]. It has been comprehended that the regular consumption of Brahmi oil reduces the chance of various diseases like Alzheimer's disease and amnesia [64]. Bhattacharya et al. (2000) found that extracts of *Bacopa monnieri* enhance the activity of reactive oxygen species-scavenging enzyme catalase (CAT), glutathione peroxidase (GPX) and superoxide dismutase (SOD), in a dose-dependent manner. This study was carried out in the brain regions of rats and investigated after 14 and 21 days [65]. Shinomol and colleagues conducted an in vitro and in vivo study using 3-nitropropionic acid (NPA) (fungal toxin responsible for causing neurotoxicity in humans and animals) and *Bacopa monnieri* extract. The result obtained showed that NPA was effective in inducing the oxidative stress in dopaminergic (N27) cells and mitochondria of the striatum of rats, whereas *Bacopa monnieri* extract was found to be effective in regulating the NPA-induced oxidative reactions and reducing the Glutathione (GSH) and thiol levels [66]. Kumar and his colleagues also conducted a six-week randomized placebo-controlled trial to assess the effect of *Bacopa monnieri* extract on the cognitive functions of students studying medicine. The result obtained from the study showed significant improvement in the cognitive functioning of the students [67].

4.3. Curcuma longa

Curcuma longa is a plant of the ginger family that produces a compound known as curcumin [68]. It is known for diverse biological activities, such as its anti-cancerous, anti-inflammatory and antioxidant properties [69]. Due to these natural properties, curcumin is a potential therapeutic agent for treating different types of cancers [70]. Many studies have revealed that curcumin can suppress the expression or activity of cyclooxygenase-2 (COX-2), prostaglandin E2 (PGE2), pro-inflammatory cytokines and tumor necrosis factor-α (TNF-α) [71]. The antioxidant properties of curcumin can aid in the reduction of ROS production, the scavenging of free oxygen radicals and obstructing lipid peroxidation [72]. The consumption of curcumin via the oral route in rodents has been shown to ameliorate cystic fibrosis and block tumor progression; still, the evaluation of humans is pending [70]. A study reported that curcumin induces a cellular stress response in human fibroblasts via redox signaling and the phosphatidylinositol 3-kinase/Akt (Protein Kinase B; PKB) pathway. This provides evidence that curcumin-triggered cellular antioxidant defenses can serve as an effective approach to anti-ageing intervention [73].

Moreover, it has been reported to increase the life span of fruit flies, mice and nematodes [74–76]. In fact, curcumin has been stated to improve and regulate the symptoms of age-related diseases such as atherosclerosis, cancer and diabetes [77,78]. Other than this, curcumin has been reported to show protective activity against chemotherapy-induced side effects and radiation-induced dermatitis in breast cancer patients [79,80]. Some studies have claimed that curcumin has anti-ageing potential because it can delay cellular senescence [81]. Cox et al. conducted a study to assess the effects of solid lipid curcumin on mood and cognition in healthy adults aged 60–85. In this study, subjects were examined for the effects of solid lipid curcumin formulation, i.e., 400 mg of Longvida® for acute (1 and 3 h after a single dose), chronic (4 weeks) and acute-on-chronic (1 and 3 h after a single dose following regular treatment) dosing. The results obtained showed significant improvements in the working memory for both acute and chronic dosing. Additionally, it also decreased physical fatigue (measured per Chalder Fatigue Scale) as well as total and LDL cholesterol [82].

4.4. Emblica officinalis

Emblica officinalis, also known as Amla, is a member of the Phyllanthaceae family [83]. The churn of Amla is known for reducing cholesterol level and improving memory potential [84]. The consumption of Amla in the diet is effective in lowering the cholesterol level in the brain as well as in the body [85]. It has also been stated as a beneficial functional food for treating Alzheimer's disease [86]. Draelos and colleagues conducted a double-blind study to evaluate the skin-lightening potential of a topical formulation comprising *E. officinalis* extract, glycolic acid and kojic acid. The study revealed that the topical formulation was 4% better than hydroquinone, due to which researchers claimed that the topical formulation could be an effective natural alternative for mild to moderate facial dyschromia [87]. Accumulation of free radicals in different tissues is associated with various stress-induced conditions leading to the progression of the process of ageing [88]. Tannoids obtained from *E. officinalis* also show a protective effect because of their antioxidant potential against the tardive dyskinesia rat model [89]. Moreover, the extract of *E. officinalis* shows antidepressant properties by inhibiting the activity of Gamma Amino Butyric Acid (GABA) and Monoamine oxidase-A (MAO-A) in consort with antioxidant activity in mice models [90].

4.5. Ginkgo biloba

Ginkgo biloba, also known as Gingko, is a functional food which improves the availability of oxygen in the tissues [91]. The leaves of Ginkgo have been reported to play a significant role in maintaining the blood flow and glucose level in the brain [92]. Moreover, it also improves the mental functioning of the brain [93]. Ascorbic acid, catechin, shikimic acid, lactone derivatives (ginkgolides) and isorhamnetin are some of the flavone glycosides, which are active scavengers of free radicals and are obtained from the extract of ginkgo leaves [94]. Huang conducted a study to assess the effect of *Gingko biloba* extract on the liver of the aged rat. The result revealed that administration of *Gingko biloba* extract reduced the level of liver metalloproteinase as well as malondialdehyde, and improved the SOD activity to minimize the oxidative stress [95]. Another study has revealed that the administration of *Gingko biloba* extract improves the cognitive function in aged female rats [96]. Even clinical studies have been conducted to assess the effect of *Gingko biloba* extract in the treatment of Alzheimer's disease and cognitive function. Extensive analysis has revealed that the consumption of *Gingko biloba* extract improves the cognitive functioning of individuals who have mild dementia [97].

4.6. Glycyrrhiza glabra

Glycyrrhiza glabra, also known as licorice, is a member of the Fabaceae family [98]. The rhizomes, as well as roots of this plant, serve as a brain tonic which helps in regulating the blood sugar level [99]. Glycyrrhizin is the prime bioactive molecule obtained from this plant rich in antioxidants, which protects the brain from oxidative damage, maintains the normal functioning of the nervous system and improves the memory of the individual [100]. *Glycyrrhiza glabra* has a phenolic compound named "liquorice" which has antioxidant potential, due to which it is effective in the chelating of metal ions and the scavenging of free radicals [101]. It has been reported that *G. glabra* enhances the memory in the murine model of scopolamine-induced dementia [102]. Dhingra and colleagues also reported improvements in the memory of mice administered with *Glycyrrhiza glabra*. Three different doses, i.e., 75, 150 and 300 mg/kg p.o. of *Glycyrrhiza glabra* extracts, were administered for seven consecutive days. The result obtained showed that a dose of 150 mg/kg was effective in enhancing memory in the mice model [103].

4.7. Panax ginseng

Panax ginseng, also known as ginseng, is highly known for its medicinal value [104]. The bioactive molecule ginsenoside is obtained from the roots of this plant [105]. This bioactive molecule improves the resistance of the body against anxiety, fatigue, stress and trauma, and modulates the immune function [106]. Moreover, it also shows anti-stress properties and improves learning performance and memory [104]. A study reported an increase in the life span of juvenile mice with leukaemia upon the administration of ginseng [107]. Another study on *Panax ginseng* reported that it is able to decrease lipid peroxidation and improve antioxidant potential by reducing oxidative stress [108].

Moreover, double-blind clinical trials have confirmed that the consumption of ginseng improves the psychomotor performance of the individuals [109]. *Panax ginseng* has also been reported to have anti-melanogenic potential, and is associated with the activation of the foxo3a gene, also stated as the longevity gene [110]. Certain studies have reported that *Panax ginseng* prevents skin ageing. Furthermore, a randomized, placebo-controlled, double-blind study was conducted to assess the potential of both *Panax ginseng* and ginsenosides in preventing skin ageing. The result obtained from the study showed a significant reduction in wrinkle formation, and no participant showed an adverse reaction to the treatment [111].

5. Plant-Based Metabolites with Anti-Ageing and Medicinal Properties

5.1. Polyphenols

Plants are prime producers of secondary metabolites, especially polyphenolic compounds, and these are abundantly found in vegetables, fruits, cereals and beverages [112]. Polyphenols have intrigued researchers globally owing to their inherent properties, such as antioxidant potential, and their anticarcinogenic and anti-inflammatory action [113]. These characteristics enable polyphenolic compounds to be useful in the amelioration of various diseases, such as cancer, asthma, microbial infections, diabetes and cardiovascular diseases [114]. Studies have been conducted on numerous polyphenolic compounds, such as resveratrol, proanthocyanins and silymarin. They have been evaluated for their action on animal models subjected to DNA damage, oxidative stress and UV-induced skin irritation [115]. Moreover, these polyphenols, consolidated with sun protection cosmetic products, can effectively shield the skin from UV radiation-associated skin problems and aid in reducing the incidence of skin cancer [116]. Some polyphenols with therapeutic properties have been described below.

Resveratrol (Stilbenes) is a natural polyphenolic compound with antioxidant potential, and is present in the skin of peanuts and grapes [117]. In the last two decades, it has been a prime area of extensive research owing to its application as an anti-ageing ingredient [118]. Additionally, it exhibits anti-inflammatory action and radical scavenging properties, and can act as a chelating agent [119]. Studies have found it to be effective in the treatment of various diseases, including Alzheimer's and cardiovascular disease [120]. Moreover, Bhat et al. stated that resveratrol possesses cancer chemo-preventive potential [121]. It also has a protective action against human skin, which was confirmed via the study conducted on HaCat cells exposed to nitric oxide free radical donor sodium nitroprusside [122]. Giardina and colleagues conducted an in vitro study on skin fibroblast to assess the efficacy of resveratrol on the proliferation and inhibition of collagen activity. The result obtained showed a dose-related increase in the proliferation rate of cells and substantial inhibition of collagenase activity [123]. Although it has been claimed that resveratrol has the potential to combat ageing at the cellular level and could be a breakthrough in anti-ageing and geriatric medicine, data supporting this claim in the human context are quite limited [124–126]. It has been well comprehended that resveratrol modulates mitochondrial biogenesis via stimulating Peroxisome proliferator-activated receptor gamma coactivator 1-alpha (PGC-1α), which further slows down the process of ageing and circumvents the chronic diseases [127,128].

Flavonoids (Phlorizin): Few plants have been found to synthesize phlorizin, a type of flavonoid [129]. It has been immensely exploited by pharmaceutical industries for more than a century, while also serving as a platform to evaluate physiological functioning [115]. Several studies have been conducted on the nutritional benefits of phlorizin. In a recent study, the anti-aging effects of phlorizin and phloretin were tested on murine senile osteoporosis models. The study revealed that phlorizin helped in the management of the ratio of receptor activator of nuclear factor kappa-B ligand (RANKL) to osteoprotegerin (OPG), which is a biochemical marker of osteoporosis. Phlorizin also reduced the population of osteoclast cells expressing tartrate-resistant acid phosphatase (TRAP) [130]. Phlorizin is found at high concentrations in unripe apples. A preliminary study on human volunteers revealed the beneficial effects of unripe apples containing phlorizin in mitigating post-prandial hyperglycemia. The study was carried out on six healthy individuals and revealed that the consumption of unripe apples caused statistically significant reductions in post-prandial glucose response, as well as increased urinary glucose [131]. Mela and colleagues conducted a study to evaluate the effects of eight plant extracts as well as their combinations (apple (AE, 2.0 g), mulberry fruit (MFE, 1.5 g), elderberry (EE, 2.0 g), mulberry leaf (MLE, 1.0 g), turmeric (TE, 0.18 g), white bean (WBE, 3.0 g), EE + TE and AE + TE) on post-prandial insulin (PPI) and glucose (PPG) response. The results obtained from the study revealed that extracts of AE, MLE and MFE were effective in reducing PPI and PPG response [132]. Hyperglycemia has been reported to accelerate the aging process, which describes the potential of phlorizin in mitigating the effects of ageing, thereby improving the quality of life [133]. Many other plant extracts have emerged as potent sources of compounds with antioxidant potential [134]. Metabolites such as silymarin, genistein and apigenin have been found to impact the symptoms of skin ageing positively [91]. Still, no clinical or human trials have been conducted to unveil the real anti-ageing potential of phlorizin.

Apple Polyphenols: Apple is enriched with phytochemicals, especially polyphenols that exhibit immense antioxidant potential [135]. A wide range of polyphenolic compounds is found in apples, such as rutin, chlorogenic acid, catechin phloretin, epicatechin and proanthocyanidin B2 [136]. The daily consumption of apples has been portrayed to reduce the incidence of the occurrence of hypercholesterolemia and cardiovascular diseases [137]. Research studies have suggested that consuming apples can considerably lower the risk of lung cancer, especially in females [138]. Different studies have proven that apple is effective in impeding low-density lipoprotein (LDL) oxidation [137]. A study was conducted to evaluate the effects of apple polyphenols on the gene expression of CcO (cytochrome c oxidase) subunits III, CAT (catalase), Mth (methuselah), Rpn11, SOD and VIb. The result obtained from the study revealed that apple polyphenols increased the life span of fruit flies by 10%. Moreover, the downregulation of Mth, the upregulation of gene CAT, SOD1 and SOD2, and no significant change in the gene expression of CcO subunits, Rpn11 or VIb, were observed in the fruit flies [139]. Furthermore, concentrated apple juice has neuroprotective potential, confirmed via the studies conducted on normal aged mice and genetically compromised mice. Still, the anti-ageing potential of apple and its underlining mechanisms remain indefinable [51].

Blueberry Extract: Polyphenols are more abundantly found in blueberries than in other fruits and vegetables [140]. The high antioxidant potential of blueberry extracts has been associated with the amelioration of ageing symptoms [141]. Studies suggest that the regular consumption of blueberries can potentially enhance memory-related issues in elderly populations [142]. It has been stated that the consumption of blueberry extract slows down age-related functional and physiological deficits [143]. Galli and colleagues have found that supplementation with blueberry extract reversed the age-linked decline in the heat shock protein (HSP) of the hippocampal in rats [144]. Additionally, blueberries have been found to be effective in improving motor and cognitive behavior in aged rat models [145]. The life-prolonging potential of blueberry extracts has also been studied in fruit flies to understand the underlying mechanism. The results obtained from the study revealed that the incorporation of 5 mg/mL of blueberry extract into the diet significantly increased the lifespan of fruit flies by 10% [146].

Tea Catechins and Theaflavins: Tea has emerged as the most preferred beverage in the Asian subcontinent [147]. The beneficial aspects associated with the consumption of tea can be attributed to its inherent compounds, namely theaflavins and catechins [148]. Studies have shown the reduced oxidation of DNA molecules via regular intake of green or black tea [149]. Other in vivo studies on Drosophila have reported positive results concerning the increase in average life span by theaflavins and catechins [150]. Various published reports have stated that the consumption of oral tea polyphenols, as well as topical treatment with green tea, inhibits UV radiation- or chemical-induced skin tumorigenesis in various animal models [151]. Tea catechins and theaflavins possess both anti-inflammatory and anticarcinogenic properties [148]. Elmets and his team conducted a study to assess the effect of tea polyphenol extract on parameters linked with acute UV injury. For this, the skin of volunteers was first treated with green tea extract or its constituents, and treated sites were subjected to two minimal erythema doses of solar simulated radiation. Later, the skin was examined for the biochemical, clinical and histologic characteristics of UV-induced DNA damage. The results revealed that tea extract has a dose-dependent inhibitory effect on erythema response induced by UV irradiation. The histologic evaluation also showed a reduced number of Langerhans and sunburn cells [152].

Moreover, tea polyphenol extracts also reduced the DNA damage in the skin. Therefore, researchers stated that tea polyphenol extract could serve as a natural alternative for photoprotection [152]. Chiu and colleagues conducted a study to assess the effect of a combination therapy course of topical and oral green tea on the histological and clinical characteristics of photo-ageing. For this study, 40 women with rational photo-ageing were randomized either to a placebo regimen or a combination of 300 mg tea oral supplements (consumed twice daily) and 10% green tea cream for eight weeks. The results obtained from the study did not show any significant differences in the clinical characteristics of photo-ageing for the placebo or green tea-treated group. However, a histologic improvement in elastic tissue content was observed in the treated participants [153].

Black Rice Anthocyanins: Black rice is abundant in antioxidants, the supplementation of which has been proven to relieve symptoms in patients who have Alzheimer's [10]. It also has an anticarcinogenic and anti-inflammatory effect [154]. It is also rich in anthocyanins, namely peonidin-3-glucoside and cyanidin-3-o glucoside [155]. Zuo and colleagues conducted a study of the potential of black rice in extending the lifespan of fruit flies. For determination, the effects on the gene expressions of CAT, Mth, Rpn11, SOD1 and SOD2 were evaluated. The result obtained from the study revealed that the consumption of 30 mg/dL of black rice anthocyanins prolonged the lifespan by 14% of the fruit flies. Moreover, the downregulated gene expression of Mth and the upregulated gene expression of CAT, Rpn11, SOD1 and SOD2 was recorded [156]. Huang et al. also conducted a study on a subacute ageing mice model to assess the effect of black rice anthocyanins, and found that black rice anthocyanins exhibit anti-ageing, anti-fatigue and anti-hypoxic properties [157].

5.2. Carotenoids

Carotenoids are vitamin A derivates, such as lycopene and β-carotene, which are known to possess high antioxidant potential as well as photoprotective characteristics [158]. β-carotene and lycopene can moderately improve skin texture [159].

β-Carotene is obtained from various plant sources, such as carrots, mangoes, papaya and pumpkins, among others [160]. It has emerged as a significant carotenoid owing to its characteristics, such as pro-vitamin-A activity, lipid radical scavenging activity and single oxygen quenching properties [161]. β-Carotene has been reported to avert erythema induced by UV rays and possess excellent photoprotection properties [162]. Reports have suggested the association of cellular ageing with low β-Carotene levels in plasma. A study conducted on 68 old-age subjects showed that β-carotene might modulate telomerase activity in older adults [163]. On the other hand, there are well-known ill effects of supplementary beta carotene for smokers, leading to the progression of lung cancer. A pioneering study in 1994 was published in the New England Journal of Medicine by the alpha tocopherol, beta carotene cancer prevention study group. This study reported that there was an unexpected observation of a greater incidence of lung cancer in men receiving supplementary beta-carotene, as opposed to those who did not [164].

Lycopene is a red carotene, carotenoid and phytochemical present in numerous fruits and vegetables such as papayas, watermelons, tomatoes, carrots and others [4]. It possesses a high single oxygen quenching potential, but lacks vitamin A activity [165]. Moreover, a study confirmed the role of lycopene in attenuating oxidative damage in tissues. Upon exposure to UV light, it was observed that more skin lycopene was destroyed in contrast to β-carotene [166]. Products of lycopene have also been reported to be effective against cancerous cells, in addition to their potential to significantly reduce MMP-1 activity, which is known to degrade collagen [167]. Both lycopene and β-carotene, dominant carotenoids found in human tissues and blood, are known to regulate skin properties [168]. In a very recently published paper, Cheng and co-workers reported that lycopene induces the base excision repair pathway in vitro in A549 cells. This study has opened a molecular pathway, which needs further investigation in vivo and in animal models [169].

5.3. Vitamins

Vitamin C is commonly known as ascorbic acid, and is a highly water-soluble vitamin [170]. This colorless compound has high antioxidant potential owing to its strong reducing nature [171]. The photosensitive ascorbic acid works best in a hydrophilic environment [172]. This crystalline compound is not synthesized in humans; therefore, it has to be taken in the regular diet [173]. Diets should be supplemented with vitamin C-rich sources, such as oranges, broccoli, brussels sprouts, green peppers, strawberries, kiwifruit and grapefruit, to avoid the vitamin C deficiency associated health problems like cardiovascular diseases, scurvy, and others [174]. Ascorbic acid has a high antioxidant potential and free radical-scavenging properties, which helps in preventing the oxidation of tissues, cell membranes and macromolecules (DNA and proteins) by free radicals [173].

Vitamin E is a fat-soluble membrane-bound compound which has high free radical-scavenging as well as antioxidant potential [175]. This nonenzymatic antioxidant is found in wheat germ oil, safflower oil, sunflower oil, vegetables, peanuts, corn, almonds, soy and meat [176]. A deficiency of vitamin E in the body may lead to the development of various health conditions in infants, such as dryness, papular erythema, depigmentation and oedema [177]. Vitamin E consumption helps in combating skin ageing symptoms due to its efficacy in preventing the peroxidation of lipids and the cross-connection of collagen fibers [4]. Vitamin E has been proven to relieve sunburn and UV-associated skin damage [178].

Both vitamins C and E work synergistically. For instance, when UV-induced molecules oxidize the cellular constituents, a chain reaction of lipid peroxidation starts in the membrane rich in polyunsaturated fatty acids. During this, d-α-tocopherol (antioxidant) gets oxidized to the tocopheroxyl radical and regenerates itself through ascorbic acid [179,180]. Different food sources such as corn, seeds, vegetable oils (sunflower oil and safflower oil) and soy are rich in tocopherol [4]. Moreover, the consumption of vitamin E from natural sources help against lipid peroxidation and collagen cross-linking, as both are associated with skin ageing. Additionally, topically applied vitamin E has also been reported to reduce chronic UVB-induced skin damage, erythema, sunburned cells and photocarcinogenesis [181,182]. A deficiency of vitamin E is also associated with a syndrome of edema with seborrheic changes, as well as depigmentation and dryness in premature infants [183]. Ekanayake-Mudiyanselage and Thiele, upon analyzing their study, stated that the level of vitamin E is dependent on the density of sebaceous glands in the skin. The oral supplementation of α-tocopherol for three weeks has been shown to cause a substantial increase in vitamin E levels in the sebaceous gland, especially on the face [184]. In a comparative study, the oral consumption of both vitamin C and E has been shown to improve the photoprotective effect in contrast to monotherapies [185]. Another study was conducted on 33 participants who received 100 or 180 mg vitamin C or placebo per day for four weeks. The result obtained from the study revealed that orally consumed vitamin C improved the radical scavenging activity of the skin by 22% (for 100 mg) and 37% (for 180 mg) from the baseline [87]. In the study by the alpha-tocopherol and beta carotene cancer prevention study group, it was found that vitamin E has insignificant effects on the prevention of lung cancer [164].

Nutraceuticals, functional foods and dietary supplements encompass a large group of compounds which are well known to improve health [186]. Functional foods have gained global attention owing to their impact on improving the symptoms of skin ageing [187]. Notably, fruits constitute an essential source of active metabolites used to curb skin ageing symptoms, as they are enriched with phenolic compounds, carotenoids and ascorbic acid, and possess high antioxidant potential [188]. The various plants and their components with anti-ageing potential are listed in Table 1.

Table 1. Fruits and vegetable extracts and their phytochemicals with antiageing effects.

Common Name	Scientific Name	Study Conducted Region	Active Compounds	Biological Activities	Dose and Duration	Study Type	Experimental Models	References
Sweet orange	Citrus sinensis L.	Italy	Anthocyanins, flavanones, hydroxycinnamic acid and ascorbic acid	NF-B and AP-1 translocation and procaspase-3 cleavage	15 and 30 µg/mL for 7 h	In vitro	Human keratinocytes (HaCaT cell line)	[189]
Indian gooseberry	Emblica officinalis L.	Japan	Ascorbic acid, gallic Acid, elaeocarpusin	Inhibited type-1 collagen collagenase, increase TIMP-1 level; Cellular proliferation inhibition and procollagen 1 protection against UVB-induced depletion by inhibition of UVB-induced MMP-1	(0–40 g/mL) for 48 h	In vitro	NB1RGB human skin fibroblasts	[190]
Indian gooseberry	Emblica officinalis	India	Ascorbic acid	Promotion of procollagen content and inhibition of matrix metalloproteinase levels in skin fibroblast	10–40 µg/mL for 24 h	In vitro	Fibroblast cell line (HS68 cell)	[191]
Cucumber	Cucumis sativus L.	India	Ascorbic acid	In vitro inhibition of hyaluronidase, elastase and MMP-1	20.98 and 6.14 µg/mL	In vitro assay	ND	[192]
Bitter gourd	Momordica charantia L.	China	Resveratrol	Anti-oxidative stress enhancement and UTH1, SKN7, SOD1 and SOD2 yeast gene expression regulation	1–3 µM for 12 h	In vitro	Yeast	[193]
Litchi, Rambutan, Tamarind	Litchi chinensis; Nephelium lappaceum L.; Tamarindus indica	Thailand	Ferulic acid, gallic acid, epigallocatechin	Suppression of melanin production in B16F10 melanoma cells through inhibition of tyrosinase and TRP-2; effectiveness for elastase and collagenase inhibition	0.05, 0.01 and 0.007 mg/mL for 72 h	In vitro	Human skin fibroblasts	[194]
Mandarin orange	Citrus reticulata Blanco	India	D-Limonene, n-Hexadecanoic acid	Collagenase and elastase inhibition, anti-enzymatic activity	NS	In vitro assay	ND	[195]
Snake fruit	Salacca zalacca (Gaertr.) Voss	Indonesia	Chlorogenic acid	MMP-1 inhibition	NS	In silico	ND	[196]
Mandarin, Grapes	Citrus sunki Hort. ex Tanaka, Citrus unshiu Marcov, Citrus sinensis Osbeck, Citrus reticulata Blanco and Vitis vinifera L.	Republic of Korea	Narirutin, hesperidin, ascorbic acid	Increase in the expression levels of antioxidant enzymes; Reduction in skin thickness and wrinkle formation while elevating collagen level in an ultraviolet light B-exposed hairless mouse model	33, 100, 300 mg/kg for 10 weeks	In vitro and in vivo	Cell culture and mice	[197]
Carrot	Daucus carota L.	South Korea	Carrot glycoprotein	Neutralization of reactive oxygen, cell membrane protection	0.3, 0.5, 1 mg/mL	In vitro	Cell culture	[198]
Safflower Seed Oil	Carthamus tinctorius	France	Phenol	Inhibition in the collagenase assay, inhibition in the elastase assay	NS	In vitro assay	ND	[199]
Chinese quince	Chaenomeles sinensis	Japan	β-1,4-xyloglucan	Inhibition of the activity of dermal extracellular matrix proteases: Elastase and Collagenase	NS	In vitro assay	ND	[200]
Almonds	Prunus dulcis	California	α-tocopherol	Decreased wrinkle severity in postmenopausal females	340 kcal/day of almonds (58.9 g) for 16 weeks	Observational study	Human subjects	[201]

Table 1. Cont.

Common Name	Scientific Name	Study Conducted Region	Active Compounds	Biological Activities	Dose and Duration	Study Type	Experimental Models	References
Maidenhair tree	Ginkgo biloba L.	China	kaempferol 3-O-β-D-glucopyranoside, isorhamnetin-3-O-glucoside, myricetin, ginkgolide A, bilobalide	Inhibition of ROS and MMP-1 degradation in human dermal fibroblasts	0.1, 0.2 mg/mL for 24 h	In vitro	Human dermal fibroblasts	[202]
Turmeric	Curcuma longa	India	Curcumin	Reduction in levels of C-reactive protein (CRP) an anti-ageing inflammatory marker	200 mg and 400 mg of Curcumin/kg bodyweight for six months	In vivo	Rat	[203]
Asian ginseng	Panax ginseng	Korea	Gingenoside	Promotion in collagen synthesis through the activation of transforming growth factor-β (TGF-β) in human skin fibroblast cells	0.05% PGLE for eight weeks	In vitro and In vivo	In vitro and human volunteer	[204]
Korean ginseng, mountain hawthorn	Panax ginseng Meyer and Crataegus pinnatifida	Republic of Korea	Ginsenoside	Protective effect against UVB-exposed photo-ageing of the skin by regulating procollagen type 1 and MMP-1 expression in NHDFs	100 μg/mL for 12 weeks	In vitro and Observational study	Human dermal fibroblasts, healthy human skin	[205]
Licorice	Glycyrrhiza glabra L.	Croatia	Glabridin and isoliquiritigenin	Tyrosinase and elastase inhibitory activity	NS	In vitro assay	ND	[101]
Siberian ginseng, touch-me-not	Eleutherococcus senticosus	Republic of Korea	Phlorizin	miR135b suppression improves the microenvironment and increases the proliferative potential of basal epidermal cells	NS	In vitro	Human keratinocytes	[206]
Marula	Sclerocarya birrea	South Africa	Quinic acid, catechin, epigallocatechin gallate and epicatechin gallate	Exhibited collagenase inhibition activities	100, 200 μg/mL	In vitro assay	ND	[207]
Lemon	Citrus limon	Japan	Eriocitrin (Polyphenols)	Increase in ageing-related scores (e.g., periophthalmic lesions) and delay in locomotor atrophy	4 mL and 6 mL/day/mouse	In vivo	Mice	[208]
Black rice	Zizania aquatica	China	Cyanidin-3-O-glucoside	Increases superoxide dismutase (SOD) and catalase (CAT), while decreases MDA and the activity of monoamine oxidase (MAO)	15, 30 and 60 mg/kg	In vivo	Mice	[209]
Green tea	Camellia sinensis L.	China	Epigallocatechin-3-gallate	Extension of lifespan through mitohormesis	50–300 μM for six days	In vivo	Caenorhabditis elegans	[210]
Orange Pekoe black tea	Camellia sinensis L.	Sri Lanka	Epigallocatechin gallate	Inhibition of elastase activity	NS	In vitro assay	ND	[211]
Banana	Musa spaientum	Korea	Corosolic acid	Inhibitory effects on MMPs activities	NS	In vitro assay	ND	[212]
Rice	Oryza sativa	Indonesia	Vanillin and coumaric acid	Elastase inhibitory activity	NS	In vitro assay	ND	[213]

NS: not specified; ND: not defined.

6. Concluding Remarks

Ageing is a complex and progressive biological process, which gets affected by environmental and genetic factors. Nowadays, ageing is also linked with the consumption of an imbalanced diet deficient in many essential nutrients. Lately, nutraceuticals have gained appreciation and are being considered as a crucial element in improving life and providing antioxidant-containing molecules. Various vegetables and fruits contain antioxidant molecules with beneficial properties that can help in delaying the process of ageing. Moreover, these nutraceuticals do not show unwanted symptoms; instead, they have a beneficial impact on the digestive system. Therefore, nutraceuticals as food supplements have promising potential in combating as well as delaying the ageing process. The benefits associated with nutraceuticals prompts their incorporation into the diet for health benefits and long life. The current review meticulously summarizes the anti-ageing effects of plant-based supplements and plant-derived metabolites. Since most of the data have been obtained in vitro, caution is advised for inferring the clinical applicability of in vitro-tested molecules. Referencing, examining and confirming the human trial data is highly recommended.

Author Contributions: Conceptualization, R.S. (Reena Singh) and K.K.; Manuscript writing, D.S.D. and S.B.; Manuscript editing, D.S.D., S.B., R.S. (Ruchi Sharma), K.B., D.K., C.C. and E.N.; Critical revising, R.S. (Reena Singh) and K.K. All authors have read and agreed to the published version of the manuscript.

Funding: This research was funded by the University of Hradec Kralove (Faculty of Science VT2019-2021) and Ministry of Health (No. NV19-09-00578).

Conflicts of Interest: The authors declare no conflict of interest.

References

1. Jin, K.; Rose, M.R. Modern Biological Theories of Aging. *Aging Dis.* **1988**, *1*, 220–221. [CrossRef]
2. Zhang, S.; Duan, E. Fighting against Skin Aging: The Way from Bench to Bedside. *Cell Transplant.* **2018**, *27*, 729–738. [CrossRef] [PubMed]
3. Bocheva, G.; Slominski, R.M.; Slominski, A.T. Neuroendocrine aspects of skin aging. *Int. J. Mol. Sci.* **2019**, *20*, 2798. [CrossRef] [PubMed]
4. Schagen, S.K.; Zampeli, V.A.; Makrantonaki, E.; Zouboulis, C.C. Discovering the link between nutrition and skin aging. *Dermatoendocrinology* **2012**, *4*, 298–307. [CrossRef] [PubMed]
5. Lobo, V.; Patil, A.; Phatak, A.; Chandra, N. Free radicals, antioxidants and functional foods: Impact on human health. *Pharmacogn. Rev.* **2010**, *4*, 118–126. [CrossRef]
6. Alam, I.; Almajwal, A.M.; Alam, W.; Alam, I.; Ullah, N.; Abulmeaaty, M.; Razak, S.; Khan, S.; Pawelec, G.; Paracha, P.I. The immune-nutrition interplay in aging-Facts and controversies. *Nutr. Healthy Aging* **2019**, *5*, 73–95. [CrossRef]
7. Rathore, H.; Prasad, S.; Sharma, S. Mushroom nutraceuticals for improved nutrition and better human health: A review. *PharmaNutrition* **2017**, *5*, 35–46. [CrossRef]
8. Da Costa, J.P. A current look at nutraceuticals–Key concepts and future prospects. *Trends Food Sci. Technol.* **2017**, *62*, 68–78. [CrossRef]
9. Chauhan, B.; Kumar, G.; Kalam, N.; Ansari, S.H. Current concepts and prospects of herbal nutraceutical: A review. *J. Adv. Pharm. Technol. Res.* **2013**, *4*, 4–8.
10. Liu, Z.; Ren, Z.; Zhang, J.; Chuang, C.C.; Kandaswamy, E.; Zhou, T.; Zuo, L. Role of ROS and nutritional antioxidants in human diseases. *Front. Physiol.* **2018**, *9*, 477. [CrossRef]
11. Conlon, M.A.; Bird, A.R. The impact of diet and lifestyle on gut microbiota and human health. *Nutrients* **2015**, *7*, 17–44. [CrossRef] [PubMed]
12. Eming, S.A.; Martin, P.; Tomic-Canic, M. Wound repair and regeneration: Mechanisms, signaling, and translation. *Sci. Transl. Med.* **2014**, *6*, 265sr6. [CrossRef] [PubMed]
13. Salam, N.; Rane, S.; Das, R.; Faulkner, M.; Gund, R.; Kandpal, U.; Lewis, V.; Mattoo, H.; Prabhu, S.; Ranganathan, V.; et al. T cell ageing: Effects of age on development, survival & function. *Indian J. Med. Res.* **2013**, *138*, 595–608. [PubMed]

14. Amarya, S.; Singh, K.; Sabharwal, M. Ageing Process and Physiological Changes. In *Gerontology*; InTech: London, UK, 2018.
15. Prohaska, T.R.; Keller, M.L.; Leventhal, E.A.; Leventhal, H. Impact of symptoms and aging attribution on emotions and coping. *Health Psychol.* **1987**, *6*, 495–514. [CrossRef]
16. Heinemann, L.A.J.; Zimmermann, T.; Vermeulen, A.; Thiel, C.; Hummel, W. A new «aging males» symptoms' rating scale. *Aging Male* **1999**, *2*, 105–114. [CrossRef]
17. Maddy, A.J.; Tosti, A. Hair and nail diseases in the mature patient. *Clin. Dermatol.* **2018**, *36*, 159–166. [CrossRef]
18. Sarbacher, C.A.; Halper, J.T. Connective tissue and age-related diseases. In *Subcellular Biochemistry*; Springer: New York, NY, USA, 2019; pp. 281–310.
19. Patel, I.; West, S.K. Presbyopia: Prevalence, impact, and interventions. *Community Eye Health J.* **2007**, *20*, 40–41.
20. Boostani, R.; Karimzadeh, F.; Nami, M. A comparative review on sleep stage classification methods in patients and healthy individuals. *Comput. Methods Progr. Biomed.* **2017**, *140*, 77–91. [CrossRef]
21. Locantore, P.; Del Gatto, V.; Gelli, S.; Paragliola, R.M.; Pontecorvi, A. The Interplay between Immune System and Microbiota in Osteoporosis. *Mediat. Inflamm.* **2020**, *2020*, 3686749. [CrossRef]
22. Trexler, E.T.; Smith-Ryan, A.E.; Norton, L.E. Metabolic adaptation to weight loss: Implications for the athlete. *J. Int. Soc. Sports Nutr.* **2014**, *11*, 7. [CrossRef]
23. Wood, R.L. Accelerated cognitive aging following severe traumatic brain injury: A review. *Brain Inj.* **2017**, *31*, 1270–1278. [CrossRef] [PubMed]
24. Sarnak, M.J. A patient with heart failure and worsening kidney function. *Clin. J. Am. Soc. Nephrol.* **2014**, *9*, 1790–1798. [CrossRef]
25. De Martinis, M.; Sirufo, M.M.; Ginaldi, L. Allergy and aging: An Old/new emerging health issue. *Aging Dis.* **2017**, *8*, 162–175. [CrossRef]
26. Santoro, N.; Epperson, C.N.; Mathews, S.B. Menopausal Symptoms and Their Management. *Endocrinol. Metab. Clin. N. Am.* **2015**, *44*, 497–515. [CrossRef] [PubMed]
27. Booth, F.W.; Roberts, C.K.; Laye, M.J. Lack of exercise is a major cause of chronic diseases. *Compr. Physiol.* **2012**, *2*, 1143–1211. [CrossRef]
28. Da Costa, J.P.; Vitorino, R.; Silva, G.M.; Vogel, C.; Duarte, A.C.; Rocha-Santos, T. A synopsis on aging—Theories, mechanisms and future prospects. *Ageing Res. Rev.* **2016**, *29*, 90–112. [CrossRef] [PubMed]
29. De, A.; Ghosh, C. Basics of aging theories and disease related aging-an overview. *PharmaTutor* **2017**, *5*, 16–23.
30. Weinert, B.T.; Timiras, P.S. Invited review: Theories of aging. *J. Appl. Physiol.* **2003**, *95*, 1706–1716. [CrossRef]
31. Gladyshev, V.N. The free radical theory of aging is dead. Long live the damage theory! *Antioxid. Redox Signal.* **2014**, *20*, 727–731. [CrossRef]
32. Sailaja Rao, P.; Kalva, S.; Yerramilli, A.; Mamidi, S. Free Radicals and Tissue Damage: Role of Antioxidants. *Free Radic. Antioxid.* **2011**, *1*, 2–7. [CrossRef]
33. Phaniendra, A.; Jestadi, D.B.; Periyasamy, L. Free Radicals: Properties, Sources, Targets, and Their Implication in Various Diseases. *Indian J. Clin. Biochem.* **2015**, *30*, 11–26. [CrossRef] [PubMed]
34. Di Meo, S.; Venditti, P. Evolution of the Knowledge of Free Radicals and Other Oxidants. *Oxid. Med. Cell. Longev.* **2020**, *2020*, 9829176. [CrossRef] [PubMed]
35. Pham-Huy, L.A.; He, H.; Pham-Huy, C. Free radicals, antioxidants in disease and health. *Int. J. Biomed. Sci.* **2008**, *4*, 89–96. [PubMed]
36. Aruoma, O.I. Nutrition and health aspects of free radicals and antioxidants. *Food Chem. Toxicol.* **1994**, *32*, 671–683. [CrossRef]
37. Dröge, W. Free radicals in the physiological control of cell function. *Physiol. Rev.* **2002**, *82*, 47–95. [CrossRef]
38. Floyd, R.A.; Carney, J.M. Free radical damage to protein and DNA: Mechanisms involved and relevant observations on brain undergoing oxidative stress. *Ann. Neurol.* **1992**, *32*, S22–S27. [CrossRef]
39. Kumar, H.; Bhardwaj, K.; Nepovimova, E.; Kuča, K.; Singh Dhanjal, D.; Bhardwaj, S.; Bhatia, S.K.; Verma, R.; Kumar, D. Antioxidant Functionalized Nanoparticles: A Combat against Oxidative Stress. *Nanomaterials* **2020**, *10*, 1334. [CrossRef]
40. Thanan, R.; Oikawa, S.; Hiraku, Y.; Ohnishi, S.; Ma, N.; Pinlaor, S.; Yongvanit, P.; Kawanishi, S.; Murata, M. Oxidative stress and its significant roles in neurodegenerative diseases and cancer. *Int. J. Mol. Sci.* **2014**, *16*, 193–217. [CrossRef]

41. Sharma, P.; Jha, A.B.; Dubey, R.S.; Pessarakli, M. Reactive Oxygen Species, Oxidative Damage, and Antioxidative Defense Mechanism in Plants under Stressful Conditions. *J. Bot.* **2012**, *2012*, 217037. [CrossRef]
42. Ozcan, A.; Ogun, M. Biochemistry of Reactive Oxygen and Nitrogen Species. In *Basic Principles and Clinical Significance of Oxidative Stress*; InTech: London, UK, 2015.
43. Pourahmad, J.; Salimi, A.; Seydi, E. Role of Oxygen Free Radicals in Cancer Development and Treatment. In *Free Radicals and Diseases*; InTech: London, UK, 2016.
44. Jamshidi-kia, F.; Wibowo, J.P.; Elachouri, M.; Masumi, R.; Salehifard-Jouneghani, A.; Abolhasanzadeh, Z.; Lorigooini, Z. Battle between plants as antioxidants with free radicals in human body. *J. Herbmed Pharmacol.* **2020**, *9*, 191–199. [CrossRef]
45. Santo, A.; Zhu, H.; Li, Y.R. Free radicals: From health to disease. *React. Oxyg. Species* **2016**, *2*, 245–263. [CrossRef]
46. Liguori, I.; Russo, G.; Curcio, F.; Bulli, G.; Aran, L.; Della-Morte, D.; Gargiulo, G.; Testa, G.; Cacciatore, F.; Bonaduce, D.; et al. Oxidative stress, aging, and diseases. *Clin. Interv. Aging* **2018**, *13*, 757–772. [CrossRef] [PubMed]
47. Nissanka, N.; Moraes, C.T. Mitochondrial DNA damage and reactive oxygen species in neurodegenerative disease. *FEBS Lett.* **2018**, *592*, 728–742. [CrossRef] [PubMed]
48. Cantó, C.; Auwerx, J. Caloric restriction, SIRT1 and longevity. *Trends Endocrinol. Metab.* **2009**, *20*, 325–331. [CrossRef]
49. Armandola, E. Caloric Restriction and Life Expectancy: Highlights of the 5th European Molecular Biology Organization Interdisciplinary Conference on Science and Society—Time & Aging: Mechanisms and Meanings; November 5–6, 2004; Heidelberg, Germany. *Med. Gen. Med.* **2004**, *6*, 16.
50. Gutierrez, J.; Ballinger, S.W.; Darley-Usmar, V.M.; Landar, A. Free radicals, mitochondria, and oxidized lipids: The emerging role in signal transduction in vascular cells. *Circ. Res.* **2006**, *99*, 924–932. [CrossRef]
51. Peng, C.; Wang, X.; Chen, J.; Jiao, R.; Wang, L.; Li, Y.M.; Zuo, Y.; Liu, Y.; Lei, L.; Ma, K.Y.; et al. Biology of ageing and role of dietary antioxidants. *BioMed Res. Int.* **2014**, *2014*, 831841. [CrossRef]
52. Hornsby, P.J. Telomerase and the aging process. *Exp. Gerontol.* **2007**, *42*, 575–581. [CrossRef]
53. Schmidt, J.C.; Cech, T.R. Human telomerase: Biogenesis, trafficking, recruitment, and activation. *Genes Dev.* **2015**, *29*, 1095–1105. [CrossRef] [PubMed]
54. Kalmbach, K.H.; Fontes Antunes, D.M.; Dracxler, R.C.; Knier, T.W.; Seth-Smith, M.L.; Wang, F.; Liu, L.; Keefe, D.L. Telomeres and human reproduction. *Fertil. Steril.* **2013**, *99*, 23–29. [CrossRef]
55. Kasote, D.M.; Katyare, S.S.; Hegde, M.V.; Bae, H. Significance of antioxidant potential of plants and its relevance to therapeutic applications. *Int. J. Biol. Sci.* **2015**, *11*, 982–991. [CrossRef] [PubMed]
56. Chen, L.; Deng, H.; Cui, H.; Fang, J.; Zuo, Z.; Deng, J.; Li, Y.; Wang, X.; Zhao, L. Inflammatory responses and inflammation-associated diseases in organs. *Oncotarget* **2018**, *9*, 7204–7218. [CrossRef] [PubMed]
57. Liao, L.Y.; He, Y.F.; Li, L.; Meng, H.; Dong, Y.M.; Yi, F.; Xiao, P.G. A preliminary review of studies on adaptogens: Comparison of their bioactivity in TCM with that of ginseng-like herbs used worldwide Milen Georgiev, Ruibing Wang. *Chin. Med.* **2018**, *13*, 57. [CrossRef] [PubMed]
58. Bhatia, N.; Jaggi, A.S.; Singh, N.; Anand, P.; Dhawan, R. Adaptogenic potential of curcumin in experimental chronic stress and chronic unpredictable stress-induced memory deficits and alterations in functional homeostasis. *J. Nat. Med.* **2011**, *65*, 532–543. [CrossRef] [PubMed]
59. Singh, M.K.; Jain, G.; Das, B.K.; Patil, U.K. Biomolecules from Plants as an Adaptogen. *Med. Aromat. Plants* **2017**, *6*, 307. [CrossRef]
60. Aguiar, S.; Borowski, T. Neuropharmacological review of the nootropic herb Bacopa monnieri. *Rejuvenation Res.* **2013**, *16*, 313–326. [CrossRef]
61. Jain, P.K.; Das, D.; Kumar Jain, P. Pharmacognostic Comparison of Bacopa Monnieri, Cyperus Rotundus and Emblica Officinalis. *Innovare J. Ayurvedic Sci.* **2016**, *4*, 16–26.
62. Tewari, I.; Sharma, L.; Lal Gupta, G. Synergistic antioxidant activity of three medicinal plants Hypericum perforatum, Bacopa monnieri, and Camellia Sinensis. *Indo Am. J. Pharm. Res.* **2014**, *4*, 2563–2568.
63. Vollala, V.R.; Upadhya, S.; Nayak, S. Effect of Bacopa monniera Linn. (brahmi) extract on learning and memory in rats: A behavioral study. *J. Vet. Behav. Clin. Appl. Res.* **2010**, *5*, 69–74. [CrossRef]
64. Simpson, T.; Pase, M.; Stough, C. Bacopa monnieri as an Antioxidant Therapy to Reduce Oxidative Stress in the Aging Brain. *Evid. Based Complement. Altern. Med.* **2015**, *2015*, 615384. [CrossRef]

65. Bhattacharya, S.K.; Bhattacharya, A.; Kumar, A.; Ghosal, S. Antioxidant activity of Bacopa monniera in rat frontal cortex, striatum and hippocampus. *Phyther. Res.* **2000**, *14*, 174–179. [CrossRef]
66. Shinomol, G.K.; Srinivas Bharath, M.M. Muralidhara Neuromodulatory propensity of bacopa monnieri leaf extract against 3-nitropropionic acid-induced oxidative stress: In vitro and in vivo evidences. *Neurotox. Res.* **2012**, *22*, 102–114. [CrossRef]
67. Kumar, N.; Abichandani, L.G.; Thawani, V.; Gharpure, K.J.; Naidu, M.U.R.; Venkat Ramana, G. Efficacy of Standardized Extract of Bacopa monnieri (Bacognize®) on Cognitive Functions of Medical Students: A Six-Week, Randomized Placebo-Controlled Trial. *Evid. Based Complement. Altern. Med.* **2016**, *2016*. [CrossRef]
68. Kocaadam, B.; Şanlier, N. Curcumin, an active component of turmeric (Curcuma longa), and its effects on health. *Crit. Rev. Food Sci. Nutr.* **2017**, *57*, 2889–2895. [CrossRef] [PubMed]
69. Prasad, S.; Aggarwal, B.B. Turmeric, the golden spice: From traditional medicine to modern medicine. In *Herbal Medicine: Biomolecular and Clinical Aspects: Second Edition*; CRC Press: Boca Raton, FL, USA, 2011; pp. 263–288. ISBN 9781439807163.
70. Tomeh, M.A.; Hadianamrei, R.; Zhao, X. A review of curcumin and its derivatives as anticancer agents. *Int. J. Mol. Sci.* **2019**, *20*, 1033. [CrossRef] [PubMed]
71. Desai, S.J.; Prickril, B.; Rasooly, A. Mechanisms of Phytonutrient Modulation of Cyclooxygenase-2 (COX-2) and Inflammation Related to Cancer. *Nutr. Cancer* **2018**, *70*, 350–375. [CrossRef] [PubMed]
72. Engwa, G.A. Free Radicals and the Role of Plant Phytochemicals as Antioxidants Against Oxidative Stress-Related Diseases. In *Phytochemicals-Source of Antioxidants and Role in Disease Prevention*; InTech: London, UK, 2018.
73. Lima, C.F.; Pereira-Wilson, C.; Rattan, S.I.S. Curcumin induces heme oxygenase-1 in normal human skin fibroblasts through redox signaling: Relevance for anti-aging intervention. *Mol. Nutr. Food Res.* **2011**, *55*, 430–442. [CrossRef]
74. Soh, J.W.; Marowsky, N.; Nichols, T.J.; Rahman, A.M.; Miah, T.; Sarao, P.; Khasawneh, R.; Unnikrishnan, A.; Heydari, A.R.; Silver, R.B.; et al. Curcumin is an early-acting stage-specific inducer of extended functional longevity in Drosophila. *Exp. Gerontol.* **2013**, *48*, 229–239. [CrossRef]
75. Shen, L.-R.; Parnell, L.D.; Ordovas, J.M.; Lai, C.-Q. Curcumin and aging. *BioFactors* **2013**, *39*, 133–140. [CrossRef]
76. Lee, K.S.; Lee, B.S.; Semnani, S.; Avanesian, A.; Um, C.Y.; Jeon, H.J.; Seong, K.M.; Yu, K.; Min, K.J.; Jafari, M. Curcumin extends life span, improves health span, and modulates the expression of age-associated aging genes in drosophila melanogaster. *Rejuvenation Res.* **2010**, *13*, 561–570. [CrossRef]
77. He, Y.; Yue, Y.; Zheng, X.; Zhang, K.; Chen, S.; Du, Z. Curcumin, inflammation, and chronic diseases: How are they linked? *Molecules* **2015**, *20*, 9183–9213. [CrossRef] [PubMed]
78. Olszanecki, R.; Jawien, J.; Gajda, M.; Mateuszuk, L.; Gebska, A.; Korabiowska, M.; Chlopicki, S.; Korbut, R. Effect of curcumin on atherosclerosis in apoE-LDLR-double knockout mice. *J. Physiol. Pharmacol.* **2005**, *4*, 627–635.
79. Swamy, A.V.; Gulliaya, S.; Thippeswamy, A.; Koti, B.C.; Manjula, D.V. Cardioprotective effect of curcumin against doxorubicin-induced myocardial toxicity in albino rats. *Indian J. Pharmacol.* **2012**, *44*, 73–77. [CrossRef] [PubMed]
80. Ryan, J.L.; Heckler, C.E.; Ling, M.; Katz, A.; Williams, J.P.; Pentland, A.P.; Morrow, G.R. Curcumin for radiation dermatitis: A randomized, double-blind, placebo-controlled clinical trial of thirty breast cancer patients. *Radiat. Res.* **2013**, *180*, 34–43. [CrossRef] [PubMed]
81. Ray Hamidie, R.D.; Yamada, T.; Ishizawa, R.; Saito, Y.; Masuda, K. Curcumin treatment enhances the effect of exercise on mitochondrial biogenesis in skeletal muscle by increasing cAMP levels. *Metabolism* **2015**, *64*, 1334–1347. [CrossRef] [PubMed]
82. Cox, K.H.M.; Pipingas, A.; Scholey, A.B. Investigation of the effects of solid lipid curcumin on cognition and mood in a healthy older population. *J. Psychopharmacol.* **2015**, *29*, 642–651. [CrossRef]
83. Yadav, S.S.; Singh, M.K.; Singh, P.K.; Kumar, V. Traditional knowledge to clinical trials: A review on therapeutic actions of Emblica officinalis. *Biomed. Pharmacother.* **2017**, *93*, 1292–1302. [CrossRef]
84. Kapoor, M.P.; Suzuki, K.; Derek, T.; Ozeki, M.; Okubo, T. Clinical evaluation of Emblica Officinalis Gatertn (Amla) in healthy human subjects: Health benefits and safety results from a randomized, double-blind, crossover placebo-controlled study. *Contemp. Clin. Trials Commun.* **2020**, *17*, 100499. [CrossRef]

85. Wilson, D.W.; Nash, P.; Singh, H.; Griffiths, K.; Singh, R.; De Meester, F.; Horiuchi, R.; Takahashi, T. The role of food antioxidants, benefits of functional foods, and influence of feeding habits on the health of the older person: An overview. *Antioxidants* **2017**, *6*, 81. [CrossRef]
86. Hasan, M.R.; Islam, M.N.; Islam, M.R. Phytochemistry, pharmacological activities and traditional uses of Emblica officinalis: A review. *Int. Curr. Pharm. J.* **2016**, *5*, 14–21. [CrossRef]
87. Lauer, A.C.; Groth, N.; Haag, S.F.; Darvin, M.E.; Lademann, J.; Meinke, M.C. Dose-dependent vitamin C uptake and radical scavenging activity in human skin measured with in vivo electron paramagnetic resonance spectroscopy. *Skin Pharmacol. Physiol.* **2013**, *26*, 147–154. [CrossRef] [PubMed]
88. Bhattacharya, A.; Ghosal, S.; Bhattacharya, S.K. Antioxidant activity of tannoid principles of Emblica officinalis (amla) in chronic stress induced changes in rat brain. *Indian J. Exp. Biol.* **2000**, *38*, 877–880. [PubMed]
89. Bhattachary, S.K.; Bhattacharya, D.; Muruganandam, A.V. Effect of Emblica officinalis tannoids on a rat model of tardive dyskinesia. *Indian J. Exp. Biol.* **2000**, *38*, 945–947. [PubMed]
90. Dhingra, D.; Joshi, P.; Gupta, A.; Chhillar, R. Possible Involvement of Monoaminergic Neurotransmission in Antidepressant-like activity of Emblica officinalis Fruits in Mice. *CNS Neurosci. Ther.* **2012**, *18*, 419–425. [CrossRef] [PubMed]
91. Isah, T. Rethinking *Ginkgo biloba* L.: Medicinal uses and conservation. *Pharmacogn. Rev.* **2015**, *9*, 140–148. [CrossRef]
92. Mashayekh, A.; Pham, D.L.; Yousem, D.M.; Dizon, M.; Barker, P.B.; Lin, D.D.M. Effects of Ginkgo biloba on cerebral blood flow assessed by quantitative MR perfusion imaging: A pilot study. *Neuroradiology* **2011**, *53*, 185–191. [CrossRef]
93. Zuo, W.; Yan, F.; Zhang, B.; Li, J.; Mei, D. Advances in the studies of Ginkgo biloba leaves extract on aging-related diseases. *Aging Dis.* **2017**, *8*, 812–826. [CrossRef]
94. Van Beek, T.A. Chemical analysis of Ginkgo biloba leaves and extracts. *J. Chromatogr. A* **2002**, *967*, 21–55. [CrossRef]
95. Huang, S.Z.; Luo, Y.J.; Wang, L.; Cai, K.Y. Effect of ginkgo biloba extract on livers in aged rats. *World J. Gastroenterol.* **2005**, *11*, 132–135. [CrossRef]
96. Belviranli, M.; Okudan, N. The effects of Ginkgo biloba extract on cognitive functions in aged female rats: The role of oxidative stress and brain-derived neurotrophic factor. *Behav. Brain Res.* **2015**, *278*, 453–461. [CrossRef]
97. Liu, H.; Ye, M.; Guo, H. An Updated Review of Randomized Clinical Trials Testing the Improvement of Cognitive Function of Ginkgo biloba Extract in Healthy People and Alzheimer's Patients. *Front. Pharmacol.* **2020**, *10*, 1688. [CrossRef] [PubMed]
98. Pastorino, G.; Cornara, L.; Soares, S.; Rodrigues, F.; Oliveira, M.B.P.P. Liquorice (Glycyrrhiza glabra): A phytochemical and pharmacological review. *Phyther. Res.* **2018**, *32*, 2323–2339. [CrossRef] [PubMed]
99. Frattaruolo, L.; Carullo, G.; Brindisi, M.; Mazzotta, S.; Bellissimo, L.; Rago, V.; Curcio, R.; Dolce, V.; Aiello, F.; Cappello, A.R. Antioxidant and anti-inflammatory activities of flavanones from glycyrrhiza glabra L. (licorice) leaf phytocomplexes: Identification of licoflavanone as a modulator of NF-kB/MAPK pathway. *Antioxidants* **2019**, *8*, 186. [CrossRef] [PubMed]
100. Grodzicki, W.; Dziendzikowska, K. The role of selected bioactive compounds in the prevention of alzheimer's disease. *Antioxidants* **2020**, *9*, 229. [CrossRef] [PubMed]
101. Ciganović, P.; Jakimiuk, K.; Tomczyk, M.; Končić, M.Z. Glycerolic licorice extracts as active cosmeceutical ingredients: Extraction optimization, chemical characterization, and biological activity. *Antioxidants* **2019**, *8*, 445. [CrossRef]
102. Balmus, I.M.; Ciobica, A. Main Plant Extracts' Active Properties Effective on Scopolamine-Induced Memory Loss. *Am. J. Alzheimers Dis. Other Demen.* **2017**, *32*, 418–428. [CrossRef]
103. Dhingra, D.; Parle, M.; Kulkarni, S.K. Memory enhancing activity of Glycyrrhiza glabra in mice. *J. Ethnopharmacol.* **2004**, *91*, 361–365. [CrossRef]
104. Rokot, N.T.; Kairupan, T.S.; Cheng, K.C.; Runtuwene, J.; Kapantow, N.H.; Amitani, M.; Morinaga, A.; Amitani, H.; Asakawa, A.; Inui, A. A Role of Ginseng and Its Constituents in the Treatment of Central Nervous System Disorders. *Evid. Based Complement. Altern. Med.* **2016**, *2016*, 2614742. [CrossRef]
105. Yu, H.; Zhao, J.; You, J.; Li, J.; Ma, H.; Chen, X. Factors influencing cultivated ginseng (Panax ginseng C. A. Meyer) bioactive compounds. *PLoS ONE* **2019**, *14*, e0223763. [CrossRef]

106. Kumar, G.P.; Khanum, F. Neuroprotective potential of phytochemicals. *Pharmacogn. Rev.* **2012**, *6*, 81–90. [CrossRef]
107. Wee, J.J.; Mee Park, K.; Chung, A.-S. Biological Activities of Ginseng and Its Application to Human Health. In *Herbal Medicine: Biomolecular and Clinical Aspects*; Benzie, I.F.F., Wachtel-Galor, S., Eds.; CRC Press/Taylor and Francis: Boca Raton, FL, USA, 2011; ISBN 978-1-4398-0713-2.
108. Lee, Y.M.; Yoon, H.; Park, H.M.; Song, B.C.; Yeum, K.J. Implications of red Panax ginseng in oxidative stress associated chronic diseases. *J. Ginseng Res.* **2017**, *41*, 113–119. [CrossRef] [PubMed]
109. Caldwell, L.K.; Dupont, W.H.; Beeler, M.K.; Post, E.M.; Barnhart, E.C.; Hardesty, V.H.; Anders, J.P.; Borden, E.C.; Volek, J.S.; Kraemer, W.J. The effects of a Korean ginseng, GINST15, on perceptual effort, psychomotor performance, and physical performance in men and women. *J. Sport. Sci. Med.* **2018**, *17*, 92–100.
110. Kim, J.; Cho, S.Y.; Kim, S.H.; Cho, D.; Kim, S.; Park, C.W.; Shimizu, T.; Cho, J.Y.; Seo, D.B.; Shin, S.S. Effects of Korean ginseng berry on skin antipigmentation and antiaging via FoxO3a activation. *J. Ginseng Res.* **2017**, *41*, 277–283. [CrossRef] [PubMed]
111. Hwang, E.; Park, S.Y.; Jo, H.; Lee, D.G.; Kim, H.T.; Kim, Y.M.; Yin, C.S.; Yi, T.H. Efficacy and Safety of Enzyme-Modified Panax ginseng for Anti-Wrinkle Therapy in Healthy Skin: A Single-Center, Randomized, Double-Blind, Placebo-Controlled Study. *Rejuvenation Res.* **2015**, *18*, 449–457. [CrossRef]
112. Shahidi, F.; Ambigaipalan, P. Phenolics and polyphenolics in foods, beverages and spices: Antioxidant activity and health effects-A review. *J. Funct. Foods* **2015**, *18*, 820–897. [CrossRef]
113. Quero, J.; Mármol, I.; Cerrada, E.; Rodríguez-Yoldi, M.J. Insight into the potential application of polyphenol-rich dietary intervention in degenerative disease management. *Food Funct.* **2020**, *11*, 2805–2825. [CrossRef]
114. Pandey, K.B.; Rizvi, S.I. Plant polyphenols as dietary antioxidants in human health and disease. *Oxid. Med. Cell. Longev.* **2009**, *2*, 270–278. [CrossRef]
115. Dunaway, S.; Odin, R.; Zhou, L.; Ji, L.; Zhang, Y.; Kadekaro, A.L. Natural antioxidants: Multiple mechanisms to protect skin from solar radiation. *Front. Pharmacol.* **2018**, *9*, 392. [CrossRef]
116. D'Orazio, J.; Jarrett, S.; Amaro-Ortiz, A.; Scott, T. UV radiation and the skin. *Int. J. Mol. Sci.* **2013**, *14*, 12222–12248. [CrossRef]
117. Adhikari, B.; Dhungana, S.K.; Waqas Ali, M.; Adhikari, A.; Kim, I.D.; Shin, D.H. Antioxidant activities, polyphenol, flavonoid, and amino acid contents in peanut shell. *J. Saudi Soc. Agric. Sci.* **2019**, *18*, 437–442. [CrossRef]
118. Camins, A.; Junyent, F.; Verdaguer, E.; Beas-Zarate, C.; Rojas-Mayorquín, A.; Ortuño-Sahagún, D.; Pallàs, M. Resveratrol: An Antiaging Drug with Potential Therapeutic Applications in Treating Diseases. *Pharmaceuticals* **2009**, *2*, 194–205. [CrossRef]
119. Salehi, B.; Mishra, A.P.; Nigam, M.; Sener, B.; Kilic, M.; Sharifi-Rad, M.; Fokou, P.V.T.; Martins, N.; Sharifi-Rad, J. Resveratrol: A double-edged sword in health benefits. *Biomedicines* **2018**, *6*, 91. [CrossRef]
120. Quadros Gomes, B.A.; Bastos Silva, J.P.; Rodrigues Romeiro, C.F.; dos Santos, S.M.; Rodrigues, C.A.; Gonçalves, P.R.; Sakai, J.T.; Santos Mendes, P.F.; Pompeu Varela, E.L.; Monteiro, M.C. Neuroprotective mechanisms of resveratrol in Alzheimer's disease: Role of SIRT1. *Oxid. Med. Cell. Longev.* **2018**, *2018*, 8152373.
121. Bhat, K.P.L.; Pezzuto, J.M. Cancer chemopreventive activity of resveratrol. *Ann. N. Y. Acad. Sci.* **2002**, *957*, 210–229. [CrossRef] [PubMed]
122. Bastianetto, S.; Dumont, Y.; Duranton, A.; Vercauteren, F.; Breton, L.; Quirion, R. Protective Action of Resveratrol in Human Skin: Possible Involvement of Specific Receptor Binding Sites. *PLoS ONE* **2010**, *5*, e12935. [CrossRef] [PubMed]
123. Giardina, S.; Michelotti, A.; Zavattini, G.; Finzi, S.; Ghisalberti, C.; Marzatico, F. Efficacy study in vitro: Assessment of the properties of resveratrol and resveratrol + N-acetyl-cysteine on proliferation and inhibition of collagen activity. *Minerva Ginecol.* **2010**, *62*, 195–201.
124. Demidenko, Z.N.; Blagosklonny, M.V. At concentrations that inhibit mTOR, resveratrol suppresses cellular senescence. *Cell Cycle* **2009**, *8*, 1901–1904. [CrossRef]
125. Xia, L.; Wang, X.X.; Hu, X.S.; Guo, X.G.; Shang, Y.P.; Chen, H.J.; Zeng, C.L.; Zhang, F.R.; Chen, J.Z. Resveratrol reduces endothelial progenitor cells senescence through augmentation of telomerase activity by Akt-dependent mechanisms. *Br. J. Pharmacol.* **2008**, *155*, 387–394. [CrossRef]

126. Giovannelli, L.; Pitozzi, V.; Jacomelli, M.; Mulinacci, N.; Laurenzana, A.; Dolara, P.; Mocali, A. Protective effects of resveratrol against senescence-associated changes in cultured human fibroblasts. *J. Gerontol. Ser. A Biol. Sci. Med. Sci.* **2011**, *66 A*, 9–18. [CrossRef]
127. López-Lluch, G.; Irusta, P.M.; Navas, P.; de Cabo, R. Mitochondrial biogenesis and healthy aging. *Exp. Gerontol.* **2008**, *43*, 813–819. [CrossRef]
128. Lagouge, M.; Argmann, C.; Gerhart-Hines, Z.; Meziane, H.; Lerin, C.; Daussin, F.; Messadeq, N.; Milne, J.; Lambert, P.; Elliott, P.; et al. Resveratrol Improves Mitochondrial Function and Protects against Metabolic Disease by Activating SIRT1 and PGC-1α. *Cell* **2006**, *127*, 1109–1122. [CrossRef] [PubMed]
129. Wang, T.; Li, Q.; Bi, K. Bioactive flavonoids in medicinal plants: Structure, activity and biological fate. *Asian J. Pharm. Sci.* **2018**, *13*, 12–23. [CrossRef] [PubMed]
130. Antika, L.D.; Lee, E.J.; Kim, Y.H.; Kang, M.K.; Park, S.H.; Kim, D.Y.; Oh, H.; Choi, Y.J.; Kang, Y.H. Dietary phlorizin enhances osteoblastogenic bone formation through enhancing β-catenin activity via GSK-3β inhibition in a model of senile osteoporosis. *J. Nutr. Biochem.* **2017**, *49*, 42–52. [CrossRef] [PubMed]
131. Makarova, E.; Górnaś, P.; Konrade, I.; Tirzite, D.; Cirule, H.; Gulbe, A.; Pugajeva, I.; Seglina, D.; Dambrova, M. Acute anti-hyperglycaemic effects of an unripe apple preparation containing phlorizin in healthy volunteers: A preliminary study. *J. Sci. Food Agric.* **2014**, *95*, 560–568. [CrossRef]
132. Mela, D.J.; Cao, X.Z.; Dobriyal, R.; Fowler, M.I.; Lin, L.; Joshi, M.; Mulder, T.J.P.; Murray, P.G.; Peters, H.P.F.; Vermeer, M.A.; et al. The effect of 8 plant extracts and combinations on post-prandial blood glucose and insulin responses in healthy adults: A randomized controlled trial. *Nutr. Metab.* **2020**, *17*, 51. [CrossRef]
133. Laiteerapong, N.; Karter, A.J.; Liu, J.Y.; Moffet, H.H.; Sudore, R.; Schillinger, D.; John, P.M.; Huang, E.S. Correlates of quality of life in older adults with diabetes: The diabetes & aging study. *Diabetes Care* **2011**, *34*, 1749–1753. [CrossRef]
134. Ayaz, M.; Sadiq, A.; Junaid, M.; Ullah, F.; Ovais, M.; Ullah, I.; Ahmed, J.; Shahid, M. Flavonoids as prospective neuroprotectants and their therapeutic propensity in aging associated neurological disorders. *Front. Aging Neurosci.* **2019**, *11*, 155. [CrossRef]
135. Zhang, Y.J.; Gan, R.Y.; Li, S.; Zhou, Y.; Li, A.N.; Xu, D.P.; Li, H.B.; Kitts, D.D. Antioxidant phytochemicals for the prevention and treatment of chronic diseases. *Molecules* **2015**, *20*, 21138–21156. [CrossRef]
136. Kschonsek, J.; Wolfram, T.; Stöckl, A.; Böhm, V. Polyphenolic compounds analysis of old and new apple cultivars and contribution of polyphenolic profile to the in vitro antioxidant capacity. *Antioxidants* **2018**, *7*, 20. [CrossRef]
137. Boyer, J.; Liu, R.H. Apple phytochemicals and their health benefits. *Nutr. J.* **2004**, *3*, 5. [CrossRef]
138. Vafa, M.R.; Haghighatjoo, E.; Shidfar, F.; Afshari, S.; Gohari, M.R.; Ziaee, A. Effects of apple consumption on lipid profile of hyperlipidemic and overweight men. *Int. J. Prev. Med.* **2011**, *2*, 94–100. [PubMed]
139. Peng, C.; Chan, H.Y.E.; Huang, Y.; Yu, H.; Chen, Z.Y. Apple polyphenols extend the mean lifespan of Drosophila melanogaster. *J. Agric. Food Chem.* **2011**, *59*, 2097–2106. [CrossRef] [PubMed]
140. Cory, H.; Passarelli, S.; Szeto, J.; Tamez, M.; Mattei, J. The Role of Polyphenols in Human Health and Food Systems: A Mini-Review. *Front. Nutr.* **2018**, *5*, 87. [CrossRef] [PubMed]
141. Kalt, W.; Cassidy, A.; Howard, L.R.; Krikorian, R.; Stull, A.J.; Tremblay, F.; Zamora-Ros, R. Recent Research on the Health Benefits of Blueberries and Their Anthocyanins. *Adv. Nutr.* **2020**, *11*, 224–236. [CrossRef]
142. Shukitt-Hale, B.; Thangthaeng, N.; Miller, M.G.; Poulose, S.M.; Carey, A.N.; Fisher, D.R. Blueberries Improve Neuroinflammation and Cognition differentially Depending on Individual Cognitive baseline Status. *J. Gerontol. Ser. A Biol. Sci. Med. Sci.* **2019**, *74*, 977–983. [CrossRef]
143. Joseph, J.A.; Shukitt-Hale, B.; Casadesus, G. Reversing the deleterious effects of aging on neuronal communication and behavior: Beneficial properties of fruit polyphenolic compounds. *Am. J. Clin. Nutr.* **2005**, *81*, 313S–316S. [CrossRef]
144. Galli, R.L.; Bielinski, D.F.; Szprengiel, A.; Shukitt-Hale, B.; Joseph, J.A. Blueberry supplemented diet reverses age-related decline in hippocampal HSP70 neuroprotection. *Neurobiol. Aging* **2006**, *27*, 344–350. [CrossRef]
145. Goyarzu, P.; Malin, D.H.; Lau, F.C.; Taglialatela, G.; Moon, W.D.; Jennings, R.; Moy, E.; Moy, D.; Lippold, S.; Shukitt-Hale, B.; et al. Blueberry supplemented diet: Effects on object recognition memory and nuclear factor-kappa B levels in aged rats. *Nutr. Neurosci.* **2004**, *7*, 75–83. [CrossRef]
146. Peng, C.; Zuo, Y.; Kwan, K.M.; Liang, Y.; Ma, K.Y.; Chan, H.Y.E.; Huang, Y.; Yu, H.; Chen, Z.Y. Blueberry extract prolongs lifespan of Drosophila melanogaster. *Exp. Gerontol.* **2012**, *47*, 170–178. [CrossRef]

147. Su, Y.L.; Leung, L.K.; Huang, Y.; Chen, Z.Y. Stability of tea theaflavins and catechins. *Food Chem.* **2003**, *83*, 189–195. [CrossRef]
148. Musial, C.; Kuban-Jankowska, A.; Gorska-Ponikowska, M. Beneficial properties of green tea catechins. *Int. J. Mol. Sci.* **2020**, *21*, 1744. [CrossRef] [PubMed]
149. Yan, Z.; Zhong, Y.; Duan, Y.; Chen, Q.; Li, F. Antioxidant mechanism of tea polyphenols and its impact on health benefits. *Anim. Nutr.* **2020**, *6*, 115–123. [CrossRef] [PubMed]
150. Li, Y.M.; Chan, H.Y.E.; Huang, Y.; Chen, Z.Y. Green tea catechins upregulate Superoxide dismutase and catalase in fruit flies. *Mol. Nutr. Food Res.* **2007**, *51*, 546–554. [CrossRef] [PubMed]
151. Oyetakinwhite, P.; Tribout, H.; Baron, E. Protective mechanisms of green tea polyphenols in skin. *Oxid. Med. Cell. Longev.* **2012**, *2012*, 560682. [CrossRef] [PubMed]
152. Elmets, C.A.; Singh, D.; Tubesing, K.; Matsui, M.; Katiyar, S.; Mukhtar, H. Cutaneous photoprotection from ultraviolet injury by green tea polyphenols. *J. Am. Acad. Dermatol.* **2001**, *44*, 425–432. [CrossRef] [PubMed]
153. Chiu, A.E.; Chan, J.L.; Kern, D.G.; Kohler, S.; Rehmus, W.E.; Kimball, A.B. Double-blinded, placebo-controlled trial of green tea extracts in the clinical and histologic appearance of photoaging skin. *Dermatol. Surg.* **2005**, *31*, 855–860. [CrossRef]
154. Shaikh, R.; Pund, M.; Dawane, A.; Iliyas, S. Evaluation of anticancer, antioxidant, and possible anti-inflammatory properties of selected medicinal plants used in indian traditional medication. *J. Tradit. Complement. Med.* **2014**, *4*, 253–257. [CrossRef]
155. Azevedo, J.; Fernandes, I.; Faria, A.; Oliveira, J.; Fernandes, A.; de Freitas, V.; Mateus, N. Antioxidant properties of anthocyanidins, anthocyanidin-3-glucosides and respective portisins. *Food Chem.* **2010**, *119*, 518–523. [CrossRef]
156. Zuo, Y.; Peng, C.; Liang, Y.; Ma, K.Y.; Yu, H.; Edwin Chan, H.Y.; Chen, Z.Y. Black rice extract extends the lifespan of fruit flies. *Food Funct.* **2012**, *3*, 1271–1279. [CrossRef]
157. Huang, J.J.; Zhao, S.M.; Jin, L.; Huang, L.J.; He, X.; Wei, Q. Anti-aging effect of black rice in subacute aging model mice. *Chin. J. Clin. Rehabil.* **2006**, *10*, 82–84.
158. Institute of Medicine (US). Panel on Dietary Antioxidants and Related Compounds β-Carotene and Other Carotenoids. In *Dietary Reference Intakes for Vitamin C, Vitamin E, Selenium, and Carotenoids*; National Academies Press (US): Washington, DC, USA, 2000.
159. Stahl, W.; Sies, H. β-Carotene and other carotenoids in protection from sunlight. *Am. J. Clin. Nutr.* **2012**, *96*, 1179S–1184S. [CrossRef] [PubMed]
160. Pritwani, R.; Mathur, P. β-carotene Content of Some Commonly Consumed Vegetables and Fruits Available in Delhi, India. *J. Nutr. Food Sci.* **2017**, *7*, 5. [CrossRef]
161. Jaswir, I.; Noviendri, D.; Hasrini, R.F.; Octavianti, F. Carotenoids: Sources, medicinal properties and their application in food and nutraceutical industry. *J. Med. Plant Res.* **2011**, *5*, 7119–7131. [CrossRef]
162. Parrado, C.; Philips, N.; Gilaberte, Y.; Juarranz, A.; González, S. Oral photoprotection: Effective agents and potential candidates. *Front. Med.* **2018**, *5*, 188. [CrossRef] [PubMed]
163. Boccardi, V.; Arosio, B.; Cari, L.; Bastiani, P.; Scamosci, M.; Casati, M.; Ferri, E.; Bertagnoli, L.; Ciccone, S.; Rossi, P.D.; et al. Beta-carotene, telomerase activity and Alzheimer's disease in old age subjects. *Eur. J. Nutr.* **2020**, *59*, 119–126. [CrossRef] [PubMed]
164. The Alpha-Tocopherol Beta Carotene Cancer Prevention Study Group. The effect of vitamin e and beta carotene on the incidence of lung cancer and other cancers in male smokers. *N. Engl. J. Med.* **1994**, *330*, 1029–1035. [CrossRef]
165. Evans, J.A.; Johnson, E.J. The role of phytonutrients in skin health. *Nutrients* **2010**, *2*, 903–928. [CrossRef]
166. Ascenso, A.; Pedrosa, T.; Pinho, S.; Pinho, F.; De Oliveira, J.M.P.F.; Marques, H.C.; Oliveira, H.; Simões, S.; Santos, C. The Effect of Lycopene Preexposure on UV-B-Irradiated Human Keratinocytes. *Oxid. Med. Cell. Longev.* **2016**, *2016*. [CrossRef]
167. Przybylska, S. Lycopene–A bioactive carotenoid offering multiple health benefits: A review. *Int. J. Food Sci. Technol.* **2020**, *55*, 11–32. [CrossRef]
168. Darvin, M.E.; Sterry, W.; Lademann, J.; Vergou, T. The role of carotenoids in human skin. *Molecules* **2011**, *16*, 10491–10506. [CrossRef]
169. Cheng, J.; Miller, B.; Balbuena, E.; Eroglu, A. Lycopene protects against smoking-induced lung cancer by inducing base excision repair. *Antioxidants* **2020**, *9*, 643. [CrossRef] [PubMed]

170. Singh, B.; Singh, J.P.; Kaur, A.; Singh, N. Phenolic composition, antioxidant potential and health benefits of citrus peel. *Food Res. Int.* **2020**, *132*, 109114. [CrossRef] [PubMed]
171. Carr, A.; Maggini, S. Vitamin C and Immune Function. *Nutrients* **2017**, *9*, 1211. [CrossRef] [PubMed]
172. Hemilä, H. Vitamin C and Infections. *Nutrients* **2017**, *9*, 339. [CrossRef] [PubMed]
173. Souyoul, S.A.; Saussy, K.P.; Lupo, M.P. Nutraceuticals: A Review. *Dermatol. Ther.* **2018**, *8*, 5–16. [CrossRef]
174. Brickley, M.; Ives, R. Vitamin C Deficiency Scurvy. In *The Bioarchaeology of Metabolic Bone Disease*; Elsevier: Amsterdam, The Netherlands, 2008; pp. 1–74.
175. Galli, F.; Azzi, A.; Birringer, M.; Cook-Mills, J.M.; Eggersdorfer, M.; Frank, J.; Cruciani, G.; Lorkowski, S.; Özer, N.K. Vitamin E: Emerging aspects and new directions. *Free Radic. Biol. Med.* **2017**, *102*, 16–36. [CrossRef]
176. Sivakanesan, R. Antioxidants for health and longevity. In *Molecular Basis and Emerging Strategies for Anti-Aging Interventions*; Springer: Singapore, 2018; pp. 323–341. ISBN 9789811316999.
177. Leonard, P.J.; Losowsky, M.S.; Pulvertaft, C.N. Vitamin-E Deficiency. *Br. Med. J.* **1966**, *1*, 1301–1302. [CrossRef]
178. Keen, M.; Hassan, I. Vitamin E in dermatology. *Indian Dermatol. Online J.* **2016**, *7*, 311. [CrossRef]
179. Fryer, M.J. Evidence for the photoprotective effects of vitamin E. *Photochem. Photobiol.* **1993**, *58*, 304–312. [CrossRef]
180. Chan, A.C.; Tran, K.; Raynor, T.; Ganz, P.R.; Chow, C.K. Regeneration of vitamin E in human platelets-PubMed. *J. Biol. Chem.* **1991**, *266*, 17290–17295.
181. Makrantonaki, E.; Zouboulis, C.C. Skin alterations and diseases in advanced age. *Drug Discov. Today Dis. Mech.* **2008**, *5*, e153–e162. [CrossRef]
182. McVean, M.; Liebler, D.C. Prevention of DNA photodamage by vitamin E compounds and sunscreens: Roles of ultraviolet absorbance and cellular uptake. *Mol. Carcinog.* **1999**, *24*, 169–176. [CrossRef]
183. Passi, S.; Morrone, A.; De Luca, C.; Picardo, M.; Ippolito, F. Blood levels of vitamin E, polyunsaturated fatty acids of phospholipids, lipoperoxides and glutathione peroxidase in patients affected with seborrheic dermatitis. *J. Dermatol. Sci.* **1991**, *2*, 171–178. [CrossRef]
184. Ekanayake-Mudiyanselage, S.; Thiele, J. Sebaceous glands as transporters of vitamin E. *Hautarzt* **2006**, *57*, 291–296. [CrossRef]
185. Eberlein-König, B.; Ring, J. Relevance of vitamins C and E in cutaneous photoprotection. *J. Cosmet. Dermatol.* **2005**, *4*, 4–9. [CrossRef]
186. Shahidi, F. Nutraceuticals, functional foods and dietary supplements in health and disease. *J. Food Drug Anal.* **2012**, *20*, 226–230.
187. Pem, D.; Jeewon, R. Fruit and vegetable intake: Benefits and progress of nutrition education interventions-narrative review article. *Iran. J. Public Health* **2015**, *44*, 1309–1321. [PubMed]
188. Petruk, G.; Del Giudice, R.; Rigano, M.M.; Monti, D.M. Antioxidants from plants protect against skin photoaging. *Oxid. Med. Cell. Longev.* **2018**, *2018*, 1454936. [CrossRef]
189. Cimino, F.; Cristani, M.; Saija, A.; Bonina, F.P.; Virgili, F. Protective effects of a red orange extract on UVB-induced damage in human keratinocytes. *Biofactors* **2007**, *30*, 129–138. [CrossRef] [PubMed]
190. Fujii, T.; Wakaizumi, M.; Ikami, T.; Saito, M. Amla (Emblica officinalis Gaertn.) extract promotes procollagen production and inhibits matrix metalloproteinase-1 in human skin fibroblasts. *J. Ethnopharmacol.* **2008**, *119*, 53–57. [CrossRef] [PubMed]
191. Adil, M.D.; Kaiser, P.; Satti, N.K.; Zargar, A.M.; Vishwakarma, R.A.; Tasduq, S.A. Effect of Emblica officinalis (fruit) against UVB-induced photo-aging in human skin fibroblasts. *J. Ethnopharmacol.* **2010**, *132*, 109–114. [CrossRef] [PubMed]
192. Nema, N.K.; Maity, N.; Sarkar, B.; Mukherjee, P.K. Cucumis sativus fruit-potential antioxidant, anti-hyaluronidase, and anti-elastase agent. *Arch. Dermatol. Res.* **2011**, *303*, 247–252. [CrossRef] [PubMed]
193. Cao, X.; Sun, Y.; Lin, Y.; Pan, Y.; Farooq, U.; Xiang, L.; Qi, J. Antiaging of cucurbitane glycosides from fruits of Momordica charantia L. *Oxid. Med. Cell. Longev.* **2018**, *2018*. [CrossRef] [PubMed]
194. Lourith, N.; Kanlayavattanakul, M.; Chaikul, P.; Chansriniyom, C.; Bunwatcharaphansakun, P. In vitro and cellular activities of the selected fruits residues for skin aging treatment. *An. Acad. Bras. Cienc.* **2017**, *89*, 577–589. [CrossRef]
195. Apraj, V.D.; Pandita, N.S. Evaluation of skin anti-aging potential of Citrus reticulata blanco peel. *Pharmacogn. Res.* **2016**, *8*, 160–168. [CrossRef]

196. Girsang, E.; Lister, I.N.E.; Ginting, C.N.; Khu, A.; Samin, B.; Widowati, W.; Wibowo, S.; Rizal, R. Chemical Constituents of Snake Fruit (Salacca zalacca (Gaert.) Voss) Peel and in silico Anti-aging Analysis. *Mol. Cell. Biomed. Sci.* **2019**, *3*, 122. [CrossRef]
197. Kim, D.B.; Shin, G.H.; Kim, J.M.; Kim, Y.H.; Lee, J.H.; Lee, J.S.; Song, H.J.; Choe, S.Y.; Park, I.J.; Cho, J.H.; et al. Antioxidant and anti-ageing activities of citrus-based juice mixture. *Food Chem.* **2016**, *194*, 920–927. [CrossRef]
198. Lee, M.J.; Jeong, N.H.; Jang, B.S. Antioxidative activity and antiaging effect of carrot glycoprotein. *J. Ind. Eng. Chem.* **2015**, *25*, 216–221. [CrossRef]
199. Zemour, K.; Labdelli, A.; Adda, A.; Dellal, A.; Talou, T.; Merah, O. Phenol Content and Antioxidant and Antiaging Activity of Safflower Seed Oil (*Carthamus Tinctorius* L.). *Cosmetics* **2019**, *6*, 55. [CrossRef]
200. Itoh, S.; Yamaguchi, M.; Shigeyama, K.; Sakaguchi, I. The Anti-Aging Potential of Extracts from Chaenomeles sinensis. *Cosmetics* **2019**, *6*, 21. [CrossRef]
201. Foolad, N.; Vaughn, A.R.; Rybak, I.; Burney, W.A.; Chodur, G.M.; Newman, J.W.; Steinberg, F.M.; Sivamani, R.K. Prospective randomized controlled pilot study on the effects of almond consumption on skin lipids and wrinkles. *Phyther. Res.* **2019**, *33*, 3212–3217. [CrossRef] [PubMed]
202. Wang, L.; Cui, J.; Jin, B.; Zhao, J.; Xu, H.; Lu, Z.; Li, W.; Li, X.; Li, L.; Liang, E.; et al. Multifeature analyses of vascular cambial cells reveal longevity mechanisms in old Ginkgo biloba trees. *Proc. Natl. Acad. Sci. USA* **2020**, *117*, 2201–2210. [CrossRef] [PubMed]
203. Shailaja, M.; Damodara Gowda, K.M.; Vishakh, K.; Suchetha Kumari, N. Anti-aging Role of Curcumin by Modulating the Inflammatory Markers in Albino Wistar Rats. *J. Natl. Med. Assoc.* **2017**, *109*, 9–13. [CrossRef] [PubMed]
204. Shin, S.; Lee, J.A.; Son, D.; Park, D.; Jung, E. Anti-Skin-Aging Activity of a Standardized Extract from Panax ginseng Leaves In Vitro and In Human Volunteer. *Cosmetics* **2017**, *4*, 18. [CrossRef]
205. Hwang, E.; Park, S.Y.; Yin, C.S.; Kim, H.T.; Kim, Y.M.; Yi, T.H. Antiaging effects of the mixture of Panax ginseng and Crataegus pinnatifida in human dermal fibroblasts and healthy human skin. *J. Ginseng Res.* **2017**, *41*, 69–77. [CrossRef] [PubMed]
206. Choi, H.R.; Nam, K.M.; Lee, H.S.; Yang, S.H.; Kim, Y.S.; Lee, J.; Date, A.; Toyama, K.; Park, K.C. Phlorizin, an active ingredient of eleutherococcus senticosus, increases proliferative potential of keratinocytes with inhibition of MiR135b and increased expression of type IV collagen. *Oxid. Med. Cell. Longev.* **2016**, *2016*. [CrossRef]
207. Shoko, T.; Maharaj, V.J.; Naidoo, D.; Tselanyane, M.; Nthambeleni, R.; Khorombi, E.; Apostolides, Z. Anti-aging potential of extracts from Sclerocarya birrea (A. Rich.) Hochst and its chemical profiling by UPLC-Q-TOF-MS. *BMC Complement. Altern. Med.* **2018**, *18*, 54. [CrossRef]
208. Shimizu, C.; Wakita, Y.; Inoue, T.; Hiramitsu, M.; Okada, M.; Mitani, Y.; Segawa, S.; Tsuchiya, Y.; Nabeshima, T. Effects of lifelong intake of lemon polyphenols on aging and intestinal microbiome in the senescence-accelerated mouse prone 1 (SAMP1). *Sci. Rep.* **2019**, *9*, 3671. [CrossRef]
209. Lu, X.; Zhou, Y.; Wu, T.; Hao, L. Ameliorative effect of black rice anthocyanin on senescent mice induced by d-galactose. *Food Funct.* **2014**, *5*, 2892–2897. [CrossRef]
210. Xiong, L.G.; Chen, Y.J.; Tong, J.W.; Gong, Y.S.; Huang, J.A.; Liu, Z.H. Epigallocatechin-3-gallate promotes healthy lifespan through mitohormesis during early-to-mid adulthood in Caenorhabditis elegans. *Redox Biol.* **2018**, *14*, 305–315. [CrossRef]
211. Ratnasooriya, W.D.; Abeysekera, W.K.S.M.; Muthunayake, T.B.S.; Ratnasooriya, C.D.T. In vitro antiglycation and cross-link breaking activities of Sri Lankan low-grown orthodox orange pekoe grade black tea (*Camellia sinensis* L). *Trop. J. Pharm. Res.* **2014**, *13*, 567–571. [CrossRef]
212. Yoo, D.S.; Min Jeon, J.; Jeong Choi, M.; Sang Lee, H.; Woo Cheon, J.; Hoi Kim, S.; Ryu Ju, S. Potential anti-wrinkle effects of m. spaientum l. leaves extract. *BioEvolution* **2015**, *2*, 56–61.
213. Widowati, W.; Fauziah, N.; Herdiman, H.; Afni, M.; Afifah, E.; Kusuma, H.S.W.; Nufus, H.; Arumwardana, S.; Rihibiha, D.D. Antioxidant and anti aging assays of Oryza sativa extracts, vanillin and coumaric acid. *J. Nat. Remedies* **2016**, *16*, 88–99. [CrossRef]

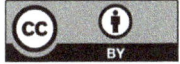

© 2020 by the authors. Licensee MDPI, Basel, Switzerland. This article is an open access article distributed under the terms and conditions of the Creative Commons Attribution (CC BY) license (http://creativecommons.org/licenses/by/4.0/).

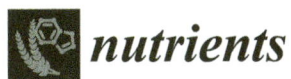

Article

Dietary Protein Intake Patterns and Inadequate Protein Intake in Older Adults from Four Countries

Alejandro Gaytán-González [1,2,*], María de Jesús Ocampo-Alfaro [3], Francisco Torres-Naranjo [1,4], Roberto Gabriel González-Mendoza [1], Martha Gil-Barreiro [3], Maritza Arroniz-Rivera [3] and Juan R. López-Taylor [1]

[1] Institute of Applied Sciences for Physical Activity and Sport, Department of Human Movement Sciences, Education, Sport, Recreation, and Dance, University Health Sciences Center, University of Guadalajara, Guadalajara 44430, Mexico; dr.francisco.torres@icloud.com (F.T.-N.); roberto.gonzalez@academicos.udg.mx (R.G.G.-M.); taylor@cucs.udg.mx (J.R.L.-T.)
[2] Department of Human Reproduction, Infantile Growth, and Development, University Health Sciences Center, University of Guadalajara, Guadalajara 44280, Mexico
[3] Geriatrics Department, Western General Hospital, Zapopan 45170, Mexico; mocampo1@prodigy.net.mx (M.d.J.O.-A.); marthagilbarreiro@yahoo.com.mx (M.G.-B.); marroniz.maritza@gmail.com (M.A.-R.)
[4] Center of Body Composition and Bone Research, Guadalajara 44600, Mexico
[*] Correspondence: alejandro.gaytan@cucs.udg.mx; Tel.: +52-1-333-619-9708

Received: 20 August 2020; Accepted: 9 October 2020; Published: 16 October 2020

Abstract: Recent interest in protein intake per meal is observed in studies that have reported the protein intake patterns in different countries; however, comparisons of these data are lacking. We aimed to compare protein intake patterns and the percentage of inadequate protein intake (IPI) per day and meal in older adults from different countries. We acquired data of protein intake in older adults from four countries (Mexico, United States of America, Germany, and United Kingdom). We compared protein intake (per day and meal), IPI per day and meal, and the number of meals with an adequate protein content among countries. The IPI per day significantly differed among countries for <0.8 and <1.0 (both $p < 0.001$), but not for <1.2 g/kg/d ($p = 0.135$). IPI per meal (<30 g/meal) did not differ among countries at breakfast ($p = 0.287$) and lunch ($p = 0.076$) but did differ at dinner ($p < 0.001$). Conversely, IPI per meal (<0.4 g/kg/meal) significantly differed among countries at breakfast, lunch, and dinner (all $p < 0.001$). The percentage of participants that ate ≥30 g/meal or ≥0.4 g/kg/meal at zero, one, and two or three meals per day significantly differed among countries (all $p < 0.05$). IPI at breakfast and lunch (<30 g/meal) was a common trait in the analyzed samples and might represent an opportunity for nutritional interventions in older adults in different countries.

Keywords: breakfast; meals; older adults; protein intake

1. Introduction

The ageing process in humans encompasses many changes that ultimately lead to undesirable clinical conditions like a higher fat deposition, osteoporosis, sarcopenia, frailty, and physical disability [1,2]. Current research on ageing focuses on decreasing the risk of developing the previously mentioned conditions and designing effective interventions to improve the patient's health [3–5].

Regarding sarcopenia, frailty, and physical disability, protein intake is one of the several factors linked to these clinical conditions [6]. A growing body of evidence suggests that daily protein intake above the recommended dietary allowance (R.D.A.) of 0.8 g/kg/d is associated with better physical performance, maintenance or even an increase in muscle mass, and decreased risk of physical disability. Therefore, it has been suggested to set the protein recommendation to a higher dose of 1.0–1.2 g/kg/d [7–10].

Additionally, it seems that other traits, like protein intake per meal and protein distribution, should be considered along with daily protein intake [11,12]. Nonetheless, the evidence is equivocal; other studies suggest that the protein intake pattern might not be an important variable to consider in terms of skeletal muscle-related outcomes (e.g., strength and functionality) [12–14]. The studies supporting the importance of protein distribution in older adults suggest that the consumption of 30 g of protein per meal or 0.4 g/kg per meal are associated with a higher skeletal muscle mass and strength and maximally stimulates muscle protein synthesis, respectively [15,16]. In this regard, some studies suggested that inadequate protein intake (<30 g/meal or <0.4 g/kg/meal) at specific meals might be a risk factor to consider as it is associated to a lower skeletal muscle mass, muscle strength, and functionality [17–19]. On the other hand, the number of meals that reach a protein content ≥30 g/meal or ≥0.4 g/kg/meal appears to be a protective factor as they are associated with a higher skeletal muscle mass, muscle strength, and lower physical disability [15,20,21]. Therefore, determining the percentage of older adults for both indicators might help visualize the magnitude of these two possible risk and protective factors.

Several studies have focused their attention on analyzing dietary protein intake patterns in older adults in different countries [14,19–27]. Nonetheless, to the best of our knowledge, direct comparisons of protein intake patterns among countries are lacking [28]. Similarly, the comparison of the percentage of older adults that did not eat enough protein per day (i.e., 0.8, 1.0, and 1.2 g/kg/d) or per meal (30 g/meal; 0.4 g/kg/meal) among countries is missing. These comparisons among countries might serve as a starting point to understand the magnitude of this situation, because comparisons would help us to determine if these different samples share common issues, allowing us to identify protein-eating patterns to be improved.

Therefore, this exploratory study aimed to (1) compare dietary protein intake patterns among older adults from four countries, (2) report and compare data of inadequate protein intake per day and per meal among older adults from four countries, and (3) analyze if these comparisons would yield similar results when the analysis was separated by sex. We hypothesized that dietary protein intake patterns would be different, but inadequate protein intake would be similar among countries. Likewise, we hypothesized that the comparisons among countries separated by sex would yield different patterns (e.g., if protein at breakfast differs among countries in women but not in men) and that the whole sample pattern would be the same in women but not in men.

2. Materials and Methods

2.1. Study Design and Data Acquisition

This is an exploratory analysis carried out with data from previously published articles where authors reported protein intake per day and meal in adults aged ≥60 years. Corresponding authors were contacted to gather demographic and protein intake data. We acquired data from two studies of two countries (Germany [14] and the United Kingdom [U.K.] [24]), from the National Health and Nutrition Examination Survey (NHANES) 2015–2016 publicly available database representing the United States of America (U.S.A.) [29], and data from our previous work in Mexico [18,20], all with cross-sectional designs.

To analyze the NHANES sample, we included data from participants with the following characteristics: (1) aged ≥60 year; (2) they were born in the U.S.A.; (3) reported an energy intake ≥600 and ≤4000 kcal/day; and (4) had complete data for age, height, and body mass. From these records (n = 1039, 50% women), we randomly selected 200 subjects (100 per sex to keep the sex proportion) to decrease the differences in sample size among groups. There were no significant differences between included and nonincluded subjects (n = 839) for age (p = 0.81), body mass (p = 0.55), height (p = 0.38), BMI (p = 0.98), nor total protein intake per day (p = 0.15). This sample was not weighted according to the NHANES complex study design as the other studies did not follow the same sampling design.

All studies independently coded the three main meals (i.e., breakfast, lunch, and dinner), and reported that they obtained participants' written informed consent and ethical approval from their local institution before any assessment. Table 1 shows an overview of the included samples.

2.2. Protein Intake Variables

When studies reported two or more days of dietary assessment, we averaged the protein intake per day and per meal, and we used these averages for further analysis. We calculated relative protein intake per day (g/kg body mass/d) and per meal (g/kg body mass/meal), meal contribution to total daily protein (%), and protein distribution coefficient of variation in addition to the absolute protein intake per day (g/d) and per meal (g/meal).

Meal contribution to total protein was calculated as:

$$\text{Meal contributrion} = PM/TP \times 100, \quad (1)$$

where *PM* is the protein reported for any given meal (g) and *TP* is the total daily protein intake (g).

The protein distribution coefficient of variation (*PDCV*) was calculated as:

$$PDCV = SDP/MP, \quad (2)$$

where *SDP* is the standard deviation of the three main meals and *MP* is the mean protein intake for the three main meals.

2.3. Inadequate Protein Intake

Inadequate protein intake (IPI) was considered as any protein consumption <0.8 (IPID-0.8), <1.0 (IPID-1.0), and <1.2 (IPID-1.2) g/kg/d [7,8] or <30 g/meal (IPIM-30) and <0.4 g/kg/meal (IPIM-0.4) [15,16]. We reported IPIM-30 and IPIM-0.4 for each main meal. We also counted the number of meals per day (coded as zero [0M], one [1M], and two or three meals [+2M]) with ≥30 g protein and ≥0.4 g protein/kg each.

Table 1. Description of studies' main characteristics.

Author (Year)	City and Country	Year of Recruitment	Sample Size (W/M)	Representativity	Setting	Recruitment	Food Assessment Tool
Gaytán-González (2020) [20]	Zapopan, Mexico	2017	187 (140/47)	Local	Community-dwelling	Users of a tertiary care hospital	One 24-h dietary recall
NHANES, 2015–2016 [29]	United States of America	2015–2016	200 (100/100)	National ‡	Community-dwelling	Random selection from the national census	Two nonconsecutive 24-h dietary recall
Gingrich (2017) [14]	Nürnberg, Germany	2016–2017	97 (48/49)	Local	Community-dwelling	Citizen registry	7-day food record
Cardon-Thomas (2018) [24]	Birmingham, United Kingdom	2014	38 (26/12)	Local	Community-dwelling	Volunteer databases	3-day food diary

NHANES: National Health and Nutrition Examination Survey; W/M: number of women and men. ‡ The complex sampling design of NHANES leads to nationally representative data; however, this is not the case for this study as the data were not weighted according to its sampling design and were composed of a smaller sample size (200 vs. 1039).

2.4. Statistics

Continuous data were expressed in mean ± standard deviation, while categorical and ordinal data in frequencies, percentages, and 95% confidence intervals. To compare the continuous variables among countries, we performed one-way ANOVAs with Scheffe test as post hoc when Levene's test suggested homogeneity of variances ($p > 0.05$). Otherwise, one-way ANOVAs with Welch's correction and Dunnett T3 test as post hoc were performed (Microsoft® Excel® 2013, Microsoft Corporation, Redmond, WA, USA). To compare the categorical and ordinal variables among countries, we used the χ^2 test of independence (GraphPad Prism 7.05, GraphPad Software Inc., La Jolla, CA, USA) and multiple t-tests for proportions with Bonferroni correction as post hoc (Statistics calculator v4.0, StatPac, Northfield, MN, USA). All comparisons were deemed significant at a p-value ≤ 0.05. Effect sizes were calculated for ANOVAs (omega squared, ω^2) and χ^2 tests of independence (phi statistic, φ). Both effect size statistics are dimensionless and range between 0 and 1. An effect size was considered small, medium, or large if ω^2 reached 0.01, 0.06, or 0.14, respectively; the respective values for φ were 0.1, 0.3, 0.5 [30,31]. Effect sizes below the "small" cut point were considered trivial [32]. The difference between the highest mean and the lowest mean was reported along with the effect size. The comparisons among countries were carried out for the whole sample and separated by sex.

3. Results

3.1. Demographic Data

There were significant differences among countries for all demographic data. Mexico showed the highest women proportion while Germany the lowest (25% difference, small effect). Age, body mass, and height comparisons showed a large effect. The oldest participants came from Mexico, Germany, and U.K. in contrast to those in U.S.A. (8-year difference). The heaviest participants belonged to U.S.A. (20 kg difference vs. Mexico), and U.S.A. and Germany showed the tallest participants (13 cm difference vs. Mexico). The B.M.I. comparison showed a medium effect with U.S.A. having the heaviest participants (3.3 units difference vs. Germany) (Table 2). A similar pattern was observed in women (Table S1) and men (Table S2).

3.2. Protein Intake

For absolute protein intake (g), U.K., U.S.A., and Germany showed the highest protein consumption per day (19 g difference vs. Mexico, medium effect). Mexico, U.S.A., and Germany showed the highest intake at breakfast (3 g difference vs. U.K., trivial effect). In comparison, U.K. and U.S.A. showed the highest intake at dinner (20 g difference vs. Mexico, large effect). There were no significant differences among countries for protein intake at lunch (Table 2).

For relative protein intake (g/kg), U.K. showed the highest intake per day (0.22 g/kg difference vs. U.S.A., small effect). Mexico showed the highest intake at breakfast (0.09 g/kg difference vs. U.S.A., medium effect). U.K. and Mexico showed the highest intake at lunch (0.15 g/kg difference vs. U.S.A., medium effect). U.K. showed the highest intake at dinner (0.29 g/kg difference vs. Mexico, large effect) (Table 2).

Analyzing the percentage of meal contribution to total protein intake, Germany, and Mexico ate most of their daily protein at lunch, whereas U.S.A. and U.K. did it at dinner. Mexico showed the highest breakfast (13% difference vs. U.K., medium effect) and lunch contribution (12% difference vs. U.S.A., medium effect), whereas U.S.A. and U.K. showed the highest dinner contribution (19% difference vs. Mexico, large effect). In terms of the PDCV, Germany showed the evenest protein distribution (−0.17 units difference vs. U.K., small effect) (Table 2). The comparisons divided by sex showed a very similar pattern to that observed of the whole sample, with slight differences in which countries differ from one another (Tables S1 and S2). However, it is remarkable that there were no significant differences among countries at breakfast and lunch (g) nor per day and breakfast (g/kg) in men (Table S2).

Table 2. Participants' main characteristics and protein intake variables by country.

	Mexico	U.S.A.	Germany	United Kingdom	p-Value	Effect Size	
n	187	200	97	38			
Women (%)	74.9 a	50.0 b	49.5 b	68.4 a,b	<0.001	0.244	S
Age (year)	79 ± 8 a	71 ± 7 b	78 ± 3 a	78 ± 5 a	<0.001	0.226	L
Body mass (kg)	63.2 ± 13.1 a	83.8 ± 19.6 b	74.1 ± 14.0 c	68.0 ± 12.0 a,c	<0.001	0.238	L
Height (cm)	153.6 ± 9.1 a	166.6 ± 10.3 b	166.1 ± 9.2 b	- †	<0.001	0.297	L
BMI (kg/m^2)	26.9 ± 5.7 a	30.1 ± 6.0 b	26.8 ± 4.0 a	- †	<0.001	0.074	M
			Absolute protein intake (g)				
Day	57 ± 20 a	74 ± 28 b	70 ± 19 b	76 ± 12 b	<0.001	0.111	M
Breakfast	17 ± 8 a	16 ± 10 a,b	16 ± 9 a,b	14 ± 6 b	0.023	0.006	T
Lunch	25 ± 12	23 ± 14	24 ± 10	29 ± 14	0.098	0.009	T
Dinner	13 ± 8 a	30 ± 17 b	22 ± 11 c	33 ± 12 b	<0.001	0.275	L
			Relative protein intake (g/kg)				
Day	0.93 ± 0.37 a	0.92 ± 0.38 a	0.97 ± 0.28 a	1.14 ± 0.25 b	<0.001	0.019	S
Breakfast	0.29 ± 0.16 a	0.20 ± 0.13 b	0.23 ± 0.12 b	0.21 ± 0.10 b	<0.001	0.077	M
Lunch	0.41 ± 0.22 a	0.28 ± 0.19 b	0.33 ± 0.14 c	0.43 ± 0.23 a,c	<0.001	0.082	M
Dinner	0.21 ± 0.14 a	0.37 ± 0.22 b	0.30 ± 0.14 c	0.50 ± 0.19 d	<0.001	0.196	L
			Daily contribution (%)				
Breakfast	32 ± 14 a	22 ± 13 b,c	23 ± 10 b	19 ± 8 c	<0.001	0.126	M
Lunch	43 ± 15 a	31 ± 16 b	35 ± 12 b	38 ± 16 a,b	<0.001	0.114	M
Dinner	23 ± 12 a	40 ± 16 b	31 ± 11 c	44 ± 15 b	<0.001	0.268	L
PDCV	0.55 ± 0.26 a	0.59 ± 0.28 a	0.43 ± 0.24 b	0.60 ± 0.18 a	<0.001	0.044	S

† Data not obtained. BMI: Body Mass Index; g/kg: grams of protein per kilogram of body mass; L: large effect size; M: medium effect size; PDCV: protein distribution coefficient of variation (dimensionless); S: small effect size; T: trivial effect size; U.S.A.: United States of America. Countries not sharing a similar letter denote significant differences among them (p ≤ 0.05) within each variable.

3.3. Inadequate Protein Intake per Day

There were significant differences among countries for IPID-0.8, IPID-1.0, but not IPID-1.2. For IPID-0.8, the highest percentage was observed in U.S.A. (43.0%) and Mexico (42.2%) (35% difference vs. U.K., small effect). For IPID-1.0, U.S.A. (61.5%), Mexico (61.5%), and Germany (60.8%) showed the highest percentages (35% difference vs. U.K., small effect). For IPID-1.2, percentages ranged from 65.8% in U.K. to 83.5% in Germany (Figure 1). A similar pattern was observed in women. However, in men, there were no significant differences among countries for any cut point (Figure S1).

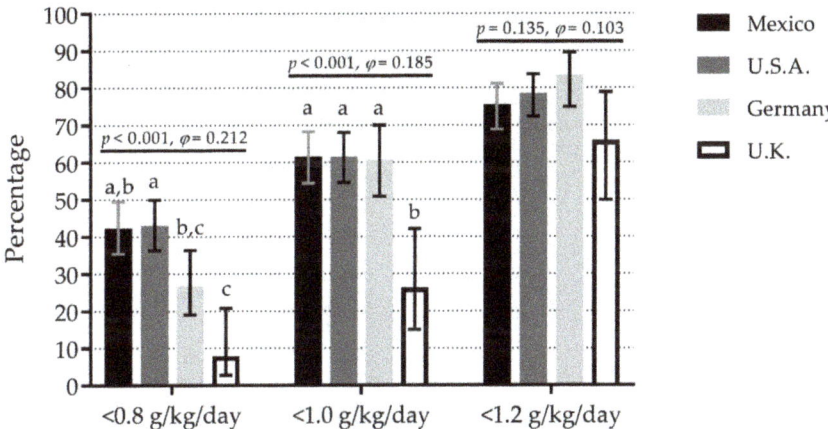

Figure 1. Comparison of inadequate protein intake per day with different cut points among four countries. Bars represent the percentage of inadequate protein intake per day; whiskers represent 95% confidence intervals. p-values and φ statistic are for comparisons among countries within cut points (χ^2 test of independence). Bars not sharing a similar letter (a, b, c) denote significant differences ($p \leq 0.05$) among countries within cut points (t-test for proportions with Bonferroni correction). g/kg/day: grams of protein per kilogram of body mass per day; U.K.: United Kingdom; U.S.A.: United States of America. Detailed data can be found in Table S3.

3.4. Inadequate Protein Intake per Meal

For IPIM-30, there were no significant differences among countries at breakfast (range 91.5% in U.S.A. to 97.4% in U.K.) and lunch (range 63.2% in U.K. to 77.0% in U.S.A.). However, there were significant differences at dinner, where Mexico (96.8%) showed the highest percentage (60% difference vs. U.K., medium effect) (Figure 2a). The pattern was very similar when comparisons were separated by sex (Figure S2a,b).

For IPIM-0.4, there were significant differences among countries for the three meals. At breakfast, U.K. (97.4%), U.S.A. (94.0%), and Germany (90.7%) showed the highest percentages (20% difference vs. Mexico, small effect). At lunch, U.S.A. (80.5%) and Germany (72.2%) showed the highest percentages (31% difference vs. Mexico, small effect). At dinner, Mexico (92.0%) showed the highest percentage (61% difference vs. U.K., medium effect) (Figure 2b). The pattern was very similar when comparisons were separated by sex (Figure S2c,d).

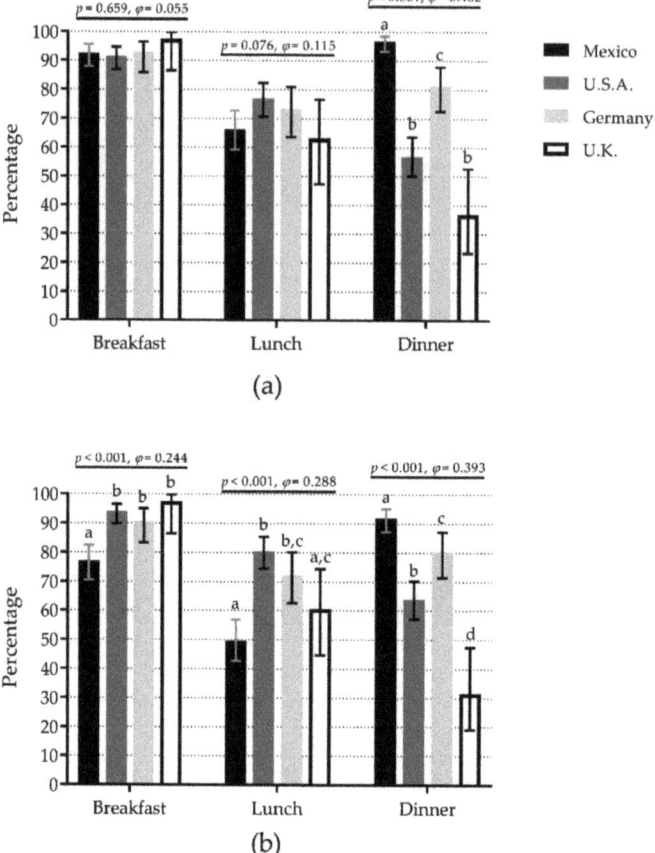

Figure 2. Comparison of inadequate protein intake per meal (breakfast, lunch, and dinner) among four countries depending on the protein content at each meal as <30 g/meal (**a**) or <0.4 g/kg body mass/meal (**b**). Bars represent the percentage of inadequate protein intake per meal; whiskers represent 95% confidence intervals. p-values and φ statistic are for comparisons among countries within meals (χ^2 test of independence). Bars not sharing a similar letter (a, b, c, d) denote significant differences ($p \leq 0.05$) among countries within meals (t-test for proportions with Bonferroni correction). U.K.: United Kingdom; U.S.A.: United States of America. Detailed data can be found in Table S3.

3.5. Number of Meals per Day with Adequate Protein Content

When the ≥30 g protein/meal criterion was used, Mexico (61.0%) and Germany (60.8%) showed the highest percentages of 0M (50% difference vs. U.K., small effect), U.K. (76.3%) showed the highest percentage of 1M (48% difference vs. Germany, small effect), whereas U.S.A. (14.5%) showed the highest percentage of +2M (10% difference vs. Mexico, small effect) (Figure 3a). The pattern was similar when comparisons were separated by sex, except there were no significant differences among countries for +2M for either sex (Figure S3a,b).

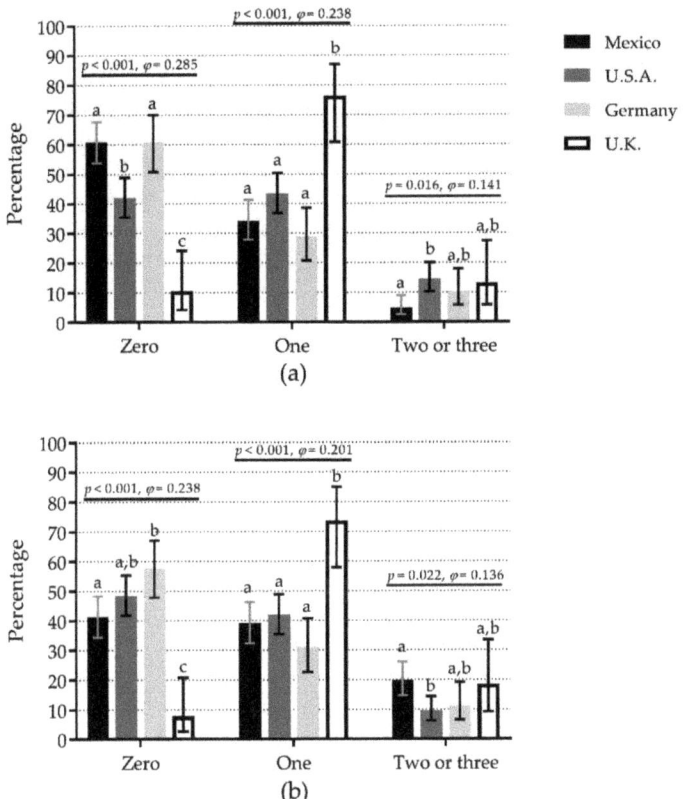

Figure 3. The number of meals per day containing ≥30 g protein (**a**) or ≥0.4 g protein/kg body mass (**b**) compared among countries. Bars represent the percentage of participants that reported the number of meals per day (zero, one, and two or three) with the mentioned protein content; whiskers represent 95% confidence intervals. p-values and φ statistic are for comparisons among countries within the number of meals (χ^2 test of independence). Bars not sharing a similar letter (a, b, c) denote significant differences ($p \leq 0.05$) among countries within the number of meals (t-test for proportions with Bonferroni correction). U.K.: United Kingdom; U.S.A.: United States of America. Detailed data can be found in Table S3.

When the ≥0.4 g protein/kg/meal criterion was used, Germany (57.7%) and U.S.A. (48.5%) showed the highest percentages of 0M (50% difference vs. U.K., small effect), whereas U.K. (73.7%) showed the highest percentage of 1M (42% difference vs. Germany, small effect). In contrast, Mexico (19.8%) showed the highest percentage of +2M (10% difference vs. U.S.A., small effect) (Figure 3b). The comparisons separated by sex showed a different pattern to that observed in the whole sample. In women, there were significant differences among countries for 0M and 1M, but not for +2M groups (Figure S3c). In men, there were significant differences among countries for 0M, but not for 1M and +2M groups (Figure S3d).

3.6. IPI Combined Results

When data from the four samples were combined (n = 522), we calculated the percentage of IPID-0.8, IPID-1.0, IPID-1.2, IPIM-30, IPIM-0.4, and the number of meals with an adequate protein content (Table 3). Briefly, we observed that there was about a 20% increase in the percentage of IPI per day every time when the cut point was increased. For both IPIM-30 and IPIM-0.4, breakfast was the meal with the highest percentage, followed by dinner and lunch. For both ≥30 g/meal and ≥0.4 g/kg/meal criteria, eating 0M was the most condition, followed by 1M and +2M.

Table 3. Combined data (n = 522) from the four samples analyzed.

	n	(%)	(95% CI)
IPID-0.8	194	(37.2)	(33.1–41.4)
IPID-1.0	307	(58.8)	(54.5–63.0)
IPID-1.2	404	(77.4)	(73.6–80.8)
IPIM-30			
Breakfast	483	(92.5)	(89.9–94.5)
Lunch	373	(71.5)	(67.4–75.2)
Dinner	388	(74.3)	(70.4–77.9)
IPIM-0.4			
Breakfast	457	(87.5)	(84.4–90.1)
Lunch	347	(66.5)	(62.3–70.4)
Dinner	390	(74.7)	(70.8–78.3)
Number of meals with ≥30 g/meal			
Zero	261	(50.0)	(45.7–54.3)
One	208	(39.8)	(35.7–44.1)
Two or three	53	(10.2)	(7.8–13.0)
Number of meals with ≥0.4 g/kg/meal			
Zero	233	(44.6)	(40.4–48.9)
One	215	(41.2)	(37.0–45.5)
Two or three	74	(14.2)	(11.4–17.4)

95% CI: 95% confidence intervals; IPID-0.8: inadequate protein intake per day (<0.8 g/kg/d); IPID-1.0: inadequate protein intake per day (<1.0 g/kg/d); IPID-1.2: inadequate protein intake per day (<1.2 g/kg/d); IPIM-30: inadequate protein intake per meal (<30 g/meal); IPIM-0.4: inadequate protein intake per meal (<0.4 g/kg/meal).

4. Discussion

To the best of our knowledge, this is the first study that compares dietary protein intake patterns and the percentage of IPI per day and per meal among countries. While there are studies where dietary protein intake patterns were reported, direct evidence about their differences was lacking. This study demonstrates that some dietary protein intake patterns in older adults significantly differed among countries, but they shared traits in IPI. For instance, three countries showed a similar percentage of IPID-1.0 (>60%) and IPID-1.2 (>75%) (Figure 1). These high percentages of IPI per day might represent a higher risk of lower physical functioning [9,10,33] and developing frailty [34,35].

Furthermore, the main finding of this study was that participants from all the analyzed samples reported a high percentage of IPIM-30 at breakfast (>90%) and lunch (>60%) (Figure 2a). This is relevant due to IPI at breakfast might also be attributable to breakfast skipping [36]. Although breakfast skipping is less studied in older adults, evidence in their younger counterparts offers insight about what to expect. For example, breakfast skipping was associated with lower skeletal muscle mass in young adults [37], which seems feasible in older adults because meal skipping might lead to malnutrition [38] and skeletal muscle loss [39]. Additionally, breakfast skipping is associated with a higher risk of developing type 2 diabetes in adults of different ages (18–83 year) [40]. Moreover, breakfast has been previously reported as a low-energy containing meal [36]. For instance, Huseinovic et al. [28] reported that breakfast composed the lowest contribution to the daily energy intake in different European countries, which we speculate might include IPIM-30. On the other hand, insufficient protein intake at lunch is also associated with lower functionality and muscle mass decline [18,19]. Both eating occasions might represent an opportunity for nutritional interventions in older adults in many countries; however, breakfast appears to be a priority due to its larger percentage of inadequate protein intake.

We observed that most differences among countries could be attributable to women because the pattern was very similar to that observed in the whole sample. However, while it appears to be a sex-derived pattern in some variables (e.g., protein at breakfast and lunch), it is important to highlight that there were more women than men in this analysis. Therefore, men could be underrepresented and different patterns attributable to different sample sizes. Further research among countries with larger men samples is recommended.

As previously mentioned, the evidence comparing eating patterns among countries is scarce, and the available studies are focused on eating occasions, meal frequency, and meal energy content, rather than protein intake per meal [28,36,41]. Therefore, it is difficult to draw comparisons with the previous evidence. However, we can see that our results are supported by drawing inferences from other studies; i.e., IPI per day may differ among countries [42,43], but IPI at breakfast appears to be high [43,44]. Although an "all countries" comparison might not be reliable, we believe it would be of interest to compare countries sharing a geographical area (e.g., North America, South America, and Western Europe) and among states/provinces within countries. It would lead to data about the magnitude of the problem in specific regions to design concrete strategies to overcome this problem.

Another important finding is that about 90%, 70%, and 74% of the participants did not eat enough protein at breakfast, lunch, and dinner, respectively (Table 3). Therefore, there is interest in strategies to increase total dietary protein intake [4,5,45]. We [20] and others [15,21,46] have previously reported that reaching an adequate protein content per meal (i.e., ≥30 g) is significantly associated with higher daily protein intake and lower proportion of IPI per day (<1.2 g/kg/d). However, this practice is not usual. We reported here that only about 15% of participants ate two or three meals with adequate protein content (Table 3). This low proportion of compliance might be attributable to the lack of appetite and some chewing difficulties commonly observed in older adults [5,6,47], thus making it challenging to reach this protein amount with simple foods [47]. Some strategies, like mincing meat [48] and food enrichment with protein [46], may help overcome the difficulties mentioned earlier. On the other hand, about 45% of the participants did not eat enough protein at any meal (Table 3), which may be a concern because their muscle protein synthesis might not be stimulated to its maximum level at any meal [11]. This low protein intake might lead to a negative protein balance, muscle loss, and possibly accelerating the functional decline in the elderly [49,50].

In this study, the combined data suggested that about 40%, 60%, and 80% of the participants showed IPI per day for the <0.8, <1.0, and <1.2 g/kg criteria (Table 3). These results are similar to those recently reported by Hengeveld et al. [51]. In their meta-analysis, they found that when protein intake was divided by the actual body weight (g/kg of actual body weight/day), the IPI was 29.1, 54.3, and 75.7%, respectively. Nevertheless, when they used the adjusted body weight (g/kg adjusted body weight/day), the percentages of IPI were lower, 21.5%, 46.7%, and 70.8%, respectively. It is important to note that Hengeveld et al. analyzed data from adults aged ≥55 year, belonging to large cohorts (n = 410 to 2660) from different countries (U.S.A., the Netherlands, U.K., Canada, Finland, and Italy) and that they performed complex statistics to came up with the previously mentioned percentages. However, despite these differences in comparison to our study, they showed similar results when the protein intake was reported with the actual body weight for the 1.0 and 1.2 g/kg/d criteria. Nonetheless, the authors suggest using the adjusted body weight to decrease the chances of over- or underestimation [25,51].

It is important to consider this study's limitations. First, meal identification varied among studies (participant-identified [18,29]; time of the day [24]; time of the day and meal composition [14]); therefore, it impedes us to analyze the specific hour when occurred. Thus, meals could be close to one another in the time of the day but were categorized differently due to cultural traits [36]. Hence, it is difficult to fully conclude differences among meals, at least at their respective timing (i.e., breakfast, lunch, and dinner) [36]. This is one of the most important limitations to consider when translating results regarding the timing of IPI and functionality in older adults [17,18]. Consequently, the number of meals per day that reach adequate protein content might offer a better approach than meal timing labelling. This number has shown significant associations with higher muscle mass, strength, and lower risk of physical disability, even in samples that showed different protein eating patterns (e.g., eating more protein at dinner [15] vs. lunch [20]). Thus, it is less likely to be affected by differences in meal labelling [36].

Second, we did not analyze snacks because its categorization is more complex than with the main meals [36]. Nevertheless, further studies should include them because some protein-rich foods (e.g., dairy) might be commonly eaten at snacks [22,43]. In addition, snacks might represent as much energy as a main meal when merged [28], and possibly, the same is true with protein intake.

Third, we had no data about the foods consumed (e.g., meat, dairy, and grains). Protein sources are important because animal protein has a higher anabolic effect than vegetable proteins; this effect is mainly attributable to higher amino acid availability in animal-based foods than those coming from plant-based foods [52]. Therefore, the inclusion of data of ingested foods and food intake patterns along the determination of IPI per day and per meal might help to understand their combined role on health-related variables and which foods are associated with a lower probability of inadequacy [19,53–55].

Fourth, there were different dietary assessment methods for all studies (Table 1), and each one addresses the information from a different approach [56,57]. Moreover, the results should be interpreted cautiously because recall methods are prone to underreporting when compared to doubly labelled water, and two studies relied on one- and 2-days dietary recalls [20,29], which may poorly represent the actual nutritional intake [58,59]. Additionally, the differences in the nutritional analysis due to different food databases must be considered. It is important to highlight that data reported in this study might differ from that in the original articles due to differences in how it was analyzed. For example, Gingrich et al. [14] calculated the PDCV for each day of the 7-day diary and then averaged them. Instead, we first averaged the 7-day protein intake, and then we calculated the PDCV. As mentioned in the methods section, all databases followed the same procedure to average protein intake and made comparisons possible.

Fifth, these results came from very localized samples and must not be deemed nationally representative (Table 1). Instead, these data should be considered a glance into how the dietary protein intake patterns are in these countries. In the case of NHANES, it is a nationally representative study; however, we analyzed a sample of the available cases (200 out of 1039), and data were not weighted according to the complex sampling design; therefore, it cannot be considered as nationally representative. Comparisons of data coming from nationally representative studies deserve further research [51]. Similarly, the combined data reported here should be regarded with caution for several reasons: (1) it came from very different samples (Tables 1 and 2); (2) there are some studies reporting protein intake per meal that were not included here, and the lack of these data surely affect the reported percentages; and (3) the percentages were not weighted. A meta-analysis of the available evidence with weighted pooled prevalence would help to overcome this limitation. We hope this work stimulates the curiosity to carry out systematic reviews with meta-analysis in this area.

The recruitment period may be another limitation. Although the recruitment years were close to one another (about 3 years), this period may yield differences in dietary patterns within countries. Similarly, the recruitment method differed among studies (Table 1). While all participants were community-dwelling, there may be differences in sociodemographic (e.g., education and income) and health-related variables (e.g., functionality and diagnosed diseases) (not included here) that may explain the differences in the outcome variables instead of the geographical localization. The addition and comparison of these variables for further studies are recommended. Additionally, mean ages ranged from 71 to 79 year; this eight-year gap might have influenced the differences observed among countries as older adults tend to eat less protein [23,25]. Finally, the differences in sample sizes in some comparisons were considerable (38 vs. 200, min vs. max), affecting the statistical tests.

5. Conclusions

Inadequate protein intake at breakfast and lunch (<30 g/meal) was a common trait in the analyzed samples, even though most dietary protein intake patterns differed among them. Therefore, these two eating occasions might represent an opportunity for nutritional interventions in older adults in different countries. Similarly, the consumption of two or three meals per day with adequate protein content is less frequent. Further research is recommended to analyze if better dietary protein intake patterns match with better functionality or other health-related variables.

Supplementary Materials: The following are available online at http://www.mdpi.com/2072-6643/12/10/3156/s1, Table S1: Women's main characteristics and protein intake variables by country. Table S2: Men's main characteristics and protein intake variables by country. Table S3: Detailed inadequate protein intake per day and meal in older adults from four countries. Figure S1: Comparison of inadequate protein intake per day with different cut points among four countries in women and men. Figure S2: Inadequate protein intake per meal (breakfast, lunch, and dinner) compared among four countries depending on the protein content for each meal as <30 g/meal or <0.4 g/kg body mass/meal in women and men. Figure S3: The number of meals per day containing ≥30 g protein or ≥0.4 g protein/kg body mass each, in women and men and compared among countries.

Author Contributions: Conceptualization, A.G.-G., M.d.J.O.-A., F.T.-N., and J.R.L.-T.; methodology, A.G.-G., M.d.J.O.-A., F.T.-N., M.A.-R., and M.G.-B.; formal analysis, A.G.-G. and R.G.G.-M.; investigation, A.G.-G.; resources, M.d.J.O.-A. and J.R.L.-T.; data curation, A.G.-G. and R.G.G.-M.; writing—original draft preparation, A.G.-G.; writing—review and editing, M.d.J.O.-A., F.T.-N., M.A.-R., R.G.G.-M., M.G.-B., and J.R.L.-T.; visualization, A.G.-G.; project administration, A.G.-G. and J.R.L.-T. All authors have read and agreed to the published version of the manuscript.

Funding: This research received no external funding.

Acknowledgments: The authors would like to thank to Danielle Cardon-Thomas and Carolyn Greig, from the School of Sport, Exercise and Rehabilitation Sciences and the MRC-Versus Arthritis Centre for Musculoskeletal Ageing Research, the University of Birmingham, UK and to Anne Gingrich and Eva Kiesswetter from the Friedrich-Alexander-Universität Erlangen-Nürnberg, Germany, for their kindly disposition to provide their data to carry out this study.

Conflicts of Interest: The authors declare no conflict of interest.

References

1. Jafarinasabian, P.; Inglis, J.E.; Reilly, W.; Kelly, O.J.; Ilich, J.Z. Aging Human Body: Changes in Bone, Muscle and Body Fat with Consequent Changes in Nutrient Intake. *J. Endocrinol.* **2017**, *234*, R37–R51. [CrossRef] [PubMed]
2. Fulop, T.; Larbi, A.; Khalil, A.; Cohen, A.A.; Witkowski, J.M. Are We Ill Because We Age? *Front. Physiol.* **2019**, *10*, 1508. [CrossRef] [PubMed]
3. Seals, D.R.; Justice, J.N.; Larocca, T.J. Physiological Geroscience: Targeting Function to Increase Healthspan and Achieve Optimal Longevity. *J. Physiol.* **2016**, *594*, 2001–2024. [CrossRef]
4. Martone, A.M.; Marzetti, E.; Calvani, R.; Picca, A.; Tosato, M.; Santoro, L.; Di Giorgio, A.; Nesci, A.; Sisto, A.; Santoliquido, A.; et al. Exercise and Protein Intake: A Synergistic Approach against Sarcopenia. *BioMed Res. Int.* **2017**, *2017*, 2672435. [CrossRef]

5. Robinson, S.M.; Reginster, J.Y.; Rizzoli, R.; Shaw, S.C.; Kanis, J.A.; Bautmans, I.; Bischoff-Ferrari, H.; Bruyère, O.; Cesari, M.; Dawson-Hughes, B.; et al. Does Nutrition Play a Role in the Prevention and Management of Sarcopenia? *Clin. Nutr.* **2018**, *37*, 1121–1132. [CrossRef] [PubMed]
6. Tieland, M.; Trouwborst, I.; Clark, B.C. Skeletal Muscle Performance and Ageing. *J. Cachexia. Sarcopenia Muscle* **2018**, *9*, 3–19. [CrossRef]
7. Landi, F.; Calvani, R.; Tosato, M.; Martone, A.M.; Ortolani, E.; Savera, G.; D'Angelo, E.; Sisto, A.; Marzetti, E. Protein Intake and Muscle Health in Old Age: From Biological Plausibility to Clinical Evidence. *Nutrients* **2016**, *8*, 295. [CrossRef]
8. Bauer, J.; Biolo, G.; Cederholm, T.; Cesari, M.; Cruz-Jentoft, A.J.; Morley, J.E.; Phillips, S.; Sieber, C.; Stehle, P.; Teta, D.; et al. Evidence-Based Recommendations for Optimal Dietary Protein Intake in Older People: A Position Paper from the PROT-AGE Study Group. *J. Am. Med. Dir. Assoc.* **2013**, *14*, 542–559. [CrossRef]
9. Coelho-Júnior, H.; Milano-Teixeira, L.; Rodrigues, B.; Bacurau, R.; Marzetti, E.; Uchida, M. Relative Protein Intake and Physical Function in Older Adults: A Systematic Review and Meta-Analysis of Observational Studies. *Nutrients* **2018**, *10*, 1330. [CrossRef]
10. Mendonça, N.; Granic, A.; Hill, T.R.; Siervo, M.; Mathers, J.C.; Kingston, A.; Jagger, C. Protein Intake and Disability Trajectories in Very Old Adults: The Newcastle 85+ Study. *J. Am. Geriatr. Soc.* **2019**, *67*, 50–56. [CrossRef]
11. Murphy, C.H.; Oikawa, S.Y.; Phillips, S.M. Dietary Protein to Maintain Muscle Mass in Aging: A Case for per-Meal Protein Recommendations. *J. Frailty Aging* **2016**, *5*, 49–58. [CrossRef] [PubMed]
12. Hudson, J.L.; Bergia, R.E.I.; Campbell, W.W. Protein Distribution and Muscle-Related Outcomes: Does the Evidence Support the Concept? *Nutrients* **2020**, *12*, 1441. [CrossRef] [PubMed]
13. Kim, I.Y.; Schutzler, S.; Schrader, A.M.; Spencer, H.J.; Azhar, G.; Wolfe, R.R.; Ferrando, A.A. Protein Intake Distribution Pattern Does Not Affect Anabolic Response, Lean Body Mass, Muscle Strength or Function over 8 Weeks in Older Adults: A Randomized-Controlled Trial. *Clin. Nutr.* **2018**, *37*, 488–493. [CrossRef] [PubMed]
14. Gingrich, A.; Spiegel, A.; Kob, R.; Schoene, D.; Skurk, T.; Hauner, H.; Siebe, C.C.; Volkert, D.; Kiesswetter, E. Amount, Distribution, and Quality of Protein Intake Are Not Associated with Muscle Mass, Strength, and Power in Healthy Older Adults without Functional Limitations—An Enable Study. *Nutrients* **2017**, *9*, 1358. [CrossRef] [PubMed]
15. Loenneke, J.P.; Loprinzi, P.D.; Murphy, C.H.; Phillips, S.M. Per Meal Dose and Frequency of Protein Consumption Is Associated with Lean Mass and Muscle Performance. *Clin. Nutr.* **2016**, *35*, 1506–1511. [CrossRef] [PubMed]
16. Moore, D.R.; Churchward-Venne, T.A.; Witard, O.; Breen, L.; Burd, N.A.; Tipton, K.D.; Phillips, S.M. Protein Ingestion to Stimulate Myofibrillar Protein Synthesis Requires Greater Relative Protein Intakes in Healthy Older versus Younger Men. *J. Gerontol. A Biol. Sci. Med. Sci.* **2015**, *70*, 57–62. [CrossRef]
17. Buckner, S.L.; Loenneke, J.P.; Loprinzi, P.D. Protein Timing during the Day and Its Relevance for Muscle Strength and Lean Mass. *Clin. Physiol. Funct. Imaging* **2017**, *38*, 332–337. [CrossRef]
18. Gaytán-González, A.; Ocampo-Alfaro, M.D.J.; Arroniz-Rivera, M.; Torres-Naranjo, F.; González-Mendoza, R.G.; Gil-Barreiro, M.; López-Taylor, J.R. Inadequate Protein Intake at Specific Meals Is Associated with Higher Risk of Impaired Functionality in Middle to Older Aged Mexican Adults. *J. Aging Res.* **2019**, *2019*, 6597617. [CrossRef]
19. Otsuka, R.; Kato, Y.; Tange, C.; Nishita, Y.; Tomida, M.; Imai, T.; Ando, F.; Shimokata, H.; Arai, H. Protein Intake per Day and at Each Daily Meal and Skeletal Muscle Mass Declines among Older Community Dwellers in Japan. *Public Health Nutr.* **2019**, *23*, 1090–1097. [CrossRef]
20. Gaytán-González, A.; Ocampo-Alfaro, M.D.J.; Torres-Naranjo, F.; Arroniz-Rivera, M.; González-Mendoza, R.G.; Gil-Barreiro, M.; López-Taylor, J.R. The Consumption of Two or Three Meals per Day with Adequate Protein Content Is Associated with Lower Risk of Physical Disability in Mexican Adults Aged 60 Years and Older. *Geriatrics* **2020**, *5*, 1. [CrossRef]
21. Hayashi, A.P.; de Capitani, M.D.; Dias, S.F.; de Souza Gonçalves, L.; Fernandes, A.L.; Jambassi-Filho, J.C.; de Santana, D.A.; Lixandrão, M.; dos Santos Pereira, R.T.; Riani, L.; et al. Number of High-Protein Containing Meals Correlates with Muscle Mass in Pre-Frail and Frail Elderly. *Eur. J. Clin. Nutr.* **2020**, *74*, 1047–1053. [CrossRef] [PubMed]

22. Tieland, M.; den Berg, K.J.B.-V.; van Loon, L.J.C.; de Groot, L.C.P.G.M. Dietary Protein Intake in Dutch Elderly People: A Focus on Protein Sources. *Nutrients* **2015**, *7*, 9697–9706. [CrossRef]
23. Rousset, S.; Mirand, P.P.; Brandolini, M.; Martin, J.-F.; Boirie, Y. Daily Protein Intakes and Eating Patterns in Young and Elderly French. *Br. J. Nutr.* **2003**, *90*, 1107–1115. [CrossRef]
24. Cardon-Thomas, D.K.; Riviere, T.; Tieges, Z.; Greig, C.A. Dietary Protein in Older Adults: Adequate Daily Intake but Potential for Improved Distribution. *Nutrients* **2017**, *9*, 184. [CrossRef] [PubMed]
25. Berner, L.A.; Becker, G.; Wise, M.; Doi, J. Characterization of Dietary Protein among Older Adults in the United States: Amount, Animal Sources, and Meal Patterns. *J. Acad. Nutr. Diet.* **2013**, *113*, 809–815. [CrossRef] [PubMed]
26. Bollwein, J.; Diekmann, R.; Kaiser, M.J.; Bauer, J.M.; Uter, W.; Sieber, C.C.; Volkert, D. Distribution but Not Amount of Protein Intake Is Associated with Frailty: A Cross-Sectional Investigation in the Region of Nürnberg. *Nutr. J.* **2013**, *12*, 109. [CrossRef] [PubMed]
27. Ten Haaf, D.S.M.; Van Dongen, E.J.I.; Nuijten, M.A.H.; Eijsvogels, T.M.H.; De Groot, L.C.P.G.M.; Hopman, M.T.E. Protein Intake and Distribution in Relation to Physical Functioning and Quality of Life in Community-Dwelling Elderly People: Acknowledging the Role of Physical Activity. *Nutrients* **2018**, *10*, 506. [CrossRef]
28. Huseinovic, E.; Winkvist, A.; Slimani, N.; Park, M.K.; Freisling, H.; Boeing, H.; Buckland, G.; Schwingshackl, L.; Weiderpass, E.; Rostgaard-Hansen, A.L.; et al. Meal Patterns across Ten European Countries-Results from the European Prospective Investigation into Cancer and Nutrition (EPIC) Calibration Study. *Public Health Nutr.* **2016**, *19*, 2769–2780. [CrossRef]
29. Centers for Disease Control and Prevention. National Health and Nutrition Examination Survey (NHANES) 2015–2016. Available online: https://wwwn.cdc.gov/nchs/nhanes/ContinuousNhanes/Default.aspx?BeginYear=2015 (accessed on 2 April 2019).
30. Volker, M.A. Reporting Effect Size Estimates in School Psychology Research. *Psychol. Sch.* **2006**, *43*, 653–672. [CrossRef]
31. Cohen, J. *Statistical Power Analysis for the Behavioral Sciences*, 2nd ed.; Lawerence Erlbaum Associates: New York, NY, USA, 1988.
32. Sullivan, G.M.; Feinn, R. Using Effect Size-or Why the p Value Is Not Enough. *J. Grad. Med. Educ.* **2012**, *4*, 279–282. [CrossRef]
33. Isanejad, M.; Mursu, J.; Sirola, J.; Kröger, H.; Rikkonen, T.; Tuppurainen, M.; Erkkilä, A.T. Dietary Protein Intake Is Associated with Better Physical Function and Muscle Strength among Elderly Women. *Br. J. Nutr.* **2016**, *115*, 1281–1291. [CrossRef] [PubMed]
34. Rahi, B.; Colombet, Z.; Gonzalez-Colaço, H.M.; Dartigues, J.F.; Boirie, Y.; Letenneur, L.; Feart, C. Higher Protein but Not Energy Intake Is Associated with a Lower Prevalence of Frailty among Community-Dwelling Older Adults in the French Three-City Cohort. *J. Am. Med. Dir. Assoc.* **2016**, *17*, 672.e7–672.e11. [CrossRef] [PubMed]
35. Coelho-Júnior, H.J.; Rodrigues, B.; Uchida, M.; Marzetti, E. Low Protein Intake Is Associated with Frailty in Older Adults: A Systematic Review and Meta-Analysis of Observational Studies. *Nutrients* **2018**, *10*, 1334. [CrossRef] [PubMed]
36. Leech, R.M.; Worsley, A.; Timperio, A.; McNaughton, S.A. Understanding Meal Patterns: Definitions, Methodology and Impact on Nutrient Intake and Diet Quality. *Nutr. Res. Rev.* **2015**, *28*, 1–21. [CrossRef]
37. Yasuda, J.; Asako, M.; Arimitsu, T.; Fujita, S. Skipping Breakfast Is Associated with Lower Fat-Free Mass in Healthy Young Subjects: A Cross-Sectional Study. *Nutr. Res.* **2018**, *60*, 26–32. [CrossRef] [PubMed]
38. Wong, M.M.H.; So, W.K.W.; Choi, K.C.; Cheung, R.; Chan, H.Y.L.; Sit, J.W.H.; Ho, B.; Li, F.; Lee, T.Y.; Chair, S.Y. Malnutrition Risks and Their Associated Factors among Home-Living Older Chinese Adults in Hong Kong: Hidden Problems in an Affluent Chinese Community. *BMC Geriatr.* **2019**, *19*, 138. [CrossRef] [PubMed]
39. Deutz, N.E.P.; Ashurst, I.; Ballesteros, M.D.; Bear, D.E.; Cruz-Jentoft, A.J.; Genton, L.; Landi, F.; Laviano, A.; Norman, K.; Prado, C.M. The Underappreciated Role of Low Muscle Mass in the Management of Malnutrition. *J. Am. Med. Dir. Assoc.* **2019**, *20*, 22–27. [CrossRef]
40. Ballon, A.; Neuenschwander, M.; Schlesinger, S. Breakfast Skipping Is Associated with Increased Risk of Type 2 Diabetes among Adults: A Systematic Review and Meta-Analysis of Prospective Cohort Studies. *J. Nutr.* **2019**, *149*, 106–113. [CrossRef]

41. Hutchison, A.T.; Heilbronn, L.K. Metabolic Impacts of Altering Meal Frequency and Timing-Does When We Eat Matter? *Biochimie* **2016**, *124*, 187–197. [CrossRef]
42. Ten Haaf, D.S.M.; de Regt, M.F.; Visser, M.; Witteman, B.J.M.; de Vries, J.H.M.; Eijsvogels, T.M.H.; Hopman, M.T.E. Insufficient Protein Intake Is Highly Prevalent among Physically Active Elderly. *J. Nutr. Health Aging* **2018**, *22*, 1112–1114. [CrossRef]
43. Smeuninx, B.; Greig, C.A.; Breen, L. Amount, Source and Pattern of Dietary Protein Intake across the Adult Lifespan: A Cross-Sectional Study. *Front. Nutr.* **2020**, *7*, 25. [CrossRef]
44. Ruiz Valenzuela, R.E.; Ponce, J.A.; Morales-Figueroa, G.G.; Muro, K.A.; Carreón, V.R.; Alemán-Mateo, H. Insufficient Amounts and Inadequate Distribution of Dietary Protein Intake in Apparently Healthy Older Adults in a Developing Country: Implications for Dietary Strategies to Prevent Sarcopenia. *Clin. Interv. Aging* **2013**, *8*, 1143–1148. [CrossRef]
45. Tessier, A.J.; Chevalier, S. An Update on Protein, Leucine, Omega-3 Fatty Acids, and Vitamin D in the Prevention and Treatment of Sarcopenia and Functional Decline. *Nutrients* **2018**, *10*, 1099. [CrossRef]
46. Van Til, A.J.; Naumann, E.; Cox-Claessens, I.J.H.M.; Kremer, S.; Boelsma, E.; van der Schueren, M.A.E. Effects of the Daily Consumption of Protein Enriched Bread and Protein Enriched Drinking Yoghurt on the Total Protein Intake in Elderly in a Rehabilitation Centre: A Single Blind Randomised Controlled Trial. *J. Nutr. Health Aging* **2015**, *19*, 525–530. [CrossRef]
47. Host, A.; McMahon, A.T.; Walton, K.; Charlton, K. Factors Influencing Food Choice for Independently Living Older People—A Systematic Literature Review. *J. Nutr. Gerontol. Geriatr.* **2016**, *35*, 67–94. [CrossRef]
48. Pennings, B.; Groen, B.B.L.; van Dijk, J.-W.; de Lange, A.; Kiskini, A.; Kuklinski, M.; Senden, J.M.G.; van Loon, L.J.C. Minced Beef Is More Rapidly Digested and Absorbed than Beef Steak, Resulting in Greater Postprandial Protein Retention in Older Men. *Am. J. Clin. Nutr.* **2013**, *98*, 121–128. [CrossRef]
49. Beasley, J.M.; Wertheim, B.C.; LaCroix, A.Z.; Prentice, R.L.; Neuhouser, M.L.; Tinker, L.F.; Kritchevsky, S.; Shikany, J.M.; Eaton, C.; Chen, Z.; et al. Biomarker-Calibrated Protein Intake and Physical Function in the Women's Health Initiative. *J. Am. Geriatr. Soc.* **2013**, *61*, 1863–1871. [CrossRef]
50. Houston, D.K.; Tooze, J.A.; Garcia, K.; Visser, M.; Rubin, S.; Harris, T.B.; Newman, A.B.; Kritchevsky, S.B. Protein Intake and Mobility Limitation in Community-Dwelling Older Adults: The Health ABC Study. *J. Am. Geriatr. Soc.* **2017**, *65*, 1705–1711. [CrossRef]
51. Hengeveld, L.M.; Boer, J.M.A.; Gaudreau, P.; Heymans, M.W.; Jagger, C.; Mendonça, N.; Ocké, M.C.; Presse, N.; Sette, S.; Simonsick, E.M.; et al. Prevalence of Protein Intake below Recommended in Community-dwelling Older Adults: A Meta-analysis across Cohorts from the PROMISS Consortium. *J. Cachexia. Sarcopenia Muscle* **2020**. [CrossRef]
52. Berrazaga, I.; Micard, V.; Gueugneau, M.; Walrand, S. The Role of the Anabolic Properties of Plant-versus Animal-Based Protein Sources in Supporting Muscle Mass Maintenance: A Critical Review. *Nutrients* **2019**, *11*, 1825. [CrossRef]
53. Hengeveld, L.M.; Pelgröm, A.D.A.; Visser, M.; Boer, J.M.A.; Haveman-Nies, A.; Wijnhoven, H.A.H. Comparison of Protein Intake per Eating Occasion, Food Sources of Protein and General Characteristics between Community-Dwelling Older Adults with a Low and High Protein Intake. *Clin. Nutr. ESPEN* **2019**, *29*, 165–174. [CrossRef]
54. Gingrich, A.; Spiegel, A.; Gradl, J.E.; Skurk, T.; Hauner, H.; Sieber, C.C.; Volkert, D.; Kiesswetter, E. Daily and Per-Meal Animal and Plant Protein Intake in Relation to Muscle Mass in Healthy Older Adults without Functional Limitations: An Enable Study. *Aging Clin. Exp. Res.* **2019**, *31*, 1271–1281. [CrossRef] [PubMed]
55. Murakami, K.; Livingstone, M.B.E.; Sasaki, S. Meal-Specific Dietary Patterns and Their Contribution to Overall Dietary Patterns in the Japanese Context: Findings from the 2012 National Health and Nutrition Survey, Japan. *Nutrition* **2019**, *59*, 108–115. [CrossRef]
56. Biró, G.; Hulshof, K.F.A.M.; Ovesen, L.; Amorim Cruz, J.A. Selection of Methodology to Assess Food Intake. *Eur. J. Clin. Nutr.* **2002**, *56* (Suppl. 2), S25–S32. [CrossRef]
57. Burrows, T.L.; Ho, Y.Y.; Rollo, M.E.; Collins, C.E. Validity of Dietary Assessment Methods When Compared to the Method of Doubly Labeled Water: A Systematic Review in Adults. *Front. Endocrinol.* **2019**, *10*, 850. [CrossRef]
58. Ma, Y.; Olendzki, B.C.; Pagoto, S.L.; Hurley, T.G.; Magner, R.P.; Ockene, I.S.; Schneider, K.L.; Merriam, P.A.; Hébert, J.R. Number of 24-Hour Diet Recalls Needed to Estimate Energy Intake. *Ann. Epidemiol.* **2009**, *19*, 553–559. [CrossRef] [PubMed]

59. Basiotis, P.P.; Welsh, S.O.; Cronin, F.J.; Kelsay, J.L.; Mertz, W. Number of Days of Food Intake Records Required to Estimate Individual and Group Nutrient Intakes with Defined Confidence. *J. Nutr.* **1987**, *117*, 1638–1641. [CrossRef] [PubMed]

Publisher's Note: MDPI stays neutral with regard to jurisdictional claims in published maps and institutional affiliations.

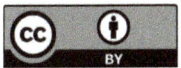
© 2020 by the authors. Licensee MDPI, Basel, Switzerland. This article is an open access article distributed under the terms and conditions of the Creative Commons Attribution (CC BY) license (http://creativecommons.org/licenses/by/4.0/).

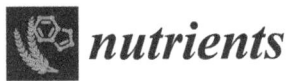

Article

Impact of Hyperhomocysteinemia and Different Dietary Interventions on Cognitive Performance in a Knock-in Mouse Model for Alzheimer's Disease

Hendrik Nieraad [1,*], Natasja de Bruin [1], Olga Arne [1], Martine C. J. Hofmann [1], Mike Schmidt [1], Takashi Saito [2,3], Takaomi C. Saido [2], Robert Gurke [1,4], Dominik Schmidt [1], Uwe Till [5], Michael J. Parnham [1] and Gerd Geisslinger [1,4]

- [1] Fraunhofer Institute for Molecular Biology and Applied Ecology IME, Branch for Translational Medicine and Pharmacology TMP, Theodor-Stern-Kai 7, 60596 Frankfurt am Main, Germany; Natasja.Debruin@ime.fraunhofer.de (N.d.B.); Olga.Arne@ime.fraunhofer.de (O.A.); Martine.Hofmann@ime.fraunhofer.de (M.C.J.H.); mikeschmidt8@hotmail.com (M.S.); gurke@med.uni-frankfurt.de (R.G.); D.Schmidt@med.uni-frankfurt.de (D.S.); Michael.Parnham@ime.fraunhofer.de (M.J.P.); geisslinger@em.uni-frankfurt.de (G.G.)
- [2] Laboratory for Proteolytic Neuroscience, RIKEN Center for Brain Science, Wako, Saitama 351-0198, Japan; takashi.saito.aa@riken.jp (T.S.); saido@brain.riken.jp (T.C.S.)
- [3] Department of Neurocognitive Science, Institute of Brain Science, Nagoya City University Graduate School of Medical Sciences, Nagoya, Aichi 467-8601, Japan
- [4] *pharmazentrum frankfurt*/ZAFES, Institute of Clinical Pharmacology, Goethe University, Theodor-Stern-Kai 7, 60590 Frankfurt am Main, Germany
- [5] Former Institute of Pathobiochemistry, Friedrich-Schiller-University Jena, Nonnenplan 2, 07743 Jena, Germany; uwe.till.erfurt@web.de
- [*] Correspondence: Hendrik.Nieraad@ime.fraunhofer.de

Received: 26 August 2020; Accepted: 20 October 2020; Published: 23 October 2020

Abstract: Background: Hyperhomocysteinemia is considered a possible contributor to the complex pathology of Alzheimer's disease (AD). For years, researchers in this field have discussed the apparent detrimental effects of the endogenous amino acid homocysteine in the brain. In this study, the roles of hyperhomocysteinemia driven by vitamin B deficiency, as well as potentially beneficial dietary interventions, were investigated in the novel App^{NL-G-F} knock-in mouse model for AD, simulating an early stage of the disease. Methods: Urine and serum samples were analyzed using a validated LC-MS/MS method and the impact of different experimental diets on cognitive performance was studied in a comprehensive behavioral test battery. Finally, we analyzed brain samples immunohistochemically in order to assess amyloid-β (Aβ) plaque deposition. Results: Behavioral testing data indicated subtle cognitive deficits in App^{NL-G-F} compared to C57BL/6J wild type mice. Elevation of homocysteine and homocysteic acid, as well as counteracting dietary interventions, mostly did not result in significant effects on learning and memory performance, nor in a modified Aβ plaque deposition in 35-week-old App^{NL-G-F} mice. Conclusion: Despite prominent Aβ plaque deposition, the App^{NL-G-F} model merely displays a very mild AD-like phenotype at the investigated age. Older App^{NL-G-F} mice should be tested in order to further investigate potential effects of hyperhomocysteinemia and dietary interventions.

Keywords: hyperhomocysteinemia; vitamin B deficiency; Alzheimer's disease; amyloid beta-peptides; disease models; animal; memory and learning tests

1. Introduction

After decades of research, there is still a huge unmet medical need for novel interventions to treat dementia-like disorders. In 2019 more than 50 million people were affected by dementia and the number could increase to about 152 million by 2050 [1]. Alzheimer's disease (AD) is the most common type of dementia, accounting for 2/3 of all cases [2]. More than 400 failures in drug development during the last decades [3] have led to the consideration of alternative intervention options, e.g., repurposing, combinatory approaches and preventive treatments [4].

The complex pathology of the disease is characterized by several hallmarks, such as prominent extracellular amyloid plaques [5,6]. According to the amyloid cascade hypothesis, an alteration of amyloid-β (Aβ) metabolism is the central pillar of AD pathology and crucially influences and initiates other hallmarks [7]. In AD, initial pathologic processes progress decades before the first cognitive symptoms appear in patients, a stage entitled preclinical Alzheimer's [8]. Disruptions in amyloid metabolism, as one of the first chronological hallmarks, potentially represent a relevant target for preventive interventions in AD.

In order to further elucidate disease mechanisms and identify novel treatment options, the group of Takaomi Saido at the RIKEN Center for Brain Science has developed a new generation of AD mouse models. These knock-in (KI) mice provide advantages compared to transgenic models, which are based on massive amyloid-β protein precursor (AβPP) overexpression with the result of artificial phenotypes due to overproduction of other AβPP fragments aside from Aβ. In the App^{NL-G-F} model, the murine AβPP sequence is humanized and three mutations are introduced. Swedish (NL), Arctic (G) and Beyreuther/Iberian mutations (F) increase the total amount of Aβ and the Aβ42/Aβ40 ratio, show pro-inflammatory effects and finally result in a three times faster memory impairment [9].

Elevated levels of the endogenous amino acid homocysteine (HCys), called hyperhomocysteinemia, have been described as another hallmark of AD [10]. HCys is increased significantly in AD patients, whereas levels of different B-vitamins are reduced compared to controls [11,12]. A remaining question is whether hyperhomocysteinemia is merely a marker or whether it contributes causally to AD pathology, thereby providing options for therapeutic intervention. Some authors describe the role of plasma HCys as an independent risk factor for memory deficits and AD [13,14]. Consequently, B-vitamin supplementation as a HCys-modifying intervention was proposed previously [15]. According to Smith et al., B-vitamins lowered HCys levels and subsequently slowed the rate of brain atrophy and cognitive decline in patients [16,17]. However, a causal link between hyperhomocysteinemia and Alzheimer's disease, called the "homocysteine hypothesis", has been a source of controversy for years. Kennedy teased out the equivocal results of numerous studies in detail [18]. Several studies neither support an association of HCys with AD nor an improvement of cognitive performance by B-vitamin treatment [19,20]. Meta-analyses were conducted to assess this topic, challenging the homocysteine hypothesis and amelioration of cognitive functions by the use of folate and other B-vitamins [21,22]. In the context of an international consensus statement, researchers assessed the homocysteine hypothesis as being plausible and considered hyperhomocysteinemia a modifiable risk factor for dementia. Furthermore, they recommended considering polyunsaturated fatty acids (PUFAs) in addition to B-vitamins for future trials [23]. PUFAs such as docosahexaenoic acid (DHA) and eicosapentaenoic acid (EPA) are also suggested to be linked to AD pathology and HCys metabolism [24,25], i.e., elevated HCys impairs the formation of PUFAs and leads to a lower availability of PUFAs in the brain. B-vitamin treatment might only be successful when PUFA plasma concentrations are in the upper normal range [26]. A more recent systematic review points out that the evidence for nutrient supplementation remains limited and indicates that more research is needed to assess preventive measures in dementia [27].

Transsulfuration and re-methylation are major metabolic pathways for HCys (Figure 1), being dependent on an adequate supply of B-vitamins, particularly B6, B12 and folate [28]. As illustrated, the relevant B-vitamins play key roles in intrinsically decreasing HCys levels and therefore correlate negatively with HCys. Vitamin B12 and folate are crucial in providing methyl groups in the context of the re-methylation cycle, whereas the transsulfuration pathway depends on vitamin B6 as an essential enzymatic cofactor. Disturbed HCys metabolism (Figure 1) is likely to be linked to AD pathology by direct and indirect neurotoxic pathways [24]. Neurotoxicity is caused by excitotoxicity via

N-methyl-D-aspartate receptor (NMDA) activation and by increased levels of reactive oxygen species promoting oxidative stress. Furthermore, excess HCys and subsequently a lack of methionine and S-Adenosyl-L-methionine (SAM), as well as elevated S-Adenosyl-L-homocysteine (SAH), are associated with a reduced methylation capacity and the inhibition of methylation reactions, which is suggested to exacerbate amyloid and tau pathologies in AD. Moreover, HCys results in an activated immune system, damages cerebral vessels and disrupts the blood-brain-barrier [24,29]. Both homocysteine and its oxidative metabolite homocysteic acid (HCA) are considered neurotoxic [30,31], but HCA is suggested to be the more potent species [32–34] and might contribute to dementia through oxidative stress and excitotoxicity by NMDA activation. Both mechanisms have been considered relevant for AD pathology [5,24].

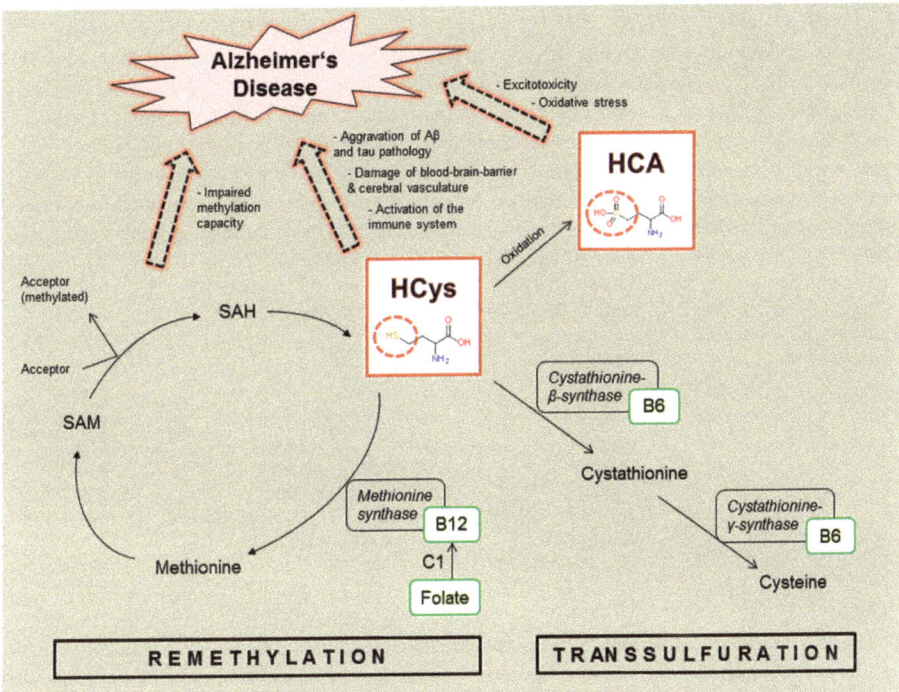

Figure 1. Homocysteine (HCys) and homocysteic acid (HCA): metabolic role and link to Alzheimer's disease; involved enzymes (black boxes) linked to relevant B-vitamins (green boxes) functioning as coenzymes or methyl donor (C1); SAM = S-Adenosyl-L-methionine; SAH = S-Adenosyl-L-homocysteine.

The present exploratory animal study concentrates on the role of hyperhomocysteinemia, driven by vitamin B deficiency, in the context of AD. Therefore, we used the novel and not yet fully characterized App^{NL-G-F} knock-in mouse as a model of the disease. The App^{NL-G-F} mouse is expected to display a mildly impaired phenotype, simulating the very early preclinical period of AD pathology and thus should provide the possibility of assessing preventive interventions adequately. A versatile behavioral test battery should firstly assess potential deterioration of cognitive performance by hyperhomocysteinemia. Secondly, behavioral testing should clarify whether special diets enhance cognition and potentially could serve as preventive measures for AD. Here, we compared B-vitamins and PUFAs with a more complex micronutrient mixture similar to Fortasyn® Connect [35]. HCys and HCA levels were measured in urine and serum using a validated LC-MS/MS method (liquid chromatography-tandem mass spectrometry) and the quantity of Aβ plaques in the brains was assessed.

2. Materials and Methods

A detailed description of all experimental procedures including the single behavioral testing systems, analytical methodologies and quality parameters of the current study can be found in Appendix A.

2.1. Animals and Experimental Diets

All experimental procedures were carried out in compliance with the '3R' and in accordance with the Principles of Laboratory Animal Care (National Institutes of Health publication no. 86-23, revised 1985), the DIRECTIVE 2010/63/EU and the regulations of GV-SOLAS and were approved by the local Ethics Committee for Animal Research in Darmstadt, Germany (approval number: F152/1011; approval date: 31.07.2017). In the current study, 16 C57BL/6J wild type mice (WT) and 96 homozygous App^{NL-G-F} knock-in (KI) mice, consisting equally of males and females, were included.

AIN93M chow served as a basis for the experimental diets and was modified, defining the different groups of App^{NL-G-F} mice (Table 1). The exact composition of the diets is summarized in Table A1. Each mouse received four grammes of diet per day, except for the period of food restriction for males during the touchscreen PAL-task. Water was available ad libitum, except for the period of temporally conditioned water access for females during the IntelliCage experiment.

Table 1. Details of the experimental groups.

Group Number	Genotype	Diet	Abbreviation
1	C57BL/6J wild type	Control	C (WT)
2	App^{NL-G-F} knock-in	Control	C (KI)
3	App^{NL-G-F} knock-in	Vitamin B deficient	B-DEF
4	App^{NL-G-F} knock-in	Vitamin B enriched	B-ENR
5	App^{NL-G-F} knock-in	PUFA supplemented	PUFA-ENR
6	App^{NL-G-F} knock-in	Vitamin B enriched and PUFA supplemented	B+PUFA-ENR
7	App^{NL-G-F} knock-in	Fortasyn® Connect-like	FC

2.2. Behavioral Testing

The testing battery we conducted consisted of diverse behavioral tests investigating different domains of cognition in the animals (Figure 2). At the age of 15 weeks, resp. 10 weeks on diet, the mice were first tested in the open field, followed by the elevated zero maze, Barnes maze and social interaction test. Finally, males were tested in a touchscreen task and females in the IntelliCage system.

Outcomes of every behavioral experiment were assessed automatically by camera or transponder detection. All experiments were performed between 8 a.m. and 3 p.m. during the light phase. After each trial, testing systems were cleaned with 70% ethanol to remove odors in the devices and to achieve comparable conditions for each animal.

2.3. Sample Collection

As illustrated in Figure 2, serum and 24-h urine of the mice were sampled after 8 and 30 weeks on experimental diets, resp. 13 and 35 weeks of age. The biological matrices were stored at −80 °C for subsequent analysis of HCys and HCA. At the end of the study, we euthanized all animals at the age of 35 weeks in order to harvest the brains. Brains were removed and post-fixed in 4% paraformaldehyde, followed by a stepwise dehydration, and embedding in paraffin. Ten μm thick sections were cut and mounted on glass slides for subsequent immunohistochemical analysis.

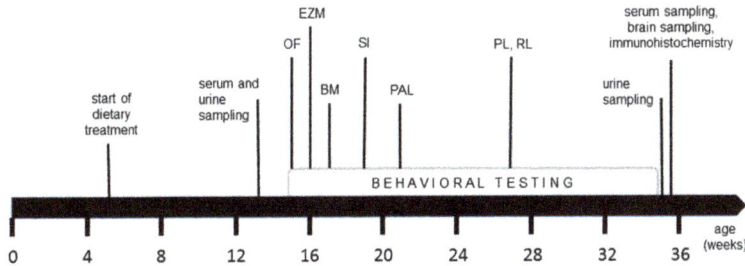

Figure 2. Time line of the study course; open field test (OF), elevated zero maze (EZM), Barnes maze (BM), social interaction test (SI), touchscreen paired associates learning (PAL) inclusive training phase, IntelliCage place learning task (PL) and reverse learning task (RL) inclusive habituation period; see Appendix A for detailed explanations of the single tests.

2.4. Biochemical and Immunohistochemical Analyses

The determination of HCA was performed as previously described in detail [36] using a combination of protein precipitation and solid phase extraction for sample preparation followed by an LC–MS/MS analysis applying a combination of a HILIC separation and tandem mass spectrometry. HCys was analyzed using protein precipitation in combination with reversed phase chromatography and tandem mass spectrometry.

Brain sections were immunohistochemically stained for amyloid-β peptides (Aβ) using an ABC/DAB protocol that is described in detail in Appendix A. After digitization of the sections, we analyzed the resulting images for the area of Aβ plaques in several regions of interest (ROI; Table A2), using ImageJ software.

2.5. Statistical Analyses

All experiments were statistically analyzed using IBM SPSS Statistics 25 (Ehningen, Germany). For each test, we conducted an outlier analysis in order to exclude extreme outliers (more than three times the interquartile range). Shapiro Wilk tests revealed whether Gaussian distribution could be assumed or not. Because of several data sets, which did not show a normal distribution, testing of statistically significant differences was computed by non-parametric Mann-Whitney-U-tests (comparison 1: C57BL/6J (group 1) versus App^{NL-G-F} control (group 2); comparison 2: App^{NL-G-F} control (group 2) versus App^{NL-G-F} on special diets (groups 3–7)). A p value lower than 0.05 was considered statistically significant. Results were expressed as median ± interquartile range (IQR). Where applicable, medians were further compared to hypothetical medians using the non-parametric one-sample Wilcoxon signed rank test.

Graphical presentation was performed using GraphPad Prism 7 software (San Diego, CA, USA).

3. Results

3.1. Homocysteine and Homocysteic Acid

LC-MS/MS analysis was performed in order to measure HCys and its oxidative metabolite HCA in serum and urine samples. Vitamin B deficiency resulted in an elevation of both HCys and HCA serum levels in males and females after 8 weeks on experimental diet (HCys male $p < 0.001$, female $p = 0.001$; HCA (pooled) $p < 0.001$) (Figure 3A,C). A consistent statistically significant difference between C57BL/6J wild type (WT) and App^{NL-G-F} knock-in (KI) mice was not observed. Dietary interventions resulted in decreased serum levels of HCys (PUFA-ENR male $p = 0.001$, female $p = 0.005$; B+PUFA-ENR male $p < 0.001$, female 0.026; FC male & female $p < 0.001$). Serum samples had to be pooled for an adequate analysis of HCA because of low sample volumes obtained by vena facialis puncture (Figure 3C).

Because of the resulting decreased number of observations, data are not depicted separately for males and females in this case. After 30 weeks on the diet, vitamin B deficient males remained significantly hyperhomocysteinemic (HCys $p = 0.001$; HCA $p = 0.001$), although to a lower extent, compared to 8 weeks on the diet, whereas females returned to baseline level due to the maintenance chow they received during the IntelliCage tasks. Analysis of 24-h urine samples delivered data that were largely comparable to the results from the serum samples. After 8 weeks on the diets (Figure 3E,G), both urinary HCys and HCA were significantly elevated because of the vitamin B deficient chow (HCys male & female $p < 0.001$; HCA male $p = 0.001$, female $p = 0.035$), whereas a genotype effect was not detectable. Experimental diets resulted in decreased amounts of HCys (PUFA-ENR female $p = 0.014$) and HCA (B-ENR female $p = 0.001$; PUFA-ENR female $p = 0.022$; FC female $p = 0.040$) in the urine compared to KI control mice. After 30 weeks on diets (Figure 3F,H), males deficient in vitamin B6, B12 and folate displayed elevated urinary amounts of HCys ($p = 0.001$) and HCA ($p = 0.003$), but to a lower extent compared to that after 8 weeks on the diets. Vitamin B deficient females showed equal quantities to the control groups due to the maintenance chow they had received during the IntelliCage tasks.

3.2. Open Field

This behavioral test aimed to evaluate locomotion, anxiety, and habituation behavior of the mice during a 30-min session in the open field boxes. The total distance moved revealed no statistically significant differences (Figure 4A). Consequently, locomotion activity was not influenced by genotype or dietary intervention. The time the animals spent in the inner zone of the box, an indicator of anxiety, was not affected by genotype or diet (Figure 4B). As a third parameter, the amount of intrasession habituation was expressed by a habituation ratio (Equation (1)):

$$\text{ratio intrasession habituation} = (5 \min(\text{final}))/((5 \min(\text{final}) + 5 \min(\text{initial}))) \tag{1}$$

A ratio lower than 0.5 indicates habituation; a ratio of 0.5 means no change in activity, i.e., that no habituation occurred as in the case of groups 2–6 in males and groups 3 and 5–6 in females. Females fed with a vitamin B deficient chow displayed the least tendency to habituate; however, effects of experimental diets did not reach statistical significance in comparison to the KI control group. Female App^{NL-G-F} control mice displayed a significantly lower level of habituation compared to the C57BL/6J WT control ($p = 0.009$), indicating an impact of the genotype (Figure 4C).

3.3. Elevated Zero Maze

We tested anxiety behavior of each mouse for a session duration of 5 min. C57BL/6J WT and App^{NL-G-F} KI control mice moved equal distances in the maze; only male App^{NL-G-F} mice fed with a vitamin B and PUFA enriched diet moved less than App^{NL-G-F} controls ($p = 0.003$) and thus displayed lower locomotion activity (Figure 5A). The time spent in the open corridors of the maze was an index for open space-induced anxiety in mice (Figure 5B). No genotype effect was observed between C57BL/6J and App^{NL-G-F} mice, whereas different dietary interventions showed a reduction of cumulative time in open corridors. Particularly, male mice fed with the combination of PUFA and vitamin B enriched chow as well as with FC-like, spent significantly less time in the open corridors (B+PUFA-ENR $p < 0.001$; FC $p = 0.021$) and thus displayed increased anxiety. In females, a reduced time in the open corridors was observed in the vitamin B deficient group ($p = 0.040$) compared to KI control mice.

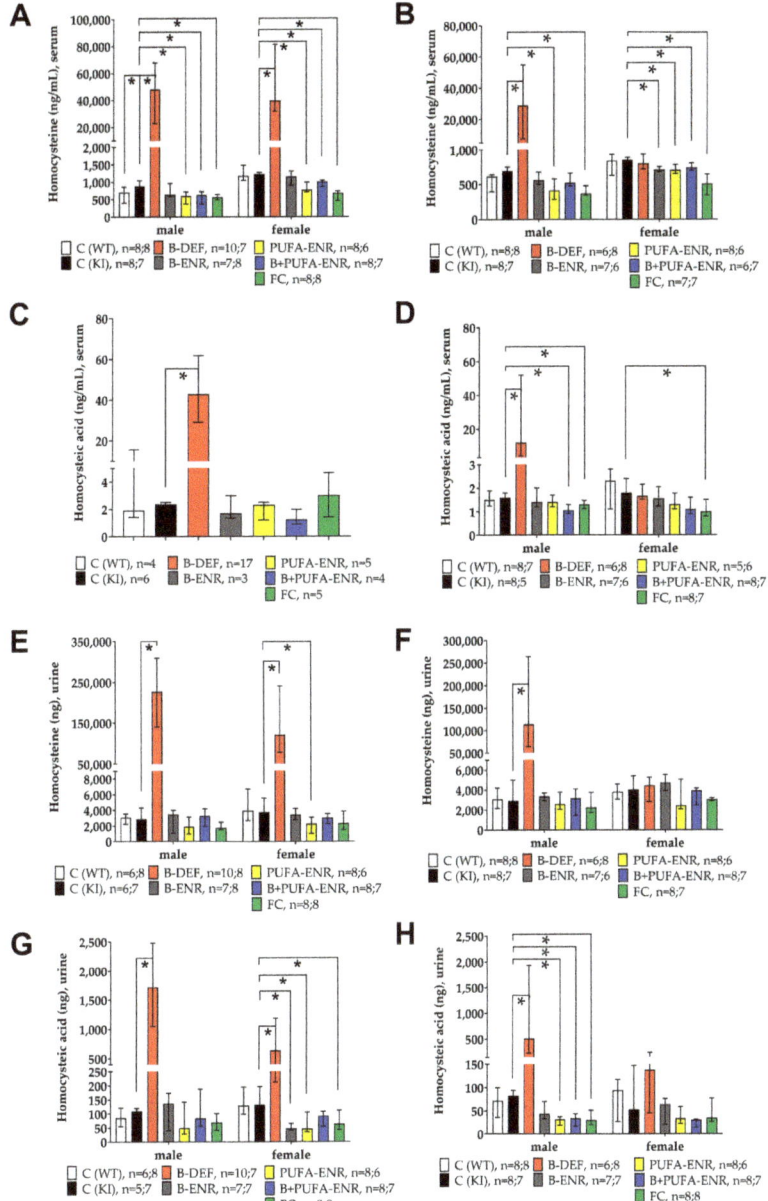

Figure 3. Homocysteine (HCys) and homocysteic acid (HCA) urine and serum levels in 13 and 35 weeks old C57BL/6J and App^{NL-G-F} mice; 8 resp. 30 weeks on experimental diet; all samples analyzed by LC-MS/MS; data presented as median ± IQR; outliers beyond threefold IQR removed; $p < 0.05$ (Mann-Whitney-U-test) considered statistically significant (*). (**A**) HCys serum levels; 8 weeks on diet. (**B**) HCys serum levels; 30 weeks on diet. (**C**) HCA serum levels; 8 weeks on diet (males and females pooled); samples pooled for analytical method due to low volumes obtained by vena facialis puncture. (**D**) HCA serum levels; 30 weeks on diet. (**E**) HCys urine levels; 8 weeks on diet. (**F**) HCys urine levels; 30 weeks on diet. (**G**) HCA urine levels; 8 weeks on diet. (**H**) HCA urine levels; 30 weeks on diet.

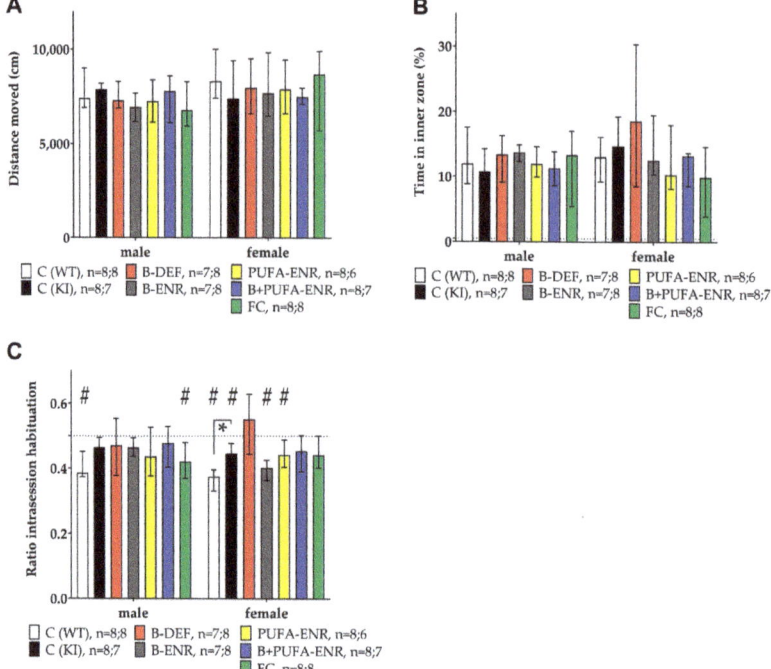

Figure 4. Open field test (30 min) in 15 weeks old C57BL/6J and App^{NL-G-F} mice; 10 weeks on experimental diet; data presented as median ± IQR; outliers beyond threefold IQR removed; $p < 0.05$ (Mann-Whitney-U-test) considered statistically significant (*). (**A**) Total distance moved. (**B**) Percentage of time spent in inner zone. (**C**) Intrasession habituation expressed as ratio between the distance moved in the final time block divided by the sum of the final and the initial time block. (#) Ratio different from 0.5 (one-sample Wilcoxon signed rank test).

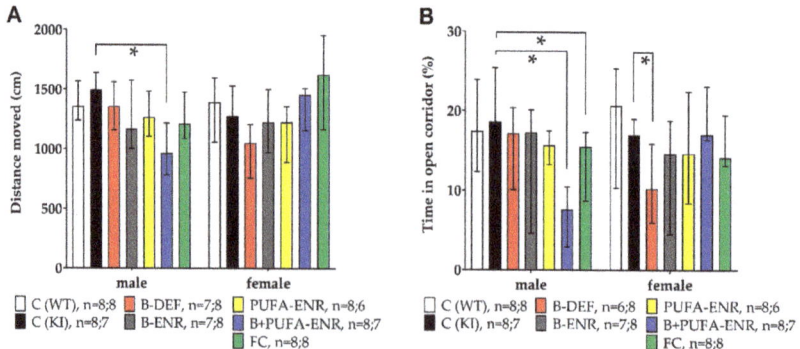

Figure 5. Elevated zero maze test (5 min) in 16 weeks old C57BL/6J and App^{NL-G-F} mice; 11 weeks on experimental diet; data presented as median ± IQR; outliers beyond threefold IQR removed; $p < 0.05$ (Mann-Whitney-U-test) considered statistically significant (*). (**A**) Total distance moved. (**B**) Percentage of time spent in open corridors.

3.4. Barnes Maze

To investigate spatial memory and learning, the Barnes maze test was implemented in this study. In the first part of the test, the acquisition phase, the mice had to learn and remember the location of the escape box at the target hole. Figure 6A shows the latencies the mice needed to reach the target hole on subsequent days of training in the acquisition phase. The graph indicates a learning curve in every group. Tests on statistical significance were carried out for day 4 and revealed no differences at this stage of the test. In the probe trial on day 5 (Figure 6B), the reference memory of the previously learned target hole was tested. At this time, female App^{NL-G-F} controls needed significantly longer to reach the target hole compared to the C57BL/6J WT control animals ($p = 0.016$). Vitamin B deficiency and corresponding hyperhomocysteinemia did not result in a worse performance at any stage of the Barnes maze test.

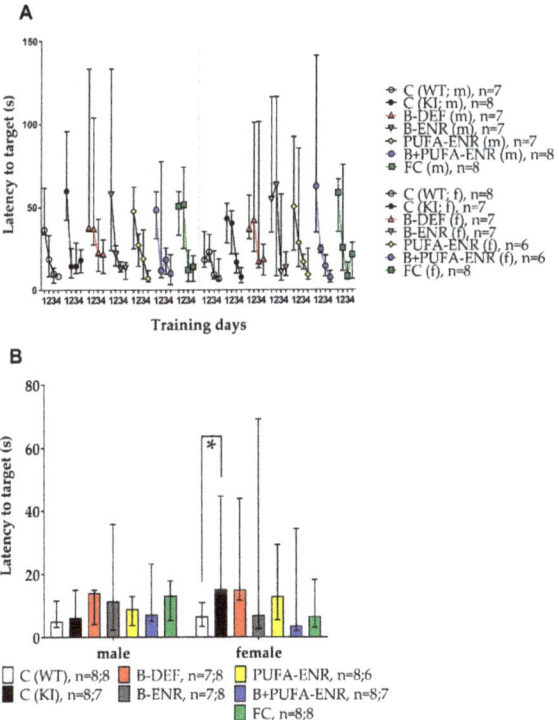

Figure 6. Barnes maze test in 17–18 weeks old C57BL/6J and App^{NL-G-F} mice; 12–13 weeks on experimental diet; data presented as median ± IQR; outliers beyond threefold IQR removed; $p < 0.05$ (Mann-Whitney-U-test) considered statistically significant (*). (**A**) Latency to target hole; training days 1–4; 180 s per trial; acquisition phase; test on statistical significance carried out for day 4. (**B**) Latency to target hole; day 5; 90 s per trial; probe trial.

3.5. Social Interaction Test

Testing social behavior proceeded in two subsequent phases. At first, we assessed sociability, describing the curiosity of the animals towards the stimulus mouse in the testing system (Equation (2)) (Figure 7A).

$$\text{ratio sociability} = (\text{time social cage})/((\text{time social cage} + \text{time empty cage})) \qquad (2)$$

No statistically significant difference was observed between C57BL/6J WT and App^{NL-G-F} control animals. Experimental diets also had no impact on the social ability of the mice. Medians were statistically unequal to 0.5 except for group 2, 4 and 6 (males) and group 2 and 3 (females). A ratio of 0.5 means that contact times with the conspecific stimulus mouse and the empty cage were equal.

In the second phase of the test, we assessed the social recognition performance of the animals (Equation (3)) (Figure 7B).

$$\text{ratio social recognition} = (\text{time novel animal})/((\text{time novel animal} + \text{time familiar animal})) \quad (3)$$

As for sociability, neither genotype nor experimental diets had an influence on social recognition in the different experimental groups. In neither phase of the test did hyperhomocysteinemia aggravate the cognitive performance of the mice. Except for group 1 (males) and group 5 and 6 (females), medians of the other groups did not differ significantly from 0.5.

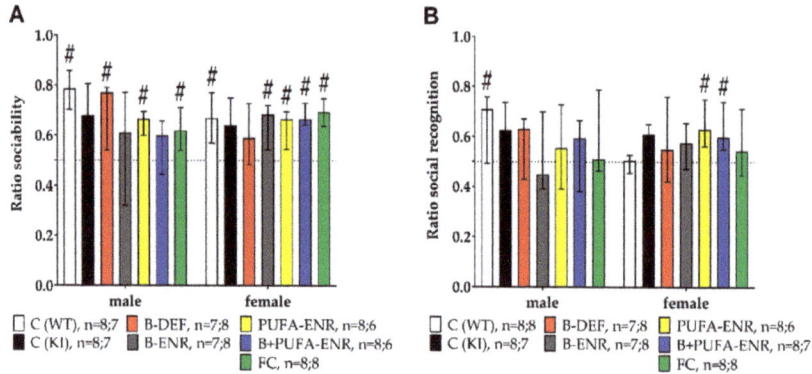

Figure 7. Social interaction test (25 min) in 19–20 weeks old C57BL/6J and App^{NL-G-F} mice; 14–15 weeks on experimental diet; data presented as median ± IQR; outliers beyond threefold IQR removed; $p < 0.05$ (Mann-Whitney-U-test) considered statistically significant (*); (#) ratio different from 0.5 (one-sample Wilcoxon signed rank test). (A) Sociability expressed as the ratio between the contact time with the stimulus mice and the sum of the contact times with the stimulus mice and the empty cage. (B) Social recognition expressed as the ratio between the contact time with novel stimulus mice and the familiar ones.

3.6. Paired Associates Learning (PAL) Task

The touchscreen PAL was used to assess potential cognitive impairment of the male mice (about five to eight months of age). Both the session duration and the number of trials completed per session, as well as the percentage of correct trials per session were analyzed (Figure 8). The resulting learning curves revealed no statistically significant difference in these parameters between C57BL/6J WT mice and App^{NL-G-F} KI mice in the final phase of the test (block 6). Hyperhomocysteinemic App^{NL-G-F} mice did not perform worse than App^{NL-G-F} control mice. Other experimental diets also had no benefit on the cognitive abilities of App^{NL-G-F} mice at this age. The C57BL/6J WT group showed a smaller variability in the touchscreen chambers in comparison to the App^{NL-G-F} KI groups. This effect was particularly observed in the parameter trials completed (Figure 8B). Vitamin B deficient animals showed a tendency to perform better at the beginning of the test (trials completed, block 1) and thus did not display a learning curve like that of App^{NL-G-F} control mice. However, no effects reached statistical significance in block 6. Animals fed with a vitamin B and PUFA combination diet did not reach the maximum number of trials per session. Therefore, the session duration scarcely also decreased over time in this group. The proportion of correct and incorrect trials was not affected.

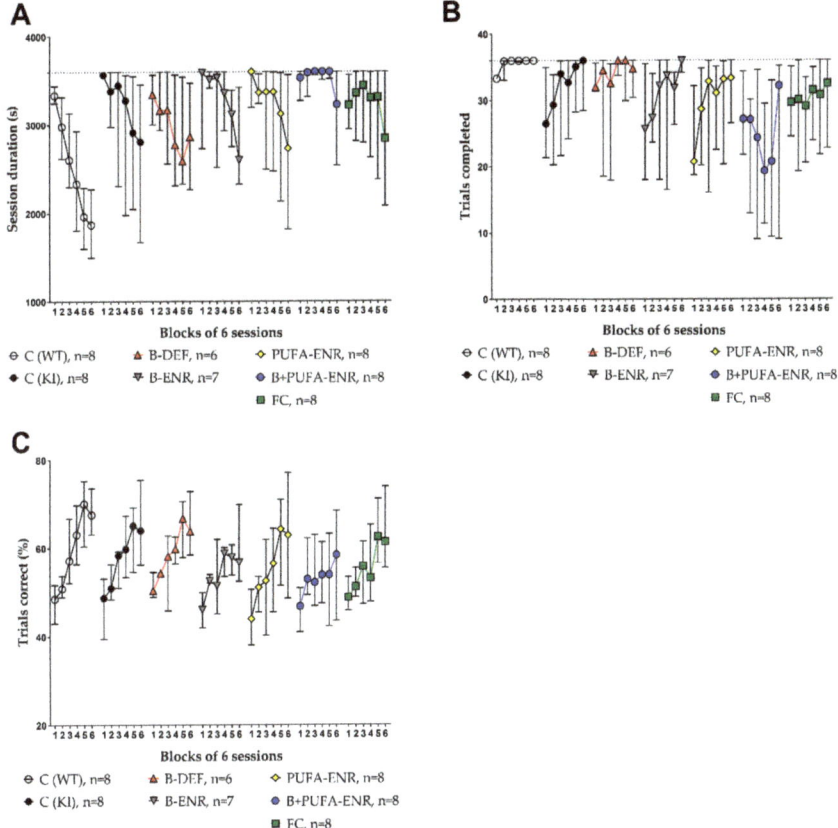

Figure 8. Touchscreen paired associates learning test (PAL) in 21–34 (incl. training phase) weeks old C57BL/6J and App^{NL-G-F} mice; 16–29 weeks on experimental diet; only males; data summarized in blocks of 6 sessions and presented as median ± IQR; outliers beyond threefold IQR removed; test on statistical significance carried out for block 6. (**A**) Session duration: time (s) needed to complete 36 trials per session; maximum 3600 s. (**B**) Amount of trials completed per session; maximum 36 trials. (**C**) Percentage of correct trials per session.

3.7. Place Learning (PL) and Reversal Learning (RL) Task

Learning and memory performance of the females at the age of about six to eight months was finally tested using two tasks in the IntelliCage system. We detected the visits of the mice to the drinking corners and analyzed the percentage of correct visits during the drinking sessions in the place learning (PL) and the reversal learning (RL) tasks. Three points in time along the course of the tasks are illustrated in Figure 9. Statistical analysis of the late phase of this course in both (Figure 9A) PL and (Figure 9B) RL (session 31; resp. 23) revealed no significant differences between App^{NL-G-F} and age-matched C57BL/6J mice. In comparison to the App^{NL-G-F} KI control group, none of the groups fed with experimental diets showed improved or impaired memory abilities.

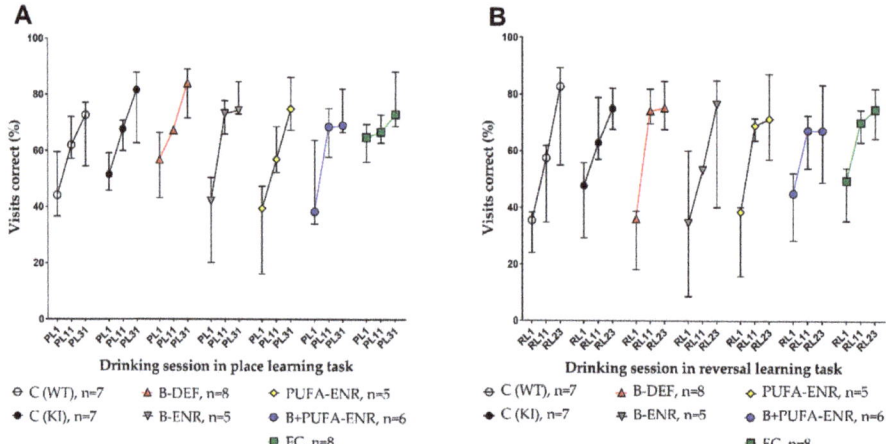

Figure 9. IntelliCage place learning (PL) and reversal learning (RL) task in 27–34 (incl. habituation period) weeks old C57BL/6J and $App^{NL\text{-}G\text{-}F}$ mice; 22–29 weeks on experimental diet; only females; data are shown for three points in time along the course of the task and presented as median ± IQR; outliers beyond threefold IQR removed; test on statistical significance carried out for the final point in time. (**A**) Percentage of correct visits during drinking sessions in the PL. (**B**) Percentage of correct visits during drinking sessions in the RL.

3.8. Immunohistochemical Analysis

Brain sections of all animals were immunohistochemically stained and analyzed in order to semi-quantify the amount of amyloid plaques. For this purpose, we assessed the area (percentage) occupied by plaques in images of several regions of interest (ROI). The positions of the different cortical and hippocampal ROI (Table A2) are marked in Figure 10.

Figure 10 illustrates examples of brain sections of a C57BL/6J WT mouse and an $App^{NL\text{-}G\text{-}F}$ KI mouse. Aβ plaques, indicated by characteristic brown staining, occurred abundantly and diffusely in the brain sections of the KI animals (Figure 10B), whereas WT mice did not show any signs of Aβ deposition at all (Figure 10A). The differences in the Aβ burden between the C57BL/6J and $App^{NL\text{-}G\text{-}F}$ genotype, as well as a potential impact of the experimental diets, were further analyzed using ImageJ software. Semi-quantification of the Aβ burden confirmed a significant difference between WT and KI control groups (Figure 11) in all ROI ($p < 0.001$; $p = 0.002$; $p < 0.001$; $p < 0.001$; $p < 0.001$; $p < 0.001$; $p < 0.001$; $p < 0.001$).

There was no statistically significant difference in the plaque area between the diet groups and the $App^{NL\text{-}G\text{-}F}$ control group in the single ROI and in total. However, the immunohistochemical results indicate prominent plaque formation in all $App^{NL\text{-}G\text{-}F}$ groups at about 8 months of age.

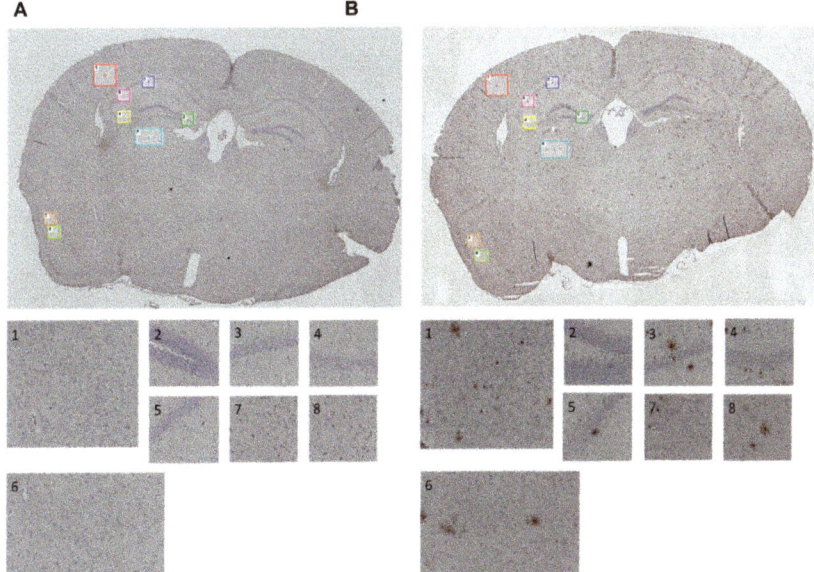

Figure 10. Immunohistochemically stained sections of mouse brains; regions of interest (ROI) in cortical and hippocampal areas are marked in whole brain images (100× magnification) and depicted separately for further semi-quantification of amyloid plaques; 35 weeks of age, 30 weeks on experimental diet. (**A**) Exemplary section of a C57BL/6J wild type animal. (**B**) Exemplary section of an App^{NL-G-F} knock-in animal.

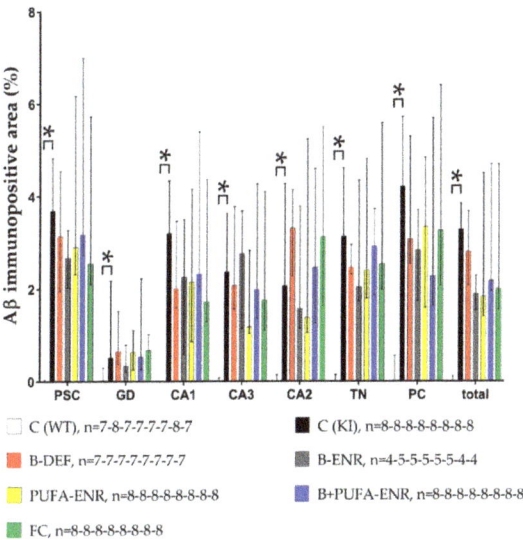

Figure 11. Semi-quantitative analysis of amyloid-β (Aβ) in immunohistochemically stained brain sections; results are shown for single regions of interest (ROI) and in total; 35 weeks of age, 30 weeks on experimental diet (males and females pooled); data presented as median ± IQR; outliers beyond threefold IQR removed; $p < 0.05$ (Mann-Whitney-U-test) considered statistically significant (*).

4. Discussion

The current preclinical study investigated the impact of an induced hyperhomocysteinemia in the App^{NL-G-F} knock-in mouse model for AD, as well as potentially preventive benefits of different micro-nutritional interventions. In order to characterize the phenotypes of the mice, we conducted a versatile behavioral test battery, accompanied by an analysis of HCys-/HCA levels and of the Aβ plaque burden. However, despite successful induction of prominent cerebral plaque deposition and hyperhomocysteinemia, merely subtle impairments were observed in the App^{NL-G-F} mice.

C57BL/6J mice, a frequently studied mouse strain and background strain of the App^{NL-G-F} knock-in (KI) model, served as an age-matched wild type (WT) control group in this study. Hence, results in these mice indicated a reference behavior and enabled subsequent assessment of the App^{NL-G-F} genotype in the KI mice. In the open field, we focused on the intrasession habituation of the mice, which is one form of learning. Intrasession habituation describes a decreasing level of exploration of a new environment over time in a single session which can typically be detected in C57BL/6J mice [37]. This is in accordance with our finding that the habituation ratio in C57BL/6J was significantly lower than 0.5 and therefore indicated intrasession habituation. As expected, C57BL/6J mice demonstrated spatial learning and memory ability on consecutive days of training in the Barnes maze [38]. In a test for sociability and social recognition [39], C57BL/6J mice preferred to spent time with a conspecific (ratio sociability > 0.5) [40]. However, they did not prefer the novel conspecific in the second part of the test (ratio social recognition = 0.5). In the touchscreen PAL [41], male WT animals completed the maximum number of all 36 trials per session, accompanied by decreasing session duration. The increase in the percentage of correct trials is in accordance with observations in a similar study [42]. In the IntelliCage setup [43,44], learning curves indicated a constant learning effect in the female WT animals.

For several reasons, we decided to use an AβPP-based KI mouse model for AD in this study. Firstly, the novel KI models provide the advantage of not overexpressing AβPP in comparison to the more established transgenic models. Consequently, artificial phenotypes due to an overproduction of AβPP fragments besides the Aβ peptide should be avoided [9]. Secondly, an increased anabolism of Aβ levels is primarily a hallmark of hereditary- or early-onset AD [3]. Hyperhomocysteinemia, which is especially prominent in older people [45], is supposed to be a risk factor for AD [24]. Therefore, elevated HCys and HCA have been regarded as a hallmark of sporadic- or late-onset AD. The late-onset form affects the vast majority of AD patients [3]. By combining both the increased Aβ anabolism as a feature of hereditary AD and the detrimental effects of excess HCys as a feature of sporadic AD, we attempted to simulate cognitive decline more comprehensively. Thirdly, in order to investigate preventive treatments, it is mandatory to use a model displaying subtle phenotypes corresponding to a very early stage of the disease. According to a review by Zahs and Ashe, AβPP-based mouse models simulate the early phase of AD and thus are adequate for preventive interventions [46]. In the current study, a very subtle phenotype, i.e., very mild cognitive deficits, was observed. For each analysis, we compared C57BL/6J WT animals with App^{NL-G-F} KI control animals. Both groups received the same control diet. KI mice displayed an impaired habituation behavior in the open field. Male mice of the two control groups habituated equally to the new environment, whereas females differed significantly. Data from the probe trial in the Barnes maze confirmed this finding: App^{NL-G-F} KI mice needed longer to locate the former target hole than WT mice. As in the open field, this effect reached statistical significance only in females. Previous clinical studies suggest that a reduced cognitive reserve in women might explain the female vulnerability to develop a more severe phenotype of AD, a disorder affecting more women than men [47,48]. Other behavioral tests did not reveal differences caused by the KI genotype. However, data from the PAL test indicated an increased variance of results (higher IQR) in the App^{NL-G-F} versus WT mice. WT animals showed a clearer performance curve with regard to the session duration and the number of trials completed along the course of the test, meaning that WT mice did not need as long as the KI mice to fulfil the 36 trials in a 1-h session. This enhanced efficiency might be the result of a higher motivation of the WT animals. Nevertheless, effects at the final stage of the test (block 6) did not indicate a significant impact of the genotype.

Other groups reported similar findings in App^{NL-G-F} mice, indicating a very subtle phenotype. Two recent publications summarized these findings in tabular overviews, considering also sex and age of the mice of the included studies [49,50]. Latif-Hernandez and colleagues showed that the behavior of App^{NL-G-F} mice was largely unaffected at the age of 3–10 months [51]. Similarities with our study can also be found in a publication by Whyte et al., who observed no differences between C57BL/6J and App^{NL-G-F} mice in different cognitive tests at the age of 6 months [52]. Sakakibara and colleagues tested App^{NL-G-F} mice at a higher age (15–18 months) and reported an intact learning ability but also recommended App^{NL-G-F} as an AD model for preventive studies [53]. One year later, Jacob et al. observed neither consequences on cognitive performance in a touchscreen task nor age-dependent changes in a phase-amplitude coupling analysis, which was used as a measure of neurophysiological functioning, in 4.5 month old App^{NL-G-F} mice. In accordance with our findings in the App^{NL-G-F} model, these mice displayed a higher variability than WT control mice [42].

The question remains whether the KI mice were too young to display clear impairments. Further investigations are required to test the combination of the App^{NL-G-F} genotype with our experimental diets in older mice. However, other groups detected significant cognitive deficits in the App^{NL-G-F} model [9,49,50,54]. As summarized elsewhere [49], the majority of studies in the field investigated only male animals. Hence, a 1:1 comparison of these studies with our results comprising both sexes is difficult. Furthermore, a review of the topic described a relatively high level of variability in AβPP KI models between different laboratories [55]. Staining results of App^{NL-G-F} brain sections showed prominent plaque deposition throughout the brain, as previously reported in similar studies [49,52], and thus indicate amyloid pathology as a central hallmark of early AD.

In order to investigate potentially detrimental effects of elevated HCys and HCA levels, one group of App^{NL-G-F} mice received a special diet deficient in vitamin B6, B12 and folate. The resulting hyperhomocysteinemic state was confirmed in serum and urine prior to the start of behavioral tests. Our behavioral testing data obtained in the social interaction test, PAL and in the IntelliCages revealed no deficits in hyperhomocysteinemic mice and therefore do not support previous findings (e.g., [56]). The open field test and Barnes maze indicated subtle deficits in habituation behavior and spatial learning and memory, but these effects did not reach statistical significance. Only the elevated zero maze revealed an increased anxiety in hyperhomocysteinemic females. This observation might be of translational relevance, because anxious behavior is also one aspect of the AD phenotype [57]. Various preclinical studies in the field indicate a significant impact of hyperhomocysteinemia on plaque burden [58,59]. Other groups reported no such effects, which is in accordance with our immunohistochemical results in the App^{NL-G-F} model [60,61]. In conclusion, despite severely elevated levels of HCys and HCA over a longer period of their life span, App^{NL-G-F} mice showed neither a modified plaque burden nor significant cognitive deficits due to hyperhomocysteinemia. A majority of preclinical data published in the field indicate behavioral deficits in animal models caused by increased HCys (e.g., [56,59,62]). However, we assume that the evidence might be biased to some extent. On the one hand, behavioral data obtained in transgenic models based on massive AβPP overexpression might be somewhat artificial because of an overproduction of other AβPP fragments aside from Aβ [9]. It should also be considered that negative results are often not published, although equally important as positive results. The publication bias, meaning the reduced publishing of negative or null results, is not restricted to the field of AD research, but is rather a general problem [63].

Hyperhomocysteinemia is referred to as a hallmark of AD [10], but its impact on the disease is still under discussion. From a translational point of view, this experimental group simulates the portion of elderly people who are deficient in B-vitamins [64]. Preclinical evidence [65] and clinical evidence [45] confirm an age-related elevation of HCys levels. An impaired vitamin status is one reason amongst others for hyperhomocysteinemia in the elderly [66]. In the present study, the lack of vitamin B6, B12 and folate in combination with 1% sulfathiazole sodium to inhibit bacterial folate synthesis in the gut [58], led to a "severe" hyperhomocysteinemic state, according to a classification used in other publications [67]. Consequently, our vitamin B deficient mice displayed high HCys serum concentrations (45,760 ng/mL ≈ 339 µmol/L) in comparison to our App^{NL-G-F} KI control (1054 ng/mL ≈ 8 µmol/L) and in comparison to elevated HCys levels in similar studies (e.g., [56,62,68]). Fuso and colleagues also reached high plasma total HCys (>400 µmol/L ≈ 54,000 ng/mL) in their study with TgCRND8 mice and explained the relatively high levels by not fasting the mice before sacrifice and by inhibiting both the re-methylation and the transsulfuration pathway [58].

Vitamin B deficient chow resulted in ~50 fold higher serum and urinary HCys and ~10–20 fold higher serum and urinary HCA compared to animals fed with control diet for 8 weeks. About 0.1% of HCys molecules were oxidized to HCA in serum (42.9 ng/mL ≈ 0.23 µmol/L) and excreted in urine (1184 ng) in 24 h. Only free HCys can be oxidized to HCA, which is suggested to be the main neurotoxic species [32–34]. In the current study, we did not measure the free form but the levels of total HCys by adding a reduction step (TCEP-solution) in the analytical method. In vivo, most HCys molecules are protein-bound or dimerized; only about 1% are available in the free thiol form [12]. Hasegawa et al. reported cognitive impairment in transgenic 3xTg-AD mice, triggered by elevated HCA in the brain [69].

We also investigated other experimental diets besides the vitamin B deficient chow discussed above. Group 4 received a vitamin B enriched diet containing a particular high content of folate, B6 and B12 compared to both the control diet and the FC-like diet. The goal of this diet was to investigate whether an additional increase, specifically of B-vitamins, in comparison to the FC-like diet could provide further benefits in the outcome of the study. Therefore, the difference in B-vitamin contents should simulate a potentially different effectiveness between FC (Souvenaid®) and existing higher dosed vitamin B preparations as human treatment options. In accordance with a recent international consensus statement [23], PUFAs (DHA + EPA) have been suggested to be beneficial for cognitive functioning in general and might be additionally linked to AD pathology [25,70]. Because single nutrient intervention studies often failed to show beneficial effects on cognitive function, it has been suggested that it might be important to investigate combinatory approaches [35]. For this purpose, we combined the high content vitamin B enrichment with the supplementation of PUFAs (group 6). Finally, group 7 received the FC-like diet, a complex mixture of ingredients (Table A1), which we implemented due to positive previous findings (e.g., [35,71]).

Supplementation of B-vitamins and PUFAs, as well as combinatory approaches and the FC-like mixture, were capable of lowering HCys and HCA below the levels of the App^{NL-G-F} control mice fed with a standard rodent chow. However, by taking both sampling points (8 and 30 weeks on diet) as well as behavioral testing data into consideration, results appear inconsistent. In the open field, anxiety-related behavior did not differ between groups fed with B-vitamins, PUFAs or a mixture and App^{NL-G-F} control animals. However, the elevated zero maze revealed increased anxiety in males fed with the combination diets. Especially the mice supplemented with both B-vitamins and PUFAs were more anxious and stayed in the closed corridors of the zero maze, but it has to be emphasized that these mice also displayed a reduced locomotion activity during the test. In the Barnes maze, experimental chow did not affect latencies to target at day 4 of training. Other researchers too did not observe benefits of PUFA-supplementation in cognitive tasks [72]. We confirmed the lack of dietary effects on cognitive performance in the social interaction test, the IntelliCage and PAL. Although not significant in the final block of 6 sessions, the session duration and trials completed indicate a worse learning curve for group 6 (B+PUFA-ENR) in the PAL test. This might be due to a lack of motivation in these mice receiving a high number of vitamins and PUFAs, which possibly lowered their affinity to the milk reward in the PAL task. One reason could be that the food restriction was not strict enough for this group. The FC-like diet did not prove beneficial in any test in comparison to the control chow. This is in accordance with some clinical studies, which do not support the benefit of the FC diet and thus indicate equivocal evidence [73,74]. In conclusion, the beneficial tendencies we observed did not mostly reach statistical significance in behavioral tests and biochemical-/immunohistochemical analyses and consequently do not suggest a clear beneficial effect of B-vitamins or PUFAs in this mouse model at the investigated age and diet duration. It is important to question here whether it is possible to observe amelioration through dietary intervention when merely a subtle behavioral deficit is induced in the KI mouse model.

Overall, this mouse model, simulating amyloid pathology without AβPP overexpression, merely displays a very mild phenotype despite massive cerebral Aβ deposition at the age of 35 weeks. The amyloid hypothesis has been questioned frequently because of the disappointing track record in clinical trials of drugs that target Aβ despite decades of extensive research in the field [7,75]. In addition, in some cases, substantial plaque deposition does not even cause dementia-like symptoms [76]. However, the window for potentially preventive measures is limited to an early stage of AD, where cerebral amyloidosis remains the central hallmark of the pathology [3]. Despite all criticism of the amyloid hypothesis, beneficial effects were recently observed using the human anti-Aβ monoclonal antibody aducanumab [77], confirming a causal role of Aβ in AD pathogenesis.

5. Conclusions

The current study only indicates a mild hyperhomocysteinemia-driven exacerbation of the AD-like phenotype, simulated in the App^{NL-G-F} knock-in mouse model. Dietary interventions consisting of B-vitamins and/or PUFAs as well as the FC-like diet as a complex micronutrient mixture were unable to modify cognitive performance in this mouse model for AD. Neither the B-vitamin deficient diet, resulting in elevated HCys and HCA levels, nor the potentially beneficial diets affected the amount of plaque deposition in the brain. In comparison with the age-matched C57BL/6J wild type control group, App^{NL-G-F} control mice displayed merely subtle behavioral deficits at the investigated age. Further investigations should clarify whether the App^{NL-G-F} genotype and the experimental diets have an impact in older animals.

Author Contributions: Conceptualization, N.d.B., U.T., M.J.P. and G.G.; Data curation, H.N. and O.A.; Formal analysis, H.N.; Funding acquisition, G.G.; Investigation, H.N., O.A., M.S. and D.S.; Methodology, N.d.B., M.C.J.H., M.S., R.G. and D.S.; Project administration, M.J.P. and G.G.; Resources, T.S. and T.C.S.; Software, H.N. and O.A.; Supervision, N.d.B. and U.T.; Validation, O.A., M.C.J.H., M.S. and R.G.; Visualization, H.N.; Writing–original draft, H.N.; Writing–review & editing, N.d.B., O.A., M.C.J.H., M.S., T.S., T.C.S., R.G., D.S., U.T., M.J.P. and G.G. All authors have given approval to the final version of the manuscript.

Funding: This research was funded by MEDICE Arzneimittel Pütter GmbH & Co. KG.

Acknowledgments: We wish to thank MEDICE Arzneimittel Pütter GmbH & Co. KG for funding this preclinical study. Furthermore, we thank RIKEN Center for Brain Science for providing the App^{NL-G-F} knock-in mice.

Conflicts of Interest: The authors declare no conflict of interest. The funders had no role in the design of the study; in the collection, analyses, or interpretation of data; in the writing of the manuscript, or in the decision to publish the results.

Appendix A

Animals

Wild type (WT) mice were purchased from Charles River Wiga GmbH (Sulzfeld, Germany), whereas the knock-in (KI) mice were kindly provided by the RIKEN Center for Brain Science (Saitama, Japan) on a C57BL/6J background and further bred at mfd Diagnostics GmbH (Wendelsheim, Germany). After their arrival at our facility at the age of four weeks, the animals were chipped with subcutaneous transponders to facilitate identification and to enable the IntelliCage task. Furthermore, additional genotyping via polymerase-chain-reaction analysis was carried out to ensure the adequate genetic background of each animal. Their allocation to the home cages was in a randomized order. All animals were housed in groups of two mice per cage (Green Line, Tecniplast, Hohenpeissenberg, Germany). In the maintenance room, constant temperature (mean: 22.7 °C) and humidity (mean: 48.6%) conditions as well as a 12/12 h dark/light cycle were provided. The pathogen-free status of the maintenance room was regularly monitored using sentinel mice. After an acclimatization phase of one week, the mice were allocated randomly to the experimental groups based on different diets. Body conditions scores were monitored, and the mice were weighed every week.

Experimental Diets

The composition of the FC-like diet was oriented towards the work of Jansen et al. All diets containing PUFAs were stored at −20 °C to minimize oxidation [35]. Due to coprophagia (the ingestion of fecal matter) in mice, the vitamin B deficient diet additionally contained the antibiotic sulfathiazole sodium (Sigma-Aldrich, Taufkirchen, Germany) to prevent bacterial folate synthesis in the gut [58]. All experimental diets were purchased from Ssniff-Spezialdiäten GmbH (Soest, Germany).

Table A1. Composition of the experimental diets.

	Control	B-DEF	B-ENR	PUFA-ENR	B+PUFA-ENR	FC
Casein	140.0	140.0	140.0	140.0	140.0	140.0
Corn starch	355.6575	345.6920	355.4795	355.6575	355.4795	328.3386
Maltodextrin	155.0	155.0	155.0	155.0	155.0	155.0
Sucrose	100.0	100.0	100.0	100.0	100.0	100.0
Dextrose	100.0	100.0	100.0	100.0	100.0	100.0
Cellulose	50.0	50.0	50.0	50.0	50.0	50.0
Mineral premix	35.0	35.0	35.0	35.0	35.0	35.0
Vitamin pre-mix (w/o B-vitamins)	10.0	10.0	10.0	10.0	10.0	10.0
Soybean oil	19.0	19.0	19.0	—	—	—
Coconut oil	9.0	9.0	9.0	11.3	11.3	11.3
Corn oil	22.0	22.0	22.0	18.7	18.7	18.7
Fish oil (eicosapentaenoic acid/docosahexaenoic acid = 1:4)	—	—	—	20.0	20.0	20.0
L-Cystine	1.8000	1.8000	1.8000	1.8000	1.8000	1.8000
Tert-butylhydroquinone	0.0080	0.0080	0.0080	0.0080	0.0080	0.0080
Choline bitartrate, 41%	2.5000	2.5000	2.5000	2.5000	2.5000	2.5000
Pyridoxine-HCl (Vit. B6)	0.0070	—	0.1000	0.0070	0.1000	0.0398
Cyanocobalamin, 0.1% (Vit. B12)	0.0250	—	0.1000	0.0250	0.1000	0.0600
Folic acid, 80%	0.0025	—	0.0125	0.0025	0.0125	0.0100
Sodium selenite • 5 H_2O, 30%	—	—	—	—	—	0.0036
Choline chloride, 43% Choline	—	—	—	—	—	6.9700
Ascorbic acid, 100% (Vit. C)	—	—	—	—	—	1.6000
DL-a-tocopheryl acetate, 50% (Vit. E)	—	—	—	—	—	4.6500
Uridine monophosphate disodium (24% H_2O)	—	—	—	—	—	10.0000
Soy lecithin	—	—	—	—	—	4.0200
Sulfathiazole sodium	—	10.0000	—	—	—	—
Sum	1000	1000	1000	1000	1000	1000

Open Field

Besides its value as a test for locomotor activity and anxiety, the open field task provides information on habituation as a form of learning [37]. For this purpose, each mouse was placed into the center of a 28.5 × 29.8 cm box (in-house manufactured, Fraunhofer IME, Schmallenberg, Germany). Animals were allowed to explore the new environment for 30 min. Total distance moved and percentage of time spent in the inner zone of the box were automatically detected by camera tracking and corresponding EthoVision XT 13 software (Noldus, Wageningen, The Netherlands). Data were analyzed additionally for time blocks of 5 min.

Elevated Zero Maze

To investigate anxiety related behavior [78], we placed each animal into the open corridor of a 60 cm diametric elevated zero maze (Ugo Basile SRL, Gemonio, Italy) for a duration of 5 min. The maze consisted of two open and two closed 5 cm wide corridors. Besides the time spent in the open corridors, the total distance moved by the mice was automatically detected by camera tracking and corresponding EthoVision XT 13 software.

Barnes Maze

The Barnes maze test is a common tool to measure spatial learning and memory [38] in AD mouse models, based on the aversion of mice to bright open spaces. We particularly preferred the Barnes maze over the Morris water maze, since it presents a less aversive alternative [79]. The apparatus (Ugo Basile SRL, Gemonio, Italy) consisted of a circular surface (diameter 100 cm) with 20 holes at the edge and an escape box positioned below one of the holes. There were four different visual cues positioned around the maze. The task required the mouse to localize the escape hole and enter the box. Initially, we transported each animal to the center of the maze in an opaque vessel to prevent an orientation before the start of the trial. The procedure was divided into two phases. First, in the acquisition phase, each mouse was subjected to two trials per day for four days (3-min limit per trial; inter-trial interval 15–30 min). The trials ended when either the mouse entered the escape box or when a duration of 180 s was over. On day 5, animals were subjected to a probe trial (90 s). During this phase, the escape box was not available anymore. Latencies to the target hole (acquisition & probe) were automatically detected by camera tracking and corresponding EthoVision XT 13 software.

Social Interaction Test

This method enables the assessment of sociability and social recognition in mice [39]. For this purpose, a three-chamber cage consisting of a central chamber and two lateral compartments (Noldus, Wageningen, Netherlands) was used. The lateral compartments included sex-matched stimulus mice in separate acrylic rod cages, which allowed social interaction without direct contact. Test animals explored the setup during three consecutive phases. During the first time block of 5 min, the mice were allowed to explore only the middle chamber. As a next step, we opened the dividers to the lateral compartments and placed a stimulus mouse into one of the rod cages (social cage). The second rod cage remained empty. The experimental mouse had a period of 10 min to explore the whole three-chamber cage and to interact with the unknown stimulus mouse. For the next 10 min, we placed an additional unknown stimulus mouse into the second rod cage. The cumulative contact time with the familiar and non-familiar conspecific was automatically detected by camera tracking and corresponding EthoVision XT 13 software.

Paired Associates Learning (PAL) Task

The ability of visuospatial associative learning was tested in males in the touchscreen PAL (touchscreen and corresponding Abet II Touch 18.7.6 software: Campden Instruments, Loughborough, UK and Lafayette Instrument Company, Lafayette, IN, USA). The task requires a lot of training, but is also a valuable tool in terms of translational cognitive research due to its similarities with the human CANTAB [41,80]. Based on the Bussey-Saksida method, animals initially were habituated to the touchscreen chambers during different pre-training phases. After completion, mice were introduced to the proper PAL task. Here, two objects were shown in two spatial locations on the screen. In each trial, only one correct association of object and location was presented, and the animal had to detect it via nose poke. As a result, a reward was delivered automatically (sugared condensed milk, 7 µL, Hochwald Foods GmbH, Thalfang, Germany). Incorrect responses were followed by an aversive light stimulus (5 s time-out period). After an inter-trial interval (20 s), the next trial was initiated by the mouse. A session ended when either 36 trials were completed, or 60 min ran out. The animals were food restricted through the whole experiment with the aim of reducing body weights to about 90% of the baseline weight before the test. This should enhance the motivation of the mice to collect the reward after each correct trial. Animal weights were monitored three times a week. For the assessment of the 36 sessions of the PAL task, the parameters' session duration, trials completed, and percentage of correct trials were analyzed. The procedure was highly standardized and the closed touchscreen chambers reduced variability due to the experimenter to a minimum.

Place Learning (PL) and Reversal Learning (RL) Task

The start of the IntelliCage experiment (IntelliCage and IntelliCagePlus 3.2.8 software: New Behavior, TSE Systems, Bad Homburg, Germany) in female mice was scheduled around the time when male mice entered the proper PAL task. Thus, males and females were largely age-matched during the last phase of the behavioral test battery (27 weeks old, resp. 22 weeks on diet). We chose not to test males in the IntelliCage setup, because males are more prone to show aggressive behavior and hierarchical fighting, potentially resulting in injuries due to the housing of male mice in large groups. The IntelliCage tasks of learning ability cover a broad cognitive spectrum by combining the analysis of spatial memory with operant conditioning [43] and provide the advantage of being both home cage and behavioral test during the time of the experiment. Animals from all experimental groups lived together in the special cage for the period of about 7 weeks. Due to this mixed group housing, the experimental diets were substituted by standard maintenance chow (ad libitum) for the duration of this behavioral test. Each apparatus had the capacity to house and detect up to 16 mice simultaneously. The experiment started with a habituation period of 1 week, followed by a pre-training phase on nose poke behavior in corners for water access for 1–2 weeks. During the following week, the animals were habituated to the two defined drinking sessions per day (5–7 a.m.; 7–9 p.m.). In the PL, only one corner per mouse yielded water access in response to nose pokes during drinking sessions (~2 weeks). Motorized doors, controlled by radio-frequency identification (RFID) transponders, opened when a mouse was detected in its adequate corner. In the RL, a different corner was designated as correct (2 weeks). Visits to the correct corners were analyzed for PL and RL. We did not weigh the animals for the duration of the experiment to avoid interference with the automated behavior recording; instead, we visually observed the mice for any sign of deficiency. The IntelliCage enabled a high throughput cognitive investigation of mice, while stress due to human intervention was reduced to a minimum.

Sample Collection

Blood was taken by carrying out a puncture of the facial vein using 5 mm Goldenrod animal lancets (MEDIpoint, Mineola, NY, USA). A maximum volume of 170 µL per 25 g mouse according to animal welfare guidelines (GV-SOLAS) was collected in serum tubes containing a clotting factor to accelerate coagulation in the subsequent 15–30 min (Sarstedt Microvette 200 Z, Nümbrecht, Germany). The tubes were centrifuged at $3200\times g$ for another 15 min at 4 °C and subsequently frozen on dry ice. For 24-h urine sampling, mice were placed into metabolic cages (Tecniplast, Hohenpeissenberg, Germany). Absolute urine volumes were documented for subsequent calculations. In order to harvest the brains, the animals were deeply anaesthetized by injecting a mixture of 200 mg/kg (body weight) ketamine (Vétoquinol GmbH, Ismaning, Germany) and 10 mg/kg (body weight) xylazine (Bayer Health Care, Leverkusen, Germany) intraperitoneally. After cessation of reflexes, blood was taken cardially and treated as described before. Mice were then perfused transcardially with 0.1 M phosphate-buffered saline (PBS) followed by 4% paraformaldehyde (Medite, Burgdorf, Germany). Brains were removed and postfixed in the same fixative for another three days followed by a stepwise dehydration in increasing ethanol concentrations (Medite) and xylene steps (Medite). Brains were then embedded in paraffin (Medite) in a heated embedding station (Thermo Fisher, Frankfurt am Main, Germany) and cut with a microtome (Thermo Fisher). 10 µm thick sections were retrieved from three different positions of the animals' brains: −1.2, −1.7 and −2.2 posterior to bregma [81]. Data of the three positions were pooled because of absent statistically significant differences. Finally, the sections were mounted on glass slides (Klinipath, Typograaf, Netherlands).

Biochemical Analysis

The determination of homocysteic acid (HCA) was performed as recently described in detail [36] with minor modifications, as the method was originally validated for the analysis of human serum and urine. Briefly, HCA was determined in murine serum and urine using a combination of protein precipitation and solid phase extraction for sample preparation followed by an LC–MS/MS analysis using a combination of a HILIC separation and tandem mass spectrometry. Samples were processed as previously described [36] by adding formic acid followed by protein precipitation using cooled acetonitrile. Samples were vortexed, centrifuged and loaded onto conditioned tables (Strata X AW SPE columns (33 μm, 30 mg / 1 mL, Phenomenex, Aschaffenburg, Germany) using the automated sample preparation system Extrahera (Biotage, Uppsala, Sweden). After washing the cartridges using water, methanol and a mixture of acetonitrile and aqueous ammonium hydroxide solution, HCA was eluted using two times a mixture of methanol and aqueous ammonium hydroxide solution. The eluate was dried and reconstituted by adding ammonium acetate solution and acetonitrile separately. Afterwards, the samples were injected into the LC-MS/MS system. The LC-MS/MS system consisted of a triple quadrupole mass spectrometer QTRAP 6500+ (Sciex, Darmstadt, Germany) equipped with a Turbo Ion Spray source operated in negative electrospray ionization mode and an Agilent 1290 Infinity LC-system with binary HPLC pump, column oven and autosampler (Agilent, Waldbronn, Germany). The chromatographic separation was performed using a Luna 3 μm HILIC 200 Å 100 × 2 mm column in combination with a KrudKatcher in-line filter (both Phenomenex, Aschaffenburg, Germany). Data acquisition was done using Analyst Software 1.6.3 and quantification was performed with MultiQuant Software 3.0.2 (both Sciex, Darmstadt, Germany), employing the internal standard method. Calibration curves were calculated by linear regression with 1/x weighting. Acceptance criteria and quality assurance measures have been applied as previously described [36].

The determination of homocysteine (HCys) was performed using protein precipitation in combination with LC–MS/MS. Briefly, 20 μL of serum or urine was pipetted to a polypropylene tube and 20 μL of 15 mg/mL aqueous TCEP-solution (tris(2-carboxyethyl)phosphine), 40 μL IS working solution (500 ng/mL HCys-d4 in methanolic TCEP solution, 1 mg/mL) and 40 μL methanolic TCEP solution, 1 mg/mL were added. Afterwards, samples were vortexed, centrifuged, transferred into another polypropylene tube, and dried using nitrogen. The dried samples were reconstituted using 50 μL of water containing 10 mM ammonium acetate buffer and 10 mM acetic acid, centrifuged again and injected into the LC-MS/MS system. The same LC-MS/MS-system and acceptance criteria as described for HCA were used. However, positive electrospray ionization mode was applied and a Luna Omega 1.6 μm Polar C18 100 × 2.1 mm column in combination with a respective pre column (both Phenomenex, Aschaffenburg, Germany) was used.

Immunohistochemical Analysis

A stepwise rehydration of the brain sections was conducted, followed by a heat-induced antigen retrieval in 10 mM citrate buffer (pH 6.0) including 0.05% Tween-20 (Sigma-Aldrich, Taufkirchen, Germany). After rinsing, sections were incubated for 5 min in 0.6% H_2O_2 (Sigma-Aldrich) in PBS (0.1 M; pH = 7.3) in order to block endogenous peroxidases. Sections were rinsed and incubated for 30 min in PBS containing 1% bovine serum albumin (PBS-B) and 5% normal goat serum (NGS, Sigma-Aldrich) to prevent unspecific binding of the antibody. After subsequent rinsing, sections were incubated overnight at 4 °C in PBS-B containing 1% NGS and the primary antibody (anti-human Aβ 82E1 mouse IgG MoAb 1:1000, IBL international, Hamburg, Germany). Rinsing was followed by an incubation with goat anti-mouse IgG H&L Biotin (1:1000, Abcam, Berlin, Germany) in PBS-B containing 1% NGS for one hour. Sections were rinsed followed by a 1-h incubation with avidin-biotin conjugate in PBS (ABC; Vectastain Elite ABC HRP Kit, Linaris, Dossenheim, Germany). After another rinsing step, sections were treated with 3,3′-diaminobenzidine tetrahydrochloride (DAB; Sigma-Aldrich) in water (0.2 mg/mL; pH = 7.6) for 10 min. The immunostaining was then developed by adding 50 µL H_2O_2 to a final concentration of 0.006%, incubating for another 10 min. The reaction was stopped by rinsing in ice-cold distilled water followed by a counterstaining using Mayer's hematoxylin (Morphisto, Frankfurt am Main, Germany). Sections were finally dehydrated and covered with Pertex (Medite). We digitized appropriate sections using a Nicon Eclipse Ni-E microscope (Nikon Instruments Europe BV, Amsterdam, Netherlands). Whole brain images were taken at a final magnification of 100x and the area occupied by plaques in several regions of interest (ROI; Table A2) was analyzed using the color segmentation plugin (Daniel Sage, Biomedical Imaging Group, EPFL, http://bigwww.epfl.ch/sage/soft/colorsegmentation/) for ImageJ software (National Institute of Health, Bethesda, MD, USA). Only animals of the first cohort were immunohistochemically investigated in this study.

Table A2. Regions of interest (ROI) in different cortical and hippocampal areas.

ROI	Brain Area	Height (µm)
1	Primary somatosensory cortex (PSC)	500 × 500
2	Gyrus dentatus (GD)	275 × 275
3	CA1	275 × 275
4	CA3	275 × 275
5	CA2	275 × 275
6	Thalamic nuclei (TN)	600 × 400
7	Piriform cortex (PC)	275 × 275
8	Piriform cortex (PC)	275 × 275

Preclinical Quality Parameters

Several aspects were considered to ensure the quality of the applied methodologies and resulting data. These points are in accordance with initiatives such as EQIPD ("European quality in preclinical data"; https://quality-preclinical-data.eu/). The aim of EQIPD is broadly to implement various quality improving measures in order to enhance the reproducibility of preclinical data [63]. In the present study, we performed a power calculation to estimate the needed group size (http://www.biomath.info/power/). The resulting total amount of 112 animals was tested in two consecutive cohorts. Nine animals were lost during the course of the whole study. In terms of translatability, we have decided to include both male and female animals in the experiments, since Alzheimer's disease affects both sexes in the clinical context, with a higher rate in women than in men [48]. In general, female animals are largely underrepresented in neuroscience research [82]. Randomization was applied at several stages along the study course. Mice were initially allocated to the home cages according to a random list (https://www.random.org/) and target holes in the Barnes maze were set randomly. Besides, drinking corners in the IntelliCages as well as the stimulus mice in the social interaction test were also assigned randomly. A within-cage randomization between groups was not applicable in this case because every mouse matched strictly to its adequate experimental diet. All animals were regularly pre-handled and transferred to the experimental rooms at least half an hour before behavioral analysis. Blinding of the experimenter in order to prevent detection bias was not performed here, because in all behavioral tests automated outcome assessment was applied (via EthoVision XT, IntelliCage and Touchsreen software). However, blinding was performed during the immunohistochemical analysis. Here, a second experimenter marked the ROI in the images without being aware of animal ID or experimental group. Furthermore, an automated animal management software as well as an electronic lab-book were used throughout the study. Standard operating procedures had been written prior to the experimental procedures.

References

1. *World Alzheimer Report 2019: Attitudes to Dementia*; Alzheimer's Disease International: London, UK, 2019.
2. Calsolaro, V.; Antognoli, R.; Okoye, C.; Monzani, F. The Use of Antipsychotic Drugs for Treating Behavioral Symptoms in Alzheimer's Disease. *Front. Pharmacol.* **2019**, *10*, 1465. [CrossRef] [PubMed]
3. Sasaguri, H.; Nilsson, P.; Hashimoto, S.; Nagata, K.; Saito, T.; De Strooper, B.; Hardy, J.; Vassar, R.; Winblad, B.; Saido, T.C. APP mouse models for Alzheimer's disease preclinical studies. *EMBO J.* **2017**, *36*, e201797397. [CrossRef] [PubMed]
4. Hara, Y.; McKeehan, N.; Fillit, H.M. Translating the biology of aging into novel therapeutics for Alzheimer disease. *Neurology* **2019**, *92*, 84–93. [CrossRef] [PubMed]
5. Sharma, P.; Srivastava, P.; Seth, A.; Tripathi, P.N.; Banerjee, A.G.; Shrivastava, S.K. Comprehensive review of mechanisms of pathogenesis involved in Alzheimer's disease and potential therapeutic strategies. *Prog. Neurobiol.* **2019**, *174*, 53–89. [CrossRef] [PubMed]
6. Masters, C.L.; Simms, G.; Weinman, N.A.; Multhaup, G.; McDonald, B.L.; Beyreuther, K. Amyloid plaque core protein in Alzheimer disease and Down syndrome. *Proc. Natl. Acad. Sci. USA* **1985**, *82*, 4245–4249. [CrossRef] [PubMed]
7. Selkoe, D.J.; Hardy, J. The amyloid hypothesis of Alzheimer's disease at 25 years. *EMBO Mol. Med.* **2016**. [CrossRef]
8. Bateman, R.J.; Xiong, C.; Benzinger, T.L.S.; Fagan, A.M.; Goate, A.; Fox, N.C.; Marcus, D.S.; Cairns, N.J.; Xie, X.; Blazey, T.M.; et al. Clinical and Biomarker Changes in Dominantly Inherited Alzheimer's Disease. *N. Engl. J. Med.* **2012**, *367*, 795–804. [CrossRef]
9. Saito, T.; Matsuba, Y.; Mihira, N.; Takano, J.; Nilsson, P.; Itohara, S.; Iwata, N.; Saido, T.C. Single App knock-in mouse models of Alzheimer's disease. *Nat. Neurosci.* **2014**, *17*, 661–663. [CrossRef]
10. Zhao, G.; He, F.; Wu, C.; Li, P.; Li, N.; Deng, J.; Zhu, G.; Ren, W.; Peng, Y. Betaine in Inflammation: Mechanistic Aspects and Applications. *Front. Immunol.* **2018**, *9*, 1–13. [CrossRef]
11. Clarke, R.; Smith, A.D.; Jobst, K.A.; Refsum, H.; Sutton, L.; Ueland, P.M. Folate, Vitamin B12, and Serum Total Homocysteine Levels in Confirmed Alzheimer Disease. *Arch. Neurol.* **1998**, *55*, 1449. [CrossRef]
12. Isobe, C.; Murata, T.; Sato, C.; Terayama, Y. Increase of total homocysteine concentration in cerebrospinal fluid in patients with Alzheimer's disease and Parkinson's disease. *Life Sci.* **2005**, *77*, 1836–1843. [CrossRef] [PubMed]
13. Seshadri, S.; Beiser, A.; Selhub, J.; Jaques, P.; Roseberg, I.H.; D'Agostino, R.B.; Wilson, P.W.F.; Wolf, P.A. Plasma Homocysteine As a Risk Factor for Dementia and Alzheimer's Disease. *N. Engl. J. Med.* **2002**, *346*, 476–483. [CrossRef] [PubMed]
14. Nurk, E.; Refsum, H.; Tell, G.S.; Engedal, K.; Vollset, S.E.; Ueland, P.M.; Nygaard, H.A.; Smith, A.D. Plasma total homocysteine and memory in the elderly: The Hordaland homocysteine study. *Ann. Neurol.* **2005**, *58*, 847–857. [CrossRef] [PubMed]
15. Morris, M.S. Homocysteine and Alzheimer's disease. *Lancet Neurol.* **2003**, *2*, 425–428. [CrossRef]
16. Smith, A.D.; Smith, S.M.; de Jager, C.A.; Whitbread, P.; Johnston, C.; Agacinski, G.; Oulhaj, A.; Bradley, K.M.; Jacoby, R.; Refsum, H. Homocysteine-Lowering by B Vitamins Slows the Rate of Accelerated Brain Atrophy in Mild Cognitive Impairment: A Randomized Controlled Trial. *PLoS ONE* **2010**, *5*, e12244. [CrossRef]
17. Douaud, G.; Refsum, H.; de Jager, C.A.; Jacoby, R.; Nichols, T.E.; Smith, S.M.; Smith, A.D. Preventing Alzheimer's disease-related gray matter atrophy by B-vitamin treatment. *Proc. Natl. Acad. Sci. USA* **2013**, *110*, 9523–9528. [CrossRef]
18. Kennedy, D. B Vitamins and the Brain: Mechanisms, Dose and Efficacy—A Review. *Nutrients* **2016**, *8*, 68. [CrossRef]
19. McMahon, J.A.; Green, T.J.; Skeaff, C.M.; Knight, R.G.; Mann, J.I.; Williams, S.M. A Controlled Trial of Homocysteine Lowering and Cognitive Performance. *N. Engl. J. Med.* **2006**, *354*, 2764–2772. [CrossRef]
20. Tabet, N.; Rafi, H.; Weaving, G.; Lyons, B.; Iversen, S.A. Behavioural and psychological symptoms of Alzheimer type dementia are not correlated with plasma homocysteine concentration. *Dement. Geriatr. Cogn. Disord.* **2006**, *22*, 432–438. [CrossRef]
21. Wald, D.S.; Kasturiratne, A.; Simmonds, M. Effect of Folic Acid, with or without Other B Vitamins, on Cognitive Decline: Meta-Analysis of Randomized Trials. *Am. J. Med.* **2010**, *123*, 522–527.e2. [CrossRef]

22. Clarke, R.; Bennett, D.; Parish, S.; Lewington, S.; Skeaff, M.; Eussen, S.J.P.M.; Lewerin, C.; Stott, D.J.; Armitage, J.; Hankey, G.J.; et al. Effects of homocysteine lowering with B vitamins on cognitive aging: Meta-analysis of 11 trials with cognitive data on 22,000 individuals. *Am. J. Clin. Nutr.* **2014**, *100*, 657–666. [CrossRef]
23. Smith, A.D.; Refsum, H.; Bottiglieri, T.; Fenech, M.; Hooshmand, B.; McCaddon, A.; Miller, J.W.; Rosenberg, I.H.; Obeid, R. Homocysteine and Dementia: An International Consensus Statement. *J. Alzheimers Dis.* **2018**, *62*, 561–570. [CrossRef] [PubMed]
24. Smith, A.D.; Refsum, H. Homocysteine, B Vitamins, and Cognitive Impairment. *Annu. Rev. Nutr.* **2016**, *36*, 211–239. [CrossRef] [PubMed]
25. Grimm, M.O.W.; Michaelson, D.M.; Hartmann, T. Omega-3 fatty acids, lipids, and apoE lipidation in Alzheimer's disease: A rationale for multi-nutrient dementia prevention. *J. Lipid Res.* **2017**, *58*, 2083–2101. [CrossRef]
26. Oulhaj, A.; Jernerén, F.; Refsum, H.; Smith, A.D.; de Jager, C.A. Omega-3 Fatty Acid Status Enhances the Prevention of Cognitive Decline by B Vitamins in Mild Cognitive Impairment. *J. Alzheimers Dis.* **2016**, *50*, 547–557. [CrossRef]
27. McCleery, J.; Abraham, R.P.; Denton, D.A.; Rutjes, A.W.S.; Chong, L.-Y.; Al-Assaf, A.S.; Griffith, D.J.; Rafeeq, S.; Yaman, H.; Malik, M.A.; et al. Vitamin and mineral supplementation for preventing dementia or delaying cognitive decline in people with mild cognitive impairment. *Cochrane Database Syst. Rev.* **2018**, *2018*. [CrossRef] [PubMed]
28. Diaz-Arrastia, R. Homocysteine and Neurologic Disease. *Arch. Neurol.* **2000**, *57*, 1422–1428. [CrossRef]
29. Obeid, R.; Herrmann, W. Mechanisms of homocysteine neurotoxicity in neurodegenerative diseases with special reference to dementia. *FEBS Lett.* **2006**, *580*, 2994–3005. [CrossRef]
30. Lipton, S.A.; Kim, W.-K.; Choi, Y.-B.; Kumar, S.; D'Emilia, D.M.; Rayudu, P.V.; Arnelle, D.R.; Stamler, J.S. Neurotoxicity associated with dual actions of homocysteine at the N-methyl-D-aspartate receptor. *Proc. Natl. Acad. Sci. USA* **1997**, *94*, 5923–5928. [CrossRef]
31. Kim, J.P.; Koh, J.; Choi, D.W. l-Homocysteate is a potent neurotoxin on cultured cortical neurons. *Brain Res.* **1987**, *437*, 103–110. [CrossRef]
32. Sommer, S.; Hunzinger, C.; Schillo, S.; Klemm, M.; Biefang-Arndt, K.; Schwall, G.; Pütter, S.; Hoelzer, K.; Schroer, K.; Stegmann, W.; et al. Molecular Analysis of Homocysteic Acid-Induced Neuronal Stress. *J. Proteome Res.* **2004**, *3*, 572–581. [CrossRef] [PubMed]
33. Görtz, P.; Hoinkes, A.; Fleischer, W.; Otto, F.; Schwahn, B.; Wendel, U.; Siebler, M. Implications for hyperhomocysteinemia: Not homocysteine but its oxidized forms strongly inhibit neuronal network activity. *J. Neurol. Sci.* **2004**, *218*, 109–114. [CrossRef] [PubMed]
34. Vladychenskaya, E.A.; Tyulina, O.V.; Boldyrev, A.A. Effect of Homocysteine and Homocysteic Acid on Glutamate Receptors on Rat Lymphocytes. *Bull. Exp. Biol. Med. Vol.* **2006**, *142*, 47–50. [CrossRef]
35. Jansen, D.; Zerbi, V.; Arnoldussen, I.A.C.; Wiesmann, M.; Rijpma, A.; Fang, X.T.; Dederen, P.J.; Mutsaers, M.P.C.; Broersen, L.M.; Lütjohann, D.; et al. Effects of Specific Multi-Nutrient Enriched Diets on Cerebral Metabolism, Cognition and Neuropathology in AβPPswe-PS1dE9 Mice. *PLoS ONE* **2013**, *8*, e75393. [CrossRef] [PubMed]
36. Gurke, R.; Schmidt, D.; Thomas, D.; Fleck, S.C.; Geisslinger, G.; Ferreirós, N. A validated LC–MS/MS method for the determination of homocysteic acid in biological samples. *J. Pharm. Biomed. Anal.* **2019**, *174*, 578–587. [CrossRef]
37. Bolivar, V.J. Intrasession and intersession habituation in mice: From inbred strain variability to linkage analysis. *Neurobiol. Learn. Mem.* **2009**, *92*, 206–214. [CrossRef]
38. Gawel, K.; Gibula, E.; Marszalek-Grabska, M.; Filarowska, J.; Kotlinska, J.H. Assessment of spatial learning and memory in the Barnes maze task in rodents—Methodological consideration. *Naunyn. Schmiedebergs. Arch. Pharmacol.* **2019**, *392*, 1–18. [CrossRef]
39. Kaidanovich-Beilin, O.; Lipina, T.; Vukobradovic, I.; Roder, J.; Woodgett, J.R. Assessment of Social Interaction Behaviors. *J. Vis. Exp.* **2011**, 2473. [CrossRef]
40. Moy, S.S.; Nadler, J.J.; Perez, A.; Barbaro, R.P.; Johns, J.M.; Magnuson, T.R.; Piven, J.; Crawley, J.N. Sociability and preference for social novelty in five inbred strains: An approach to assess autistic-like behavior in mice. *Genes Brain Behav.* **2004**, *3*, 287–302. [CrossRef]

41. Nithianantharajah, J.; McKechanie, A.G.; Stewart, T.J.; Johnstone, M.; Blackwood, D.H.; St Clair, D.; Grant, S.G.N.; Bussey, T.J.; Saksida, L.M. Bridging the translational divide: Identical cognitive touchscreen testing in mice and humans carrying mutations in a disease-relevant homologous gene. *Sci. Rep.* **2015**, *5*, 14613. [CrossRef]
42. Jacob, S.; Davies, G.; De Bock, M.; Hermans, B.; Wintmolders, C.; Bottelbergs, A.; Borgers, M.; Theunis, C.; Van Broeck, B.; Manyakov, N.V.; et al. Neural oscillations during cognitive processes in an App knock-in mouse model of Alzheimer's disease pathology. *Sci. Rep.* **2019**, *9*, 16363. [CrossRef]
43. Voikar, V.; Krackow, S.; Lipp, H.-P.; Rau, A.; Colacicco, G.; Wolfer, D.P. Automated dissection of permanent effects of hippocampal or prefrontal lesions on performance at spatial, working memory and circadian timing tasks of C57BL/6 mice in IntelliCage. *Behav. Brain Res.* **2018**, *352*, 8–22. [CrossRef]
44. Krackow, S.; Vannoni, E.; Codita, A.; Mohammed, A.H.; Cirulli, F.; Branchi, I.; Alleva, E.; Reichelt, A.; Willuweit, A.; Voikar, V.; et al. Consistent behavioral phenotype differences between inbred mouse strains in the IntelliCage. *Genes Brain Behav.* **2010**, *9*, 722–731. [CrossRef] [PubMed]
45. Agrawal, A.; Ilango, K.; Singh, P.K.; Karmakar, D.; Singh, G.P.I.; Kumari, R.; Dubey, G.P. Age dependent levels of plasma homocysteine and cognitive performance. *Behav. Brain Res.* **2015**, *283*, 139–144. [CrossRef]
46. Zahs, K.R.; Ashe, K.H. 'Too much good news'—Are Alzheimer mouse models trying to tell us how to prevent, not cure, Alzheimer's disease? *Trends Neurosci.* **2010**, *33*, 381–389. [CrossRef] [PubMed]
47. Perneczky, R.; Drzezga, A.; Diehl-Schmid, J.; Li, Y.; Kurz, A. Gender differences in brain reserve. *J. Neurol.* **2007**, *254*, 1395–1400. [CrossRef] [PubMed]
48. Mielke, M.; Vemuri, P.; Rocca, W. Clinical epidemiology of Alzheimer' disease: Assessing sex and gender differences. *Clin. Epidemiol.* **2014**, *6*, 37–48. [CrossRef] [PubMed]
49. Sakakibara, Y.; Sekiya, M.; Saito, T.; Saido, T.C.; Iijima, K.M. Amyloid-β plaque formation and reactive gliosis are required for induction of cognitive deficits in App knock-in mouse models of Alzheimer's disease. *BMC Neurosci.* **2019**, *20*, 13. [CrossRef]
50. Mehla, J.; Lacoursiere, S.G.; Lapointe, V.; McNaughton, B.L.; Sutherland, R.J.; McDonald, R.J.; Mohajerani, M.H. Age-dependent behavioral and biochemical characterization of single APP knock-in mouse (APPNL-G-F/NL-G-F) model of Alzheimer's disease. *Neurobiol. Aging* **2019**, *75*, 25–37. [CrossRef]
51. Latif-Hernandez, A.; Shah, D.; Craessaerts, K.; Saido, T.; Saito, T.; De Strooper, B.; Van der Linden, A.; D'Hooge, R. Subtle behavioral changes and increased prefrontal-hippocampal network synchronicity in APPNL−G−F mice before prominent plaque deposition. *Behav. Brain Res.* **2019**, *364*, 431–441. [CrossRef]
52. Whyte, L.S.; Hemsley, K.M.; Lau, A.A.; Hassiotis, S.; Saito, T.; Saido, T.C.; Hopwood, J.J.; Sargeant, T.J. Reduction in open field activity in the absence of memory deficits in the App NL−G−F knock-in mouse model of Alzheimer's disease. *Behav. Brain Res.* **2018**, *336*, 177–181. [CrossRef] [PubMed]
53. Sakakibara, Y.; Sekiya, M.; Saito, T.; Saido, T.C.; Iijima, K.M. Cognitive and emotional alterations in App knock-in mouse models of Aβ amyloidosis. *BMC Neurosci.* **2018**, *19*, 46. [CrossRef]
54. Masuda, A.; Kobayashi, Y.; Kogo, N.; Saito, T.; Saido, T.C.; Itohara, S. Cognitive deficits in single App knock-in mouse models. *Neurobiol. Learn. Mem.* **2016**, *135*, 73–82. [CrossRef] [PubMed]
55. Jankowsky, J.L.; Zheng, H. Practical considerations for choosing a mouse model of Alzheimer's disease. *Mol. Neurodegener.* **2017**, *12*, 89. [CrossRef]
56. Sudduth, T.L.; Powell, D.K.; Smith, C.D.; Greenstein, A.; Wilcock, D.M. Induction of Hyperhomocysteinemia Models Vascular Dementia by Induction of Cerebral Microhemorrhages and Neuroinflammation. *J. Cereb. Blood Flow Metab.* **2013**, *33*, 708–715. [CrossRef] [PubMed]
57. Teri, L.; Ferretti, L.E.; Gibbons, L.E.; Logsdon, R.G.; McCurry, S.M.; Kukull, W.A.; McCormick, W.C.; Bowen, J.D.; Larson, E.B. Anxiety in Alzheimer's Disease: Prevalence and Comorbidity. *J. Gerontol. Ser. A Biol. Sci. Med. Sci.* **1999**, *54*, M348–M352. [CrossRef]
58. Fuso, A.; Nicolia, V.; Cavallaro, R.A.; Ricceri, L.; D'Anselmi, F.; Coluccia, P.; Calamandrei, G.; Scarpa, S. B-vitamin deprivation induces hyperhomocysteinemia and brain S-adenosylhomocysteine, depletes brain S-adenosylmethionine, and enhances PS1 and BACE expression and amyloid-β deposition in mice. *Mol. Cell. Neurosci.* **2008**, *37*, 731–746. [CrossRef] [PubMed]
59. Zhang, C.-E.; Wei, W.; Liu, Y.-H.; Peng, J.-H.; Tian, Q.; Liu, G.-P.; Zhang, Y.; Wang, J.-Z. Hyperhomocysteinemia Increases β-Amyloid by Enhancing Expression of γ-Secretase and Phosphorylation of Amyloid Precursor Protein in Rat Brain. *Am. J. Pathol.* **2009**, *174*, 1481–1491. [CrossRef]

60. Kruman, I.I.; Kumaravel, T.S.; Lohani, A.; Pedersen, W.A.; Cutler, R.G.; Kruman, Y.; Haughey, N.; Lee, J.; Evans, M.; Mattson, M.P. Folic acid deficiency and homocysteine impair DNA repair in hippocampal neurons and sensitize them to amyloid toxicity in experimental models of Alzheimer's disease. *J. Neurosci.* **2002**, *22*, 1752–1762. [CrossRef]
61. Bernardo, A.; McCord, M.; Troen, A.M.; Allison, J.D.; McDonald, M.P. Impaired spatial memory in APP-overexpressing mice on a homocysteinemia-inducing diet. *Neurobiol. Aging* **2007**, *28*, 1195–1205. [CrossRef]
62. Troen, A.M.; Shea-Budgell, M.; Shukitt-Hale, B.; Smith, D.E.; Selhub, J.; Rosenberg, I.H. B-vitamin deficiency causes hyperhomocysteinemia and vascular cognitive impairment in mice. *Proc. Natl. Acad. Sci. USA* **2008**, *105*, 12474–12479. [CrossRef]
63. Bespalov, A.; Steckler, T.; Skolnick, P. Be positive about negatives–recommendations for the publication of negative (or null) results. *Eur. Neuropsychopharmacol.* **2019**, *29*, 1312–1320. [CrossRef] [PubMed]
64. Refsum, H.; Smith, A.D.; Ueland, P.M.; Nexo, E.; Clarke, R.; McPartlin, J.; Johnston, C.; Engbaek, F.; Schneede, J.; McPartlin, C.; et al. Facts and Recommendations about Total Homocysteine Determinations: An Expert Opinion. *Clin. Chem.* **2004**, *50*, 3–32. [CrossRef] [PubMed]
65. Sinha, M.; Saha, A.; Basu, S.; Pal, K.; Chakrabarti, S. Aging and antioxidants modulate rat brain levels of homocysteine and dehydroepiandrosterone sulphate (DHEA-S): Implications in the pathogenesis of Alzheimer's disease. *Neurosci. Lett.* **2010**, *483*, 123–126. [CrossRef]
66. Ueland, P.M.; Nygård, O.; Vollset, S.E.; Refsum, H. The Hordaland Homocysteine Studies. *Lipids* **2001**, *36*, S33–S39. [CrossRef] [PubMed]
67. Ernest, S.; Hosack, A.; O'Brien, W.E.; Rosenblatt, D.S.; Nadeau, J.H. Homocysteine levels in A/J and C57BL/6J mice: Genetic, diet, gender, and parental effects. *Physiol. Genom.* **2005**, *21*, 404–410. [CrossRef]
68. Zhuo, J.-M.; Praticò, D. Severe In Vivo Hyper-Homocysteinemia is not Associated with Elevation of Amyloid-β Peptides in the Tg2576 Mice. *J. Alzheimers Dis.* **2010**, *21*, 133–140. [CrossRef]
69. Hasegawa, T.; Mikoda, N.; Kitazawa, M.; LaFerla, F.M. Treatment of Alzheimer's Disease with Anti-Homocysteic Acid Antibody in 3xTg-AD Male Mice. *PLoS ONE* **2010**, *5*, e8593. [CrossRef]
70. Janssen, C.I.F.; Zerbi, V.; Mutsaers, M.P.C.; de Jong, B.S.W.; Wiesmann, M.; Arnoldussen, I.A.C.; Geenen, B.; Heerschap, A.; Muskiet, F.A.J.; Jouni, Z.E.; et al. Impact of dietary n-3 polyunsaturated fatty acids on cognition, motor skills and hippocampal neurogenesis in developing C57BL/6J mice. *J. Nutr. Biochem.* **2015**, *26*, 24–35. [CrossRef]
71. Wiesmann, M.; Zerbi, V.; Jansen, D.; Haast, R.; Lütjohann, D.; Broersen, L.M.; Heerschap, A.; Kiliaan, A.J. A Dietary Treatment Improves Cerebral Blood Flow and Brain Connectivity in Aging apoE4 Mice. *Neural Plast.* **2016**, *2016*, 1–15. [CrossRef]
72. Arendash, G.W.; Jensen, M.T.; Salem, N.; Hussein, N.; Cracchiolo, J.; Dickson, A.; Leighty, R.; Potter, H. A diet high in omega-3 fatty acids does not improve or protect cognitive performance in Alzheimer's transgenic mice. *Neuroscience* **2007**, *149*, 286–302. [CrossRef]
73. Shah, R.C.; Kamphuis, P.J.; Leurgans, S.; Swinkels, S.H.; Sadowsky, C.H.; Bongers, A.; Rappaport, S.A.; Quinn, J.F.; Wieggers, R.L.; Scheltens, P.; et al. The S-Connect study: Results from a randomized, controlled trial of Souvenaid in mild-to-moderate Alzheimer's disease. *Alzheimers Res. Ther.* **2013**, *5*, 59. [CrossRef] [PubMed]
74. Scheltens, N.M.E.; Briels, C.T.; Yaqub, M.; Barkhof, F.; Boellaard, R.; van der Flier, W.M.; Schwarte, L.A.; Teunissen, C.E.; Attali, A.; Broersen, L.M.; et al. Exploring effects of Souvenaid on cerebral glucose metabolism in Alzheimer's disease. *Alzheimers Dement. Transl. Res. Clin. Interv.* **2019**, *5*, 492–500. [CrossRef] [PubMed]
75. Panza, F.; Lozupone, M.; Logroscino, G.; Imbimbo, B.P. A critical appraisal of amyloid-β-targeting therapies for Alzheimer disease. *Nat. Rev. Neurol.* **2019**, *15*, 73–88. [CrossRef] [PubMed]
76. Aizenstein, H.J.; Nebes, R.D.; Saxton, J.A.; Price, J.C.; Mathis, C.A.; Tsopelas, N.D.; Ziolko, S.K.; James, J.A.; Snitz, B.E.; Houck, P.R.; et al. Frequent Amyloid Deposition Without Significant Cognitive Impairment Among the Elderly. *Arch. Neurol.* **2008**, *65*, 1509. [CrossRef] [PubMed]
77. Kaplon, H.; Muralidharan, M.; Schneider, Z.; Reichert, J.M. Antibodies to watch in 2020. *MAbs* **2020**, *12*, 1703531. [CrossRef] [PubMed]
78. Tucker, L.B.; McCabe, J.T. Behavior of Male and Female C57BL/6J Mice Is More Consistent with Repeated Trials in the Elevated Zero Maze than in the Elevated Plus Maze. *Front. Behav. Neurosci.* **2017**, *11*, 1–8. [CrossRef]
79. Harrison, F.E.; Reiserer, R.S.; Tomarken, A.J.; McDonald, M.P. Spatial and nonspatial escape strategies in the Barnes maze. *Learn. Mem.* **2006**, *13*, 809–819. [CrossRef] [PubMed]

80. Talpos, J.C.; Winters, B.D.; Dias, R.; Saksida, L.M.; Bussey, T.J. A novel touchscreen-automated paired-associate learning (PAL) task sensitive to pharmacological manipulation of the hippocampus: A translational rodent model of cognitive impairments in neurodegenerative disease. *Psychopharmacology* **2009**, *205*, 157–168. [CrossRef]
81. Paxinos, G.; Franklin, K.B.J. *The Mouse Brain in Stereotaxic Coordinates*, 4th ed.; Academic Press: Cambridge, MA, USA, 2013; p. 360.
82. Beery, A.K. Inclusion of females does not increase variability in rodent research studies. *Curr. Opin. Behav. Sci.* **2018**, *23*, 143–149. [CrossRef]

Publisher's Note: MDPI stays neutral with regard to jurisdictional claims in published maps and institutional affiliations.

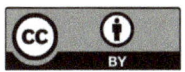

© 2020 by the authors. Licensee MDPI, Basel, Switzerland. This article is an open access article distributed under the terms and conditions of the Creative Commons Attribution (CC BY) license (http://creativecommons.org/licenses/by/4.0/).

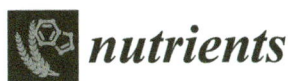

Article

Beneficial Effect of Dietary Diversity on the Risk of Disability in Activities of Daily Living in Adults: A Prospective Cohort Study

Jian Zhang [1], Ai Zhao [2], Wei Wu [1], Zhongxia Ren [1], Chenlu Yang [1], Peiyu Wang [3] and Yumei Zhang [1,*]

1. Department of Nutrition and Food Hygiene, School of Public Health, Peking University, Beijing 100191, China; zhangjian92@pku.edu.cn (J.Z.); wennie0616@163.com (W.W.); ren_zhongxia@pku.edu.cn (Z.R.); yangchenluwork@126.com (C.Y.)
2. Vanke School of Public Health, Tsinghua University, Beijing 100091, China; aizhao18@tsinghua.edu.cn
3. Department of Social Medicine and Health Education, School of Public Health, Peking University, Beijing 100191, China; wpeiyu@bjmu.edu.cn
* Correspondence: zhangyumei@bjmu.edu.cn; Tel.: +86-10-8280-1575-63

Received: 2 October 2020; Accepted: 23 October 2020; Published: 25 October 2020

Abstract: Disability in activities of daily living (ADL) is common in elderly people. Dietary diversity is associated with several age-related diseases. The evidence on dietary diversity score (DDS) and ADL disability is limited. This study was based on the China Health and Nutrition Survey. Prospective data of 5004 participants were analyzed. ADL disability was defined as the inability to perform at least one of the five self-care tasks. Cox proportional regression models were conducted to estimate the association of cumulative average DDS with the risk of ADL disability. Logistic regression models were performed to estimate the odds ratios for the average DDS, the baseline DDS, and the recent DDS prior to the end of the survey in relation to ADL disability, respectively. The results indicate that higher average DDS was associated with a decreased risk of ADL disability (T3 vs. T1: hazard ratio 0.50; 95% confidence interval 0.39–0.66). The association was stronger among participants who did not had comorbidity at baseline than those who did (P-interaction 0.035). The average DDS is the most pronounced in estimating the association of DDS with ADL disability of the three approaches. In summary, higher DDS has beneficial effects on ADL disability, and long-term dietary exposure is more preferable in the investigation of DDS and ADL.

Keywords: dietary diversity; activities of daily living; cohort study; adults

1. Introduction

The world's population is aging at a faster speed than it used to be according to a report from the World Health Organization [1]. It is predicted that the number of older people worldwide would more than double by 2050 [2]. The aging process is accompanied by declines in functional capacity and cognition [3,4]. Disability in older people is associated with low quality of life [5], increased burden on caregivers [6], rise in morbidity and mortality [7], and elevated health care costs [8], which finally put more burdens on the whole society.

Activities of daily living (ADL) is an index to represent the capability of skills essential to manage basic physical needs, comprised of the following areas: grooming/personal hygiene, dressing, toileting/continence, transferring/ambulating, and eating [9]. The prevalence of ADL disability in Chinese individuals aged 60 years and above was 10.03% in 2015 [10]. Actions aimed at preventing ADL dependence may reduce the burden on older people themselves, caregivers, and the health care system [11]. Several factors are reported to be associated with ADL disability, including gender, slow gait speed, weight loss, muscle strength, etc. [5,12]. In addition to that, diet and nutrition are found to have an impact on ADL or functional capacity. Previous prospective studies indicated that higher consumption of dairy products is associated with a lower risk of functional disability [13]. Nutrients, such as vitamin D [14] and dietary fiber [15], are also reported to be related to ADL.

Dietary diversity is an important aspect of our diet. Keeping a diverse diet is one of the key recommendations of Chinese dietary guidelines [16]. Epidemiological studies showed that a higher dietary diversity score (DDS) is inversely associated with some age-related diseases, such as diabetes [17], cognitive decline [18]. Additionally, it has been shown that adherence to a diverse diet reduced the risk of death [19,20]. However, prospective evidence on DDS and ADL disability is limited. In this study, we prospectively analyzed the effect of DDS on the risk of ADL disability in a prospective cohort study.

2. Materials and Methods

2.1. Study Population

This study was based on the China Health and Nutrition Survey (CHNS). Details about the CHNS has been described elsewhere [21]. In brief, the CHNS is an open cohort study, and participants from twelve geographically diverse areas of China were involved in this study. The CHNS was designed to understand the health and nutrition of the Chinese and how they are affected by social transformation. It was initiated in 1989, and follow-up surveys were conducted in 1991, 1993, 1997, 2000, 2004, 2006, 2009, 2011, and 2015. Data collected in phase 1997 and beyond were used in the present study. The inclusion criteria included answered the ADL survey and aged 60 years and above at the end of the survey (report of ADL disability, loss to follow-up, the phase of 2015, whichever occurred first). The exclusion criteria included absent from dietary survey, report of ADL at baseline survey, report of previously diagnosed cancer at baseline survey, and missing values on covariates. In the end, 5004 participants were included this study (Figure 1). The CHNS was approved by institutional review boards at the University of North Carolina at Chapel Hill and the National Institute of Nutrition and Food Safety, Chinese Center for Disease Control and Prevention. All participants gave written informed consent before they participated in the survey.

2.2. Dietary Survey and Dietary Diversity Score

Participants' diet intakes in the past 3 days were recorded by dietary recall and household food weight inventory. Details about the dietary survey process have been published [22]. All food items that a participant consumed in a 24 h period were divided into eight food categories (cereals and tubers, vegetables, fruits, meat, aquatic products, eggs, soybeans and nuts, and dairy products). Intake of any food from each of the food categories will add one point to DDS, with a total score of eight. Average daily DDS was calculated for each participant at each phase. Cumulative average DDS across phases before the end of the survey (report of ADL disability, loss to follow-up, the phase of 2015, whichever occurred first) was computed to represent long-term diet exposure. Subsequently, average DDS was grouped into tertiles from low to high (T1: 1.33–3.25; T2: 3.27–4.03; T3: 4.06–8.00). Besides, participants' nutrient intakes were estimated according to the Chinese food composition tables, and cumulative average daily intakes were also computed.

2.3. Ascertain of Disability in Activities of Daily Living

In phase 1997, 2000, 2004, 2006, and 2015, participants aged 55 years and above were asked whether she or he could finish some self-care tasks (standing up after sitting for a long time, dressing, toileting, bathing, and feeding). For each question, participants were asked "Do you have any difficulty doing this?": no difficulty; having some difficulty, but can still do it; need help to do it; cannot do it at all; and unknown. Participants who chose "need help to do it" or "cannot do it at all" in at least one of the five activities were defined as ADL disability [23].

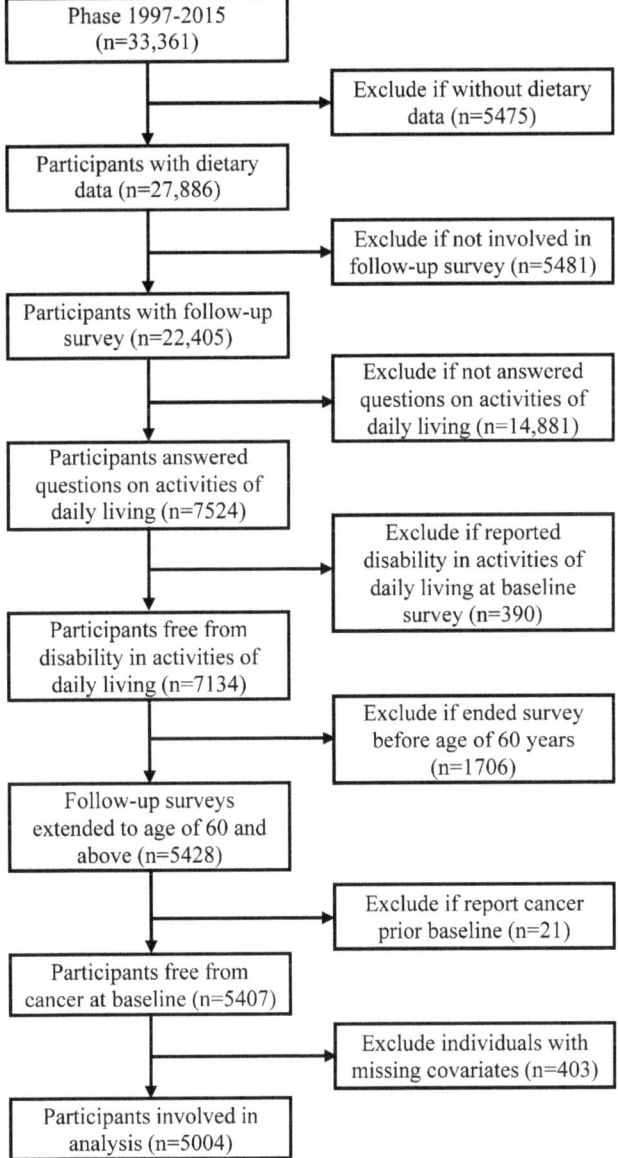

Figure 1. Flow chart of sample selection.

2.4. Covariates

Information on sociodemographic characteristics, lifestyle behaviors, and personal health and medical history were collected in the CHNS. Baseline age, gender, living region, residency, education level, per capita household income, smoking status, alcohol consumption, physical activity, body mass index (BMI), and medical history (cancer, hypertension, diabetes, stroke, and myocardial infarction) were obtained from the phase at entry.

Per capita household income was estimated at each phase, and missing values for per capita household income was replaced by the medians of each survey site. Income was grouped into tertiles and was labeled as low, middle, and high at each phase. Physical activity was measured in terms of metabolic equivalent of task (MET)-hours per week [24]. Missing values for height and weight were replaced by the means of two adjacent surveys. BMI was computed as weight (kg)/(height (m))^2. Since blood pressure was measured, participants who had been previously diagnosed with hypertension or with systolic blood pressure ≥ 140 mmHg and/or diastolic blood pressure ≥ 90 mmHg were all regarded as hypertensive patients. Other medical histories were based on the self-report from participants. Comorbidity was defined as having at least one of the four diseases (hypertension, diabetes, stroke, and myocardial infarction) at the baseline survey.

2.5. Statistics

Continuous variables were presented as means and standard deviations or medians and quartiles according to the distribution of data; categorical variables were presented as percentages. Normally distributed continuous variables were tested between groups by one-way analysis of variance, for categorical variables, chi-square tests were performed for difference across groups. To estimate the trends of nutrient intakes across DDS tertiles (T1, T2, T3), linear regression models were conducted. We assigned the midpoint values of DDS tertiles and treated the variables as continuous in the linear regression model. Values of nutrient intakes were transformed to log to reach normality.

Person years were measured from baseline survey date until the last survey date (report of ADL disability, loss to follow-up, or the phase of 2015, whichever occurred first). To assess the effect of DDS on the risk of ADL disability, hazard ratios (HRs) for DDS and ADL disability were estimated by Cox proportional hazard regression models. Multivariate models were conducted. In the first model, covariates including age at entry (continuous), gender (men or women), living region (southern or northern China), residency (urban or rural), income (low, middle, or high), and education level (primary school and below or middle school and higher) were adjusted. In the second model, smoking status (smoker or not), physical activity (≤100 or >100 MET-hours/week), BMI (continuous), and comorbidity (yes or no) were additionally adjusted.

Sensitivity analyses were performed by (1) excluding individuals whose follow-up time was less than 5 years and (2) the adjustment of alcohol consumption (regular consumer or not) and phase at entry (1997, 2000, 2004, 2006, 2009, or 2011). Subgroup analyses were conducted in participants with different baseline characteristics (gender, living region, age at entry (≤65 or >65 years old), and comorbidity).

To assess the short-term and the long-term effects of DDS on ADL disability, we analyze the DDS value reported in different surveys with the odds of ADL disability. Individuals involved in three or more dietary surveys were included. Logistic regression models were performed to estimate the odds ratios for the average DDS across phases, the baseline DDS, and the recent DDS prior to the end of the survey in relation to ADL disability, respectively.

All the statistics were conducted in R 4.0.2. All p values were two-sided, and statistical significance was defined as $p < 0.05$.

3. Results

3.1. Dietary Diversity Score and Baseline Characteristics

The average DDS among participants was 3.78 ± 1.04 (ranged from 1.33 to 8.00). Table 1 presented the baseline characteristics of participants according to DDS tertiles. Compared with individuals in the lowest tertile of DDS, those scoring higher in DDS were older when they entered the survey, had a higher proportion of men, had higher BMI, were more likely to live in southern China and urban areas, had higher education level and income, were less likely to be a smoker, and had lower physical activity. The distribution of DDS was similar in regular alcohol drinkers and the others.

Table 1. Baseline characteristics of participants according to dietary diversity score (DDS) tertiles.

Variables	DDS Tertiles [a]			p
	T1	T2	T3	
Number of participants	1663	1663	1678	
Age at entry (years)	57.6 ± 9.6	58.1 ± 9.8	60.3 ± 8.9	<0.001
Body mass index (kg/m^2)	22.2 ± 3.3	23.1 ± 3.4	24.2 ± 3.3	<0.001
Gender				
Men	44.4	48.2	49.0	0.016
Women	55.6	51.8	51.0	
Living region				
Southern China	57.7	71.9	63.5	<0.001
Northern China	42.3	28.1	36.5	
Residency				
Rural	82.9	61.3	30.5	<0.001
Urban	17.1	38.7	69.5	
Education level				<0.001
Primary school or below	86.0	70.8	40.0	
Middle school or higher	14.0	29.2	60.0	
Income [b]				
Low	51.7	26.8	9.8	<0.001
Middle	31.6	36.7	23.4	
High	16.7	36.5	66.9	
Smoking status				
Smoker	32.7	31.7	25.4	<0.001
Non-smoker	67.3	68.3	74.6	
Alcohol consumption				
Regular drinker	23.4	26.7	24.9	0.101
Others	76.6	73.3	75.1	
Physical activity (MET-hours per week)				
≤100	40.4	55.3	64.7	<0.001
>100	59.6	44.7	35.3	

MET, metabolic equivalent of task. Continuous variables were presented as means and standard deviations, and categorical variables were presented as percentages. Continuous variables were tested between groups by one-way analysis of variance, and categorical variables were tested by chi-square test. [a] DDSs were grouped into tertiles from low to high (T1, T2, T3). [b] Per capita household incomes were grouped into tertiles at each phase and was labeled as low, middle, and high, respectively.

3.2. Dietary Diversity Score and Nutrient Intakes

DDS was positively associated with intakes of protein, fat, dietary fiber, vitamin A, riboflavin, niacin, vitamin C, vitamin E, calcium, phosphorus, potassium, magnesium, iron, zinc, and selenium. Meanwhile, higher DDS was inversely associated with intakes of carbohydrate, sodium, and manganese (Table 2).

Table 2. Nutrient intakes across dietary diversity score (DDS) tertiles.

Nutrients	DDS Tertiles [a]		
	T1	T2	T3
Protein (g/d)	55.3 (45.6, 66.2)	61.1 (51.7, 71.8)	69.1 (58.2, 82.8)
Fat (g/d)	55.9 (42.8, 72.2)	73.2 (58.1, 92.3)	81.1 (64.1, 100.0)
Carbohydrate (g/d)	329.3 (265.4, 390.7)	286.4 (233.7, 340.6)	252.2 (202.0, 302.5)
Insoluble dietary fiber (g/d)	10.8 (8.0, 14.2)	9.4 (7.1, 12.5)	11.0 (8.2, 14.7)
Vitamin A (μgRE/d)	263.1 (156.0, 418.3)	391.0 (255.7, 627.4)	473.2 (323.5, 696.1)
Thiamin (mg/d)	0.9 (0.7, 1.1)	0.9 (0.7, 1.0)	0.9 (0.7, 1.1)
Riboflavin (mg/d)	0.6 (0.5, 0.7)	0.7 (0.6, 0.8)	0.8 (0.7, 1.0)
Niacin (mg/d)	12.2 (9.7, 14.8)	13.7 (11.0, 16.5)	14.5 (11.6, 17.8)
Vitamin C (mg/d)	74.6 (52.9, 100.1)	74.9 (55.2, 99.8)	80.2 (57.5, 108.0)
Vitamin E (mg/d)	26.8 (18.0, 37.3)	26.9 (19.5, 37.6)	31.0 (22.6, 41.9)
Calcium (mg/d)	315.8 (245.6, 393.1)	347.1 (275.3, 442.1)	453.8 (350.5, 591.0)

Table 2. Cont.

Nutrients	DDS Tertiles [a]		
	T1	T2	T3
Phosphorus (mg/d)	871.0 (701.7, 1058.0)	875.1 (738.6, 1027.7)	979.7 (832.6, 1158.6)
Potassium (mg/d)	1459.6 (1183.6, 1764.2)	1483.7 (1232.7, 1767.2)	1748.8 (1445.2, 2103.1)
Sodium (mg/d)	5066.2 (3869.7, 6714.2)	4781.3 (3693.8, 6378.6)	4637.7 (3532.3, 6133.1)
Magnesium (mg/d)	283.5 (227.7, 346.2)	266.1 (222.1, 318.9)	286.0 (236.3, 341.0)
Iron (mg/d)	19.5 (15.6, 24.0)	19.5 (16.1, 23.5)	20.5 (16.6, 25.0)
Zinc (mg/d)	9.6 (7.9, 11.5)	10.2 (8.5, 12.1)	10.7 (8.8, 12.8)
Selenium (μg/d)	30.9 (23.0, 39.1)	35.9 (29.4, 45.1)	46.0 (36.7, 57.6)
Copper (mg/d)	1.9 (1.5, 2.3)	1.7 (1.4, 2.1)	1.8 (1.4, 2.3)
Manganese (mg/d)	6.3 (5.0, 7.6)	5.7 (4.6, 6.9)	5.2 (4.2, 6.4)

Values are medians and quartiles. Tests for linear trend across DDS tertiles were conducted by assigning the midpoint values of DDS and treating the variables as continuous in a linear regression model, prior to that, the values of nutrient intakes were transformed to log to reach normality. All nutrients were associated with DDS tertiles with p-trend < 0.001, except for dietary fiber (p-trend = 0.041), thiamin (p-trend = 0.260), magnesium (p-trend = 0.033), and copper (p-trend = 0.138). [a] DDSs were grouped into tertiles from low to high (T1, T2, T3).

3.3. Dietary Diversity Score and Disability in Activities of Daily Living

During a median follow-up of 9 years (ranged from 2 to 18; total person years: 52,297), 601 ADL was reported. Absolute ADL rates according to DDS tertiles (from low to high: T1, T2, T3) were 14.4, 10.5, and 8.7 per 1000 person years, respectively. After the adjustment of covariates, higher DDS was associated with decreased risk of ADL disability (Table 3).

Table 3. Association between dietary diversity score (DDS) and disability in activities of daily living (ADL).

	Continuous DDS	DDS Tertiles [a]			
		T1	T2	T3	p-Trend
n of ADL disability	601	281	194	126	
n of person years	52,297	19,458	18,414	14,425	
Crude	0.86 (0.78, 0.94)	1.00	0.82 (0.68, 0.98)	0.74 (0.60, 0.91)	0.003
Model 1	0.73 (0.65, 0.82)	1.00	0.81 (0.67, 0.99)	0.53 (0.41, 0.69)	<0.001
Model 2	0.71 (0.63, 0.80)	1.00	0.80 (0.65, 0.97)	0.50 (0.39, 0.66)	<0.001

Values were hazard ratios and 95% confidence intervals unless specified. Hazard ratios were estimated by Cox proportional regression models. Multivariate models were adjusted for: Model 1: age at entry (continuous), gender (men or women), living region (southern or northern China), residency (urban or rural), income (low, middle, or high), and education level (primary school and below or middle school and higher); Model 2: additionally included smoking status (smoker or not), physical activity (≤100 or >100 metabolic equivalent of task-hours/week), body mass index (continuous), and comorbidities (no or yes). Tests for trend were performed by assigning the midpoints of each DDS tertiles and treating the value as continuous in a separate regression model. [a] DDSs were grouped into tertiles from low to high (T1, T2, T3).

3.4. Sensitivity Analyses

In the sensitivity analysis, the association of DDS with ADL disability did not change by excluding individuals whose follow-up time was less than 5 years, or additional adjustment of alcohol consumption and phase at entry (Table S1).

3.5. Subgroup Analyses

The significant association between DDS and ADL disability was observed in all subgroups based on baseline characteristics, including gender, living region, age at entry, and comorbidity. However, the association was more pronounced in participants living in southern China, participants aged over 65 years at entry, and participants without comorbidities than the others. A significant interaction term between DDS and comorbidity was observed (Figure 2).

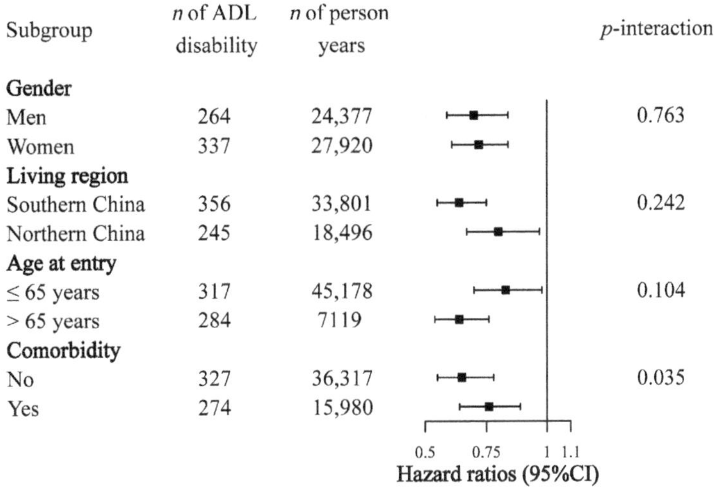

Subgroup	n of ADL disability	n of person years		p-interaction
Gender				
Men	264	24,377		0.763
Women	337	27,920		
Living region				
Southern China	356	33,801		0.242
Northern China	245	18,496		
Age at entry				
≤ 65 years	317	45,178		0.104
> 65 years	284	7119		
Comorbidity				
No	327	36,317		0.035
Yes	274	15,980		

 0.5   0.75   1 1.1
Hazard ratios (95%CI)

Figure 2. Subgroup analysis of association of continuous dietary diversity score (DDS) with disability in activities of daily living (ADL). Hazard ratios were estimated by Cox proportional regression models. Multivariate models were adjusted for age at entry (continuous), gender (men or women), living region (southern or northern China), residency (urban or rural), income (low, middle, or high), education level (primary school and below or middle school and higher), smoking status (smoker or not), physical activity (≤100 or >100 metabolic equivalent of task-hours/week), body mass index (continuous), and comorbidities (no or yes). Analyses within subgroups were adjusted for all other covariates.

3.6. Dietary Exposure Measures

We found both the average DDS across phases and the baseline DDS were associated with lower odds of ADL disability. The association was more pronounced for the average DDS. The association between the recent DDS prior to the end of the survey and ADL disability was insignificant (Figure 3).

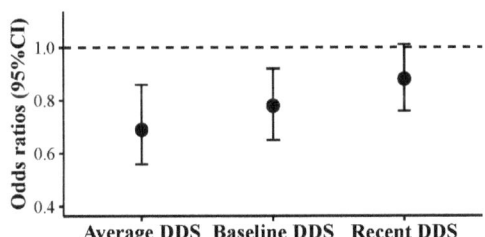

Figure 3. Dietary diversity score (DDS) at different surveys and disability in activities of daily living (ADL). Participants involved in three or more dietary surveys were included (n = 2756). Average DDS was the cumulative mean DDS from baseline to the phase prior to the end of the survey (report of disability in activities of daily living, loss to follow-up, the phase of 2015, whichever occurred first). Baseline DDS was obtained from the phase at entry. Recent DDS was obtained from the phase before the end of the survey. All DDSs were continuous. Odds ratios were estimated by logistic regression models. Models were adjusted for age at entry (continuous), gender (men or women), living region (southern or northern China), residency (urban or rural), income (low, middle, or high), education level (primary school and below or middle school and higher), smoking status (smoker or not), physical activity (≤100 or >100 metabolic equivalent of task-hours/week), body mass index (continuous), and comorbidities (no or yes).

4. Discussion

This study found that higher DDS was inversely associated with the risk of ADL disability in Chinese adults. The association was stable after the adjustment of physical activity, BMI, and comorbidity. To our best knowledge, the present study is the first one revealing the beneficial effect of dietary diversity on ADL disability.

In the western population, the Mediterranean diet is most frequently investigated when addressing the effect of dietary patterns on functional capacity. A meta-analysis showed that higher adherence to the Mediterranean diet is associated with decreased risk of frailty and functional disability in the elderly [25]. Besides, adherence to the healthy eating index may be also associated with better physical performance among elderly people [26]. In the eastern population, prospective studies found the Japanese diet was inversely associated with functional disability in Japanese individuals aged 65 years and above [27,28]. In contrast, evidence on DDS and ADL or functional capacity is relatively limited. We only observed one study that reported an insignificant relationship between DDS and higher-level functional capacity [29]. Our study found an inverse association between DDS and the risk of ADL disability based on a population-based cohort study. We believe this work will make contributions to literature on healthy aging. Besides, compared with the approach of dietary pattern assessment, the DDS approach is easier to compute, more suitable for comparison across different populations, and more appropriate to use for guiding people to follow a healthy diet. This work will contribute to the prevention of ADL disability.

Our study observed that each additional point on DDS was associated with a nearly thirty percent reduction in the risk of ADL disability. The benefits of DDS on ADL might be related to the following mechanisms. First, aging is associated with a loss of muscle mass, leading to frailty, sarcopenia, and functional disability [30]. More dietary protein is needed for the maintenance of good muscle function in the elderly [30,31]. Epidemiological studies showed that higher dietary protein may slow down the process of muscle mass loss [32–34]. Our study found individuals with higher DDS had higher intakes of protein, which may be a benefit for ADL independence. Second, it has been widely recognized that inflammation and oxidative stress played important roles in the process of aging [35,36]. We observed a positive trend between DDS and intakes of antioxidants (e.g., vitamin E, vitamin C, selenium) among the study population. Higher DDS may promote healthier aging by countering inflammation and oxidative stress. Third, aging is also caused by the loss of bone mass [37], which may increase the risk of frailty and fracture and eventually accelerate the loss of ADL independence [38–40]. In this study, we observed that participants with higher DDS enjoyed high intakes of protein, calcium, phosphorus, potassium, which were beneficial to bone health [41]. Fourth, a diverse diet has a positive effect on gut microbiota [42]. Healthy gut microbiota may promote the absorption of micronutrients and modulate individual response to dietary protein [31,43].

An interaction between DDS and comorbidity on the risk of ADL disability was observed in this study. The association of DDS with ADL disability was more pronounced among participants without comorbidity at baseline than those with comorbidity. We assumed that this might be because, among participants with comorbidity, the progression of disease played a more important role in the loss of ADL independence than the impact of diet. However, we should note that, even in individuals with comorbidity, the beneficial effect of DDS still existed.

In this study, we calculated the cumulative average DDS to address participants' long-term dietary exposure. To compare the difference between different dietary exposure measures, we estimated the OR for the average DDS across phases, the baseline DDS, and the recent DDS prior to the end of the survey in relation to ADL disability. The results indicate that when estimating the effect of DDS on ADL disability, the average DDS is the most pronounced of the three approaches, which is consistent with previous studies [44,45]. The result indicates that, in estimating the effect of dietary factors on ADL, long-term dietary exposure is more important than the recent exposure. Findings also implicated that the measure that could address the dynamic dietary exposure is more preferable to the single baseline data.

The strengths of this study include prospective design and population-based samples, which provided advantages for causal inference. Repeated dietary surveys allowed us to capture participants' long-term dietary exposure. There are several limitations. First, although comorbidities were considered in our analysis, other factors that may influence ADL (e.g., dementia, accident) were not included because of a lack of data. Second, the present study was based on a dynamic cohort study, participants joined the survey at a wide age range; however, in the subgroup and sensitivity analyses, we took participants' age at entry and phase at entry into consideration, which could partly mark up for this defect. Third, the ADL disability was self-reported. Participants might overestimate or underestimate their abilities to finish some tasks because of social desirability or misunderstanding.

5. Conclusions

In summary, this study found that higher DDS has a beneficial effect on the risk of ADL disability and long-term dietary exposure is more preferable in the investigation of DDS and ADL.

Supplementary Materials: The following are available online at http://www.mdpi.com/2072-6643/12/11/3263/s1, Table S1: Sensitivity analysis of association of dietary diversity score (DDS) with disability in activities of daily living (ADL).

Author Contributions: Conceptualization, J.Z. and A.Z.; methodology, J.Z., W.W. and Z.R.; writing—original draft preparation, J.Z. and A.Z.; writing—review and editing, C.Y., P.W. and Y.Z.; supervision, Y.Z. All authors have read and agreed to the published version of the manuscript.

Funding: This research received no external funding.

Acknowledgments: This research uses data from the CHNS. We thank the National Institute for Nutrition and Health, China Center for Disease Control and Prevention, Carolina Population Center (P2C HD050924, T32 HD007168), the University of North Carolina at Chapel Hill, the NIH (R01-HD30880, DK056350, R24 HD050924, and R01-HD38700) and the NIH Fogarty International Center (D43 TW009077, D43 TW007709) for financial support for the CHNS data collection and analysis files from 1989 to 2015 and future surveys, and the China-Japan Friendship Hospital, Ministry of Health for support for CHNS 2009, Chinese National Human Genome Center at Shanghai since 2009, and Beijing Municipal Center for Disease Prevention and Control since 2011.

Conflicts of Interest: The authors declare no conflict of interest.

References

1. World Health Organization. Ageing and Health. Available online: https://www.who.int/en/news-room/fact-sheets/detail/ageing-and-health (accessed on 22 September 2020).
2. United Nations, Department of Economic and Social Affairs, Population Division (2020). *World Population Ageing 2019 (ST/ESA/SER.A/444)*. Available online: https://www.un.org/development/desa/pd/sites/www.un.org.development.desa.pd/files/files/documents/2020/Jan/un_2019_worldpopulationageing_report.pdf (accessed on 1 October 2020).
3. Gault, M.L.; Willems, M.E. Aging, functional capacity and eccentric exercise training. *Aging Dis.* **2013**, *4*, 351–363. [CrossRef] [PubMed]
4. Morley, J.E. An Overview of Cognitive Impairment. *Clin. Geriatr. Med.* **2018**, *34*, 505–513. [CrossRef] [PubMed]
5. Carmona-Torres, J.M.; Rodriguez-Borrego, M.A.; Laredo-Aguilera, J.A.; Lopez-Soto, P.J.; Santacruz-Salas, E.; Cobo-Cuenca, A.I. Disability for basic and instrumental activities of daily living in older individuals. *PLoS ONE* **2019**, *14*, e0220157. [CrossRef] [PubMed]
6. Deyhoul, N.; Vasli, P.; Rohani, C.; Shakeri, N.; Hosseini, M. The effect of family-centered empowerment program on the family caregiver burden and the activities of daily living of Iranian patients with stroke: A randomized controlled trial study. *Aging Clin. Exp. Res.* **2020**, *32*, 1343–1352. [CrossRef]
7. Millan-Calenti, J.C.; Tubio, J.; Pita-Fernandez, S.; Gonzalez-Abraldes, I.; Lorenzo, T.; Fernandez-Arruty, T.; Maseda, A. Prevalence of functional disability in activities of daily living (ADL), instrumental activities of daily living (IADL) and associated factors, as predictors of morbidity and mortality. *Arch. Gerontol. Geriatr.* **2010**, *50*, 306–310. [CrossRef] [PubMed]
8. Fried, T.R.; Bradley, E.H.; Williams, C.S.; Tinetti, M.E. Functional disability and health care expenditures for older persons. *Arch. Intern. Med.* **2001**, *161*, 2602–2607. [CrossRef]

9. Mlinac, M.E.; Feng, M.C. Assessment of Activities of Daily Living, Self-Care, and Independence. *Arch. Clin. Neuropsychol.* **2016**, *31*, 506–516. [CrossRef]
10. Yan, M.; Qin, T.; Yin, P. Disabilities in activities of daily living and in instrumental activities of daily living among older adults in China, 2011–2015: A longitudinal cohort study. *Lancet* **2019**, *394*, S82. [CrossRef]
11. van Het Bolscher-Niehuis, M.J.; den Ouden, M.E.; de Vocht, H.M.; Francke, A.L. Effects of self-management support programmes on activities of daily living of older adults: A systematic review. *Int. J. Nurs. Stud.* **2016**, *61*, 230–247. [CrossRef]
12. Vermeulen, J.; Neyens, J.C.L.; van Rossum, E.; Spreeuwenberg, M.D.; de Witte, L.P. Predicting ADL disability in community-dwelling elderly people using physical frailty indicators: A systematic review. *BMC Geriatr.* **2011**, *11*, 33. [CrossRef]
13. Yoshida, D.; Ohara, T.; Hata, J.; Shibata, M.; Hirakawa, Y.; Honda, T.; Uchida, K.; Takasugi, S.; Kitazono, T.; Kiyohara, Y.; et al. Dairy consumption and risk of functional disability in an elderly Japanese population: The Hisayama Study. *Am. J. Clin. Nutr.* **2019**, *109*, 1664–1671. [CrossRef]
14. Alekna, V.; Kilaite, J.; Mastaviciute, A.; Tamulaitiene, M. Vitamin D Level and Activities of Daily Living in Octogenarians: Cross-Sectional Study. *Front. Endocrinol. (Lausanne)* **2018**, *9*, 326. [CrossRef] [PubMed]
15. Gopinath, B.; Flood, V.M.; Burlutksy, G.; Liew, G.; Mitchell, P. Carbohydrate nutrition variables and risk of disability in instrumental activities of daily living. *Eur. J. Nutr.* **2019**, *58*, 3221–3228. [CrossRef]
16. Chinese Nutrition Society. *Chinese Dietary Guidelines*; People's Medical Publishing House Co., LTD: Beijing, China, 2016.
17. Conklin, A.I.; Monsivais, P.; Khaw, K.T.; Wareham, N.J.; Forouhi, N.G. Dietary Diversity, Diet Cost, and Incidence of Type 2 Diabetes in the United Kingdom: A Prospective Cohort Study. *PLoS Med.* **2016**, *13*, e1002085. [CrossRef] [PubMed]
18. Otsuka, R.; Nishita, Y.; Tange, C.; Tomida, M.; Kato, Y.; Nakamoto, M.; Imai, T.; Ando, F.; Shimokata, H. Dietary diversity decreases the risk of cognitive decline among Japanese older adults. *Geriatr. Gerontol. Int.* **2017**, *17*, 937–944. [CrossRef]
19. Otsuka, R.; Tange, C.; Nishita, Y.; Kato, Y.; Tomida, M.; Imai, T.; Ando, F.; Shimokata, H. Dietary Diversity and All-Cause and Cause-Specific Mortality in Japanese Community-Dwelling Older Adults. *Nutrients* **2020**, *12*. [CrossRef]
20. Tao, L.; Xie, Z.; Huang, T. Dietary diversity and all-cause mortality among Chinese adults aged 65 or older: A community-based cohort study. *Asia Pac. J. Clin. Nutr.* **2020**, *29*, 152–160. [CrossRef] [PubMed]
21. Zhang, B.; Zhai, F.Y.; Du, S.F.; Popkin, B.M. The China Health and Nutrition Survey, 1989–2011. *Obes. Rev.* **2014**, *15* (Suppl. 1), 2–7. [CrossRef]
22. Zhai, F.; Guo, X.; Popkin, B.M.; Ma, L.; Wang, Q.; Shuigao, W.Y.; Ge, J.; Keyou, G. Evaluation of the 24-hour individual recall method in China. *Food Nutr. Bull.* **1996**, *17*, 1–7. [CrossRef]
23. Liang, Y.; Welmer, A.-K.; Wang, R.; Song, A.; Fratiglioni, L.; Qiu, C. Trends in Incidence of Disability in Activities of Daily Living in Chinese Older Adults: 1993–2006. *J. Am. Geriatr. Soc.* **2017**, *65*, 306–312. [CrossRef]
24. Ng, S.W.; Norton, E.C.; Popkin, B.M. Why have physical activity levels declined among Chinese adults? Findings from the 1991-2006 China Health and Nutrition Surveys. *Soc. Sci. Med.* **2009**, *68*, 1305–1314. [CrossRef] [PubMed]
25. Silva, R.; Pizato, N.; da Mata, F.; Figueiredo, A.; Ito, M.; Pereira, M.G. Mediterranean Diet and Musculoskeletal-Functional Outcomes in Community-Dwelling Older People: A Systematic Review and Meta-Analysis. *J. Nutr. Health Aging* **2018**, *22*, 655–663. [CrossRef]
26. Xu, B.; Houston, D.K.; Locher, J.L.; Ellison, K.J.; Gropper, S.; Buys, D.R.; Zizza, C.A. Higher Healthy Eating Index-2005 scores are associated with better physical performance. *J. Gerontol. A Biol. Sci. Med. Sci.* **2012**, *67*, 93–99. [CrossRef] [PubMed]
27. Tomata, Y.; Watanabe, T.; Sugawara, Y.; Chou, W.-T.; Kakizaki, M.; Tsuji, I. Dietary Patterns and Incident Functional Disability in Elderly Japanese: The Ohsaki Cohort 2006 Study. *J. Gerontol. Ser. A* **2014**, *69*, 843–851. [CrossRef]
28. Matsuyama, S.; Zhang, S.; Tomata, Y.; Abe, S.; Tanji, F.; Sugawara, Y.; Tsuji, I. Association between improved adherence to the Japanese diet and incident functional disability in older people: The Ohsaki Cohort 2006 Study. *Clin. Nutr.* **2020**, *39*, 2238–2245. [CrossRef] [PubMed]

29. Otsuka, R.; Kato, Y.; Nishita, Y.; Tange, C.; Nakamoto, M.; Tomida, M.; Imai, T.; Ando, F.; Shimokata, H.; Suzuki, T. Dietary diversity and 14-year decline in higher-level functional capacity among middle-aged and elderly Japanese. *Nutrition* **2016**, *32*, 784–789. [CrossRef]
30. Welch, A.A. Nutritional influences on age-related skeletal muscle loss. *Proc. Nutr. Soc.* **2014**, *73*, 16–33. [CrossRef] [PubMed]
31. Ni Lochlainn, M.; Bowyer, R.C.E.; Steves, C.J. Dietary Protein and Muscle in Aging People: The Potential Role of the Gut Microbiome. *Nutrients* **2018**, *10*. [CrossRef]
32. Landi, F.; Calvani, R.; Tosato, M.; Martone, A.M.; Picca, A.; Ortolani, E.; Savera, G.; Salini, S.; Ramaschi, M.; Bernabei, R.; et al. Animal-Derived Protein Consumption Is Associated with Muscle Mass and Strength in Community-Dwellers: Results from the Milan EXPO Survey. *J. Nutr. Health Aging* **2017**, *21*, 1050–1056. [CrossRef]
33. Houston, D.K.; Nicklas, B.J.; Ding, J.; Harris, T.B.; Tylavsky, F.A.; Newman, A.B.; Lee, J.S.; Sahyoun, N.R.; Visser, M.; Kritchevsky, S.B. Dietary protein intake is associated with lean mass change in older, community-dwelling adults: The Health, Aging, and Body Composition (Health ABC) Study. *Am. J. Clin. Nutr.* **2008**, *87*, 150–155. [CrossRef]
34. McGrath, R.; Stastny, S.; Casperson, S.; Jahns, L.; Roemmich, J.; Hackney, K.J. Daily Protein Intake and Distribution of Daily Protein Consumed Decreases Odds for Functional Disability in Older Americans. *J. Aging Health* **2019**. [CrossRef]
35. Bektas, A.; Schurman, S.H.; Sen, R.; Ferrucci, L. Aging, inflammation and the environment. *Exp. Gerontol.* **2018**, *105*, 10–18. [CrossRef]
36. Liguori, I.; Russo, G.; Curcio, F.; Bulli, G.; Aran, L.; Della-Morte, D.; Gargiulo, G.; Testa, G.; Cacciatore, F.; Bonaduce, D.; et al. Oxidative stress, aging, and diseases. *Clin. Interv. Aging* **2018**, *13*, 757–772. [CrossRef]
37. Adams, D.J.; Rowe, D.W.; Ackert-Bicknell, C.L. Genetics of aging bone. *Mamm. Genome* **2016**, *27*, 367–380. [CrossRef]
38. Ettinger, M.P. Aging bone and osteoporosis: Strategies for preventing fractures in the elderly. *Arch. Intern. Med.* **2003**, *163*, 2237–2246. [CrossRef] [PubMed]
39. Alegre-Lopez, J.; Cordero-Guevara, J.; Alonso-Valdivielso, J.L.; Fernandez-Melon, J. Factors associated with mortality and functional disability after hip fracture: An inception cohort study. *Osteoporos. Int.* **2005**, *16*, 729–736. [CrossRef]
40. Craik, R.L. Disability Following Hip Fracture. *Phys. Ther.* **1994**, *74*, 387–398. [CrossRef]
41. Cashman, K.D. Diet, nutrition, and bone health. *J. Nutr.* **2007**, *137*, 2507s–2512s. [CrossRef] [PubMed]
42. Heiman, M.L.; Greenway, F.L. A healthy gastrointestinal microbiome is dependent on dietary diversity. *Mol. Metab.* **2016**, *5*, 317–320. [CrossRef] [PubMed]
43. Rowland, I.; Gibson, G.; Heinken, A.; Scott, K.; Swann, J.; Thiele, I.; Tuohy, K. Gut microbiota functions: Metabolism of nutrients and other food components. *Eur. J. Nutr.* **2018**, *57*, 1–24. [CrossRef]
44. Yuan, C.; Fondell, E.; Ascherio, A.; Okereke, O.I.; Grodstein, F.; Hofman, A.; Willett, W.C. Long-Term Intake of Dietary Carotenoids Is Positively Associated with Late-Life Subjective Cognitive Function in a Prospective Study in US Women. *J. Nutr.* **2020**, *150*, 1871–1879. [CrossRef]
45. Hu, F.B.; Stampfer, M.J.; Rimm, E.; Ascherio, A.; Rosner, B.A.; Spiegelman, D.; Willett, W.C. Dietary fat and coronary heart disease: A comparison of approaches for adjusting for total energy intake and modeling repeated dietary measurements. *Am. J. Epidemiol.* **1999**, *149*, 531–540. [CrossRef] [PubMed]

Publisher's Note: MDPI stays neutral with regard to jurisdictional claims in published maps and institutional affiliations.

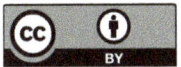

© 2020 by the authors. Licensee MDPI, Basel, Switzerland. This article is an open access article distributed under the terms and conditions of the Creative Commons Attribution (CC BY) license (http://creativecommons.org/licenses/by/4.0/).

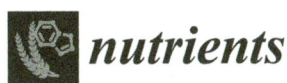

Article

Impact of the Serum Level of Albumin and Self-Assessed Chewing Ability on Mortality, QOL, and ADLs for Community-Dwelling Older Adults at the Age of 85: A 15 Year Follow up Study

Yoshiaki Nomura [1,*], Erika Kakuta [2], Ayako Okada [1], Ryoko Otsuka [1], Mieko Shimada [3], Yasuko Tomizawa [4], Chieko Taguchi [5], Kazumune Arikawa [5], Hideki Daikoku [6], Tamotsu Sato [6] and Nobuhiro Hanada [1]

1. Department of Translational Research, Tsurumi University School of Dental Medicine, Yokohama 230-8501, Japan; okada-a@tsurumi-u.ac.jp (A.O.); otsuka-ryoko@tsurumi-u.ac.jp (R.O.); hanada-n@tsurumi-u.ac.jp (N.H.)
2. Department of Oral bacteriology, Tsurumi University School of Dental Medicine, Yokohama 230-8501, Japan; kakuta-erika@tsurumi-u.ac.jp
3. Chiba Prefectural University of Health Sciences, Chiba 261-0014, Japan; mieko.shimada@cpuhs.ac.jp
4. Department of Cardiovascular Surgery, Tokyo Women's Medical University, Tokyo 162-8666, Japan; tomizawa.yasuko@twmu.ac.jp
5. Department of Preventive and Public Oral Health, Nihon University School of Dentistry at Matsudo, Matsudo 470-2101, Japan; taguchi.chieko@nihon-u.ac.jp (C.T.); arikawa.kazumune@nihon-u.ac.jp (K.A.)
6. Iwate Dental Association, Morioka 020-0045, Japan; dai-koku@nifty.com (H.D.); tamosato-dent@k-2inc.jp (T.S.)
* Correspondence: nomura-y@tsurumi-u.ac.jp; Tel.: +81-45-580-8462

Received: 9 October 2020; Accepted: 27 October 2020; Published: 29 October 2020

Abstract: Quality of life (QOL) and mortality are true endpoints of epidemiological or medical research, especially for community-dwelling older adults. Nutritional status and activities of daily living (ADLs) are associated with QOL and mortality. Good oral health status supports a good nutritional status. The aim of this study was to elucidate the complex structure of these important health-related factors. We surveyed 354 healthy older adults at the age of 85. Nutritional status was evaluated by the serum level of albumin. QOL, ADLs, self-assessed chewing ability, serum albumin level, and mortality during the 15 year follow up period were analyzed. Self-assessed chewing ability was associated with QOL and ADLs. Self-assessed chewing ability for slight-hard foods was associated with mortality in men. However, it was not associated with the serum albumin level. The serum albumin level was associated with mortality in women. These results indicate that maintaining good oral function is not enough. Nutritional instruction in accordance with oral function is indispensable for health promotion in older adults. When planning health promotion strategies for older adults, different strategies are needed for men and women.

Keywords: mortality; QOL; ADL; Serum albumin; self-assessed chewing ability

1. Introduction

Super-aging societies face many challenges, such as the use of the social security system to access optimal medical services and health services. These services are required to improve quality of life (QOL) and extend life expectancy [1–3]. QOL and life expectancy are multifactorial. Knowledge of nutrition and practice of a healthy diet are considered to be the most important factors affecting the health and quality of life of older adults [4,5]. Nutritional interventions for community-dwelling older adults are effective for the promotion of health [6–8].

Quality of life (QOL) and mortality are true endpoints of epidemiological studies or medical research. Several studies have focused on the effect of nutritional status on QOL for subjects with specific diseases [9–11]. To the best of our knowledge, no study has investigated the effect of nutritional status on QOL for the community-dwelling older adults.

The effect of nutritional status on mortality in community-dwelling older adults is well documented [12–14]. Serum level of albumin, which reflects the nutritional status, is a well-known predictor of mortality [15–20]. It is applicable for community-dwelling older adults [21,22]. In addition, nutritional status is associated with activities of daily living (ADLs). Evidence concerning nutritional status and ALD for subjects with specific conditions is also accumulating [23–25].

Oral health is an important factor in maintaining a healthy nutritional status. Oral functions, especially mastication, are associated with nutritional status. Food preferences depend on masticatory efficiency [26,27]. Overconsumption of carbohydrate-rich foods affects mortality. Excess intake of carbohydrate-rich food is associated with the consumption of excess processed food and not enough raw healthy food [28–30]. Oral functions, are key elements in maintaining a healthy nutritional status. However, a systematic review concluded that further study including demographically diverse samples is necessary [31]. For the evaluation of masticatory function, specific devices have been improved to aid in clinical diagnosis [32]. For epidemiological studies, simple questionnaires have been used. By using simple questionnaires, evidence that oral health affects mortality has been accumulated. However, the follow up period used in such studies was short and the age range of the population studied was broad.

Nutritional status and oral health may be associated with mortality, QOL, and ADLs. These variables interact with each other. Revealing the complexity of these interactions may lead to better understanding of health-related problems.

Ministry of Health and Labor in Japan directed the 8020 Data Bank Survey at four prefectures in 1997. The aim of this survey was to gather evidence that older adults with their own 20 teeth are active and healthy. In 2002, a five-year follow up study was conducted at Iwate prefecture located in the northeast of Japan. In this follow up survey, the Short form 36 (SF36) [33–35] and the Tokyo Metropolitan Institute of Gerontology Index (TMIG index) [36] were introduced. These questionnaires are validated questionnaires for the evaluation of QOL and ADL. In addition, in 2017, a follow up survey was conducted to investigate the mortality of the participants.

In this study, by using 15-year follow up data from older adults at the age of 85, we investigated the effect of nutritional status, as evaluated by serum level albumin and self-assessed chewing ability, on IADL, QOL, and mortality. The aim of this study was to elucidate the complex relationships among these important health-related factors.

2. Materials and Methods

2.1. Setting

A 15-year follow-up study was conducted with subjects aged 85 years old (from 2002 to 2017) residing in the 11 districts served by one health center in Iwate Prefecture.

2.2. Study Population and Survey Frame

In 1997, Japanese Ministry of Labor and Health directed and supported a survey of 80-year-old people residing in four areas in Japan. The details of the survey are described in our previous report [37]. In 2002, the 8020 promotion foundation, which is an affiliated organization of the Japan dental association, supported a follow up survey. Iwate Prefecture, located in the northern region of Japan, was one of the areas that participated in this survey. The sampling method was cluster sampling, and the sampling frame was a complete count survey for all subjects aged 80 years in 1997 (born in 1917) who resided in nine districts in Iwate Prefecture served by one public health center. Between

1997 and 2002, two villages were newly served by the public health center. Sixty-six subjects residing in the two areas participated in the survey conducted in 2002.

Based on residential registration, public health nurses visited homes in two districts in which subjects who participated in the survey in 1996 lived and in which 85-year-old individuals lived. Public health nurses recommended that all subjects participate in the survey. Among the 435 subjects, 349 agreed to participate, and 345 completed the survey. The surveys, including an oral examination, blood sampling, a medical interview, and a physical fitness test, were conducted at a meeting place or gymnasium owned by the local government. No institutionalized older people were included in this study. In 2017, the 8020 promotion foundation supported a follow up survey that investigated the survival rate of the participants. In October 2017, public health nurses surveyed the participants' survival and dates of death using the census register. A follow-up survey was conducted using the resident register with surviving subjects participating in the survey in 2002. Details of the follow up survey were described in our previous report [38].

2.3. Questionnaire

2.3.1. Quality of Life (QOL)

Quality of life was evaluated by the short form 36(SF-36). The Sf-36 consists of 36 items. These items are classified into 8 subscales: physical functioning (PF), role physical (RP), bodily pain (BP), general health (GH), vitality (VT), social functioning (SF), role emotional (RE), and mental health (MH).

The values of these subscales were standardized and calculated by a program provided by iHope International (Kyoto, Japan) [33–35].

2.3.2. Activities of Daily Living (ADLs)

Instrumental activity of daily living was assessed by The Tokyo Metropolitan Institute of Gerontology index of competence (TMIG index) [36]. TIMG index consists of three subscales/dimensions: self-maintenance (S.M), intellectual activity (I.A.), and social role (S.R.). These subscales consist of 5, 4, and 4 items, respectively. If subjects answered yes or able, one point was given for each item. A low IADL (≤4 points), IA (≤2 points), or SR (≤2 points) score is regarded as declining function [39,40]. The TMIG index has been widely used in epidemiological surveys [41–45].

The items included in these subscales are

S.M.: Using public transportation, shopping, preparing, meals, paying bills, managing deposits
I.A.: Filling out pension forms, reading the newspaper, reading books, becoming interested in a new story or program about health.
S.R.: Visiting friends, being called on for advice, visiting sick friends, talking to young people.

2.3.3. Self-Assessed Chewing Ability

Self-assessed chewing ability was investigated using the following question about 15 different foods: Can you chew the following 15 foods? The response was a simple dichotomous choice (yes/no). Several epidemiological studies have applied this questionnaire for the evaluation of chewing ability [37,46].

2.4. Statistical Analysis

2.4.1. Item Response Theory (IRT)

To calculate the summary score for chewing ability, a three-parameter logistic model of the item response theory (IRT) was applied. In addition, factor analysis by the major factor method with varimax rotation was carried out. Summary scores were calculated within each factor [42–49]. IRT analysis was performed using R ver3.50 with the LTR and irtoys packages.

2.4.2. Structural Equation Modeling (SEM)

Before performing structural equation modeling (SEM), factor analysis by the major factor method with varimax rotation was carried out. Based on the results of the factor analysis, latent variables were constructed. The models were modified through a comparison with the correction index to improve the fitness of the data. For the evaluation of the fitness, the root-mean-square error of approximation (RMSEA) was used for the goodness of fit index [50]. Factor analysis was carried out using SPSS Statistics ver24.0 (IBM, Tokyo, Japan) and SEM was carried out busing AMOS ver24.0 (IBM, Tokyo, Japan).

2.4.3. Generalized Linear Model

To assess the subscales and items of QOL and IADL, the generalized linear model was applied. The distribution of response and link functions was selected using Akaike's Information Criterion (AIC). The generalized linear model analysis was carried out using SPSS Statistics ver24.0 (IBM, Tokyo, Japan)

2.4.4. Survival Analysis

Survival rates were calculated using the Kaplan–Meier analysis. A log rank test was used to compare significant differences in survival curves. A Cox proportional hazards model was applied to calculate the hazard ratios. Survival analysis was carried out using SPSS Statistics ver24.0 (IBM, Tokyo, Japan)

2.5. Ethics Approval and CONSENT to Participate

Informed written consent was obtained from all of the participants at the baseline survey visit. This study was approved by the Ethics Committee of Tsurumi University School of Dental Medicine (Approval Number: 1515).

3. Results

3.1. Characteristics of the Subjects Who Participated in the Study

The study population consisted of 138 men and 205 women, who were all aged 85 in 2002. After 15 years, 12 subjects had survived. Their health status was evaluated by blood tests. The results are shown in Supplementary Table S1.

3.2. Structure of QOL, ADL, and Self-Assessed Chewing Ability of the Older Adults

3.2.1. Structure of QOL

The SF 36 consists of eight subscales. Descriptive statistics of the eight subscales are presented in Supplementary Table S2. For these subscales, factor analysis was carried out through the major factor method with varimax rotation. Factor scores were used as summary scores of the factors for the following analysis. The results are shown in Supplementary Table S3. The subscales consisted of two factors. These factors were named the function and the role. Based on this result, structural equation modeling (SEM) was carried out. The results are shown in Figure 1. Body pain (BP) and physical functioning (PF) correlated with both latent variables.

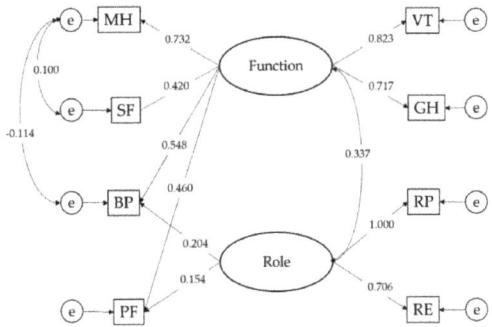

Figure 1. Structure of quality of life of the older subjects at the age of 85. The subscales of the SF 36 consisted of two latent variables, named Function and Role. All paths were statistically significant. BP and PF correlated with both latent variables. Subscales: Physical functioning (PF), Role physical (RP), Body pain (BP), General health (GH), Vitality (VT), Social functioning (SF), Role emotional (RE), Mental health (MH), e: Error variable. SF 36: 36-Item Short-Form Health Survey. REMSEA: root-mean-square error of approximation.

3.2.2. Structure of ADLs

The TIMG index consists of three subscales and has a total of 13 items. The scores of these items and the descriptive statistics of the three subscales are shown in Supplementary Tables S4 and S5. For the structure of the IADL, factor analysis and SEM were carried out in the same way as for the QOL. The results of the factor analysis are presented in Supplementary Table S6. Factor scores were used as summary scores of the factors for the following analysis. The model with SEM is shown in Figure 2. Items of the TIMG Index involved three factors. Visiting sick friends and filling out the pension form were correlated with two latent variables. Correlations between latent variables were statistically significant. However, the correlations were very weak.

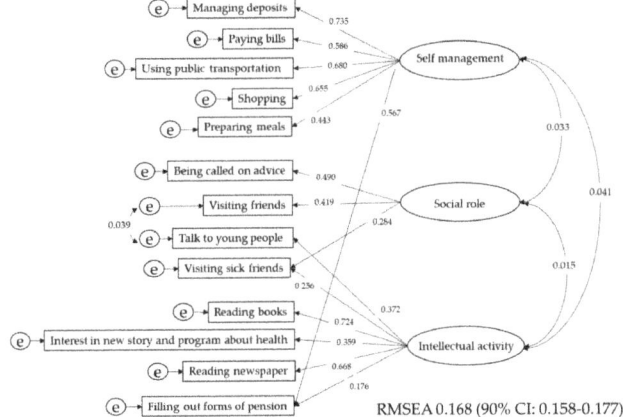

Figure 2. Structure of the ADL. Items of the TIMG Index involved 3 factors. Visiting sick friends and filling out the pension. Pension were correlated with two latent variables. Correlations between latent variables were statistically significant. However, the correlations were very weak. ADL: activity of daily living, TMIG index: The Tokyo Metropolitan Institute of Gerontology index of competence. e: Error variable. REMSEA: root-mean-square error of approximation

3.2.3. Structure of Self-Assessed Chewing Ability and Correlation with Number of Remaining Teeth

Self-assessed chewing ability was evaluated by whether participants were able to chew 15 foods. The variables were dichotomous. To calculate the summary score, the item response theory analysis (IRT) was carried out. The item response curve and item information curves are shown in Figure S1, and the model is shown in Supplementary Table S7. Similar to the QOL and IADL, a factor analysis was carried out for these 15 foods. The results are shown in Supplementary Table S8. The fifteen foods had three factors, and the factors were named easy to chew food, slightly hard to chew food, and moderate and hard to chew foods. The correlations among chewing ability, number of remaining teeth, and serum level of albumin as indicators of nutritional status were analyzed by SEM (Figure 3). The link between chewing ability and serum albumin was not statistically significant ($p = 0.692$). Other than that, all associations were statistically significant.

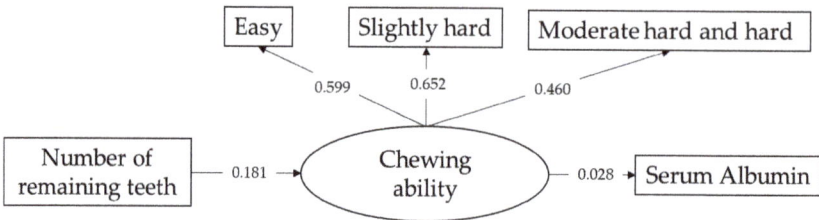

RMSEA 0.146 (90% CI: 0.123-0.170)

Figure 3. Correlations among number of remaining teeth, chewing ability, and serum level of albumin. REMSEA: root-mean-square error of approximation

3.3. Interaction of Nutritional Status, and Self-Assessed Chewing Ability with IADL and QOL

3.3.1. Correlation between Self-Assessed Chewing Ability and QOL

A generalized liner model was applied to the dimensions of QOL calculated by the factor scores presented in Section 3.2.1. The results were shown in Table 1. For both function and role, the summary score of self-assessed chewing ability was significantly correlated. However, the number of remaining teeth and serum level of albumin were not statistically significant.

Table 1. Correlations of the number of remaining teeth, serum albumin level, and self-assessed chewing ability with quality of life (QOL).

	QOL				
	Function			Role	
	Coefficient (95% CI)	p-Value	Coefficient (95% CI)	p-Value
Intercept	−0.411 (−1.839–1.018)	0.573	−0.204 (−1.671–1.262)	0.785
Number of remaining teeth	−0.002 (−0.017–0.014)	0.842	−0.006 (−0.022–0.009)	0.437
Serum Albumin (g/dL)	0.106 (−0.243–0.454)	0.553	0.060 (−0.298–0.418)	0.742
Self-assessed Chewing ability	0.336 (0.204–0.469)	<0.001	0.135 (0–0.271)	0.050

The generalized liner model was applied for the factor scores of QOL. Distribution: Normal, Link: Normal. The SF-36 consisted of eight subscales. For these subscales, the generalized linear model was applied. The results are presented in Table S9. Self-assessed chewing ability had a statistically significant correlation with PF, RP, GH, BT, and M, but not with BP, SF, or RE. The number of remaining teeth and serum level of Albumin had no correlations with the eight subscales. CI: confidence interval.

3.3.2. Correlation between Self-Assessed Chewing Ability and IADL

The TIMIG Index consists of three subscales: Self-management, Intercultural activity, and Social role. For these subscales, the generalized liner model was applied. The results were shown in Table 2. The summary score of self-assessed chewing ability calculated by IRT was significantly correlated with the three subscales. However, the number of remaining teeth and the serum level of albumin were not statistically significantly correlated with this factor.

Table 2. Correlations of the number of remaining teeth, serum albumin, and self-assessed chewing ability with the IADL.

	TMIG Index					
	Self-Management		Intercultural Activity		Social Role:	
	Coefficient (95% CI)	*p*-Value	Coefficient (95% CI)	*p*-Value	Coefficient (95% CI)	*p*-Value
Intercept	0.153 (−1.234–1.541)	0.828	0.638 (−0.785–2.062)	0.379	0.048 (−1.368–1.464)	0.947
Number of remaining teeth	−0.006 (−0.021–0.009)	0.421	0.013 (−0.002–0.028)	0.100	−0.005 (−0.020–0.010)	0.544
Serum Albumin (g/dL)	−0.015 (−0.354–0.324)	0.930	−0.160 (−0.507–0.188)	0.368	0.006 (−0.340–0.352)	0.974
Self-assessed chewing ability	0.257 (0.129–0.385)	<0.001	0.138 (0.007–0.270)	0.039	0.209 (0.079–0.340)	0.002

The generalized liner model was applied to the factor scores of the TMIG Index. Distribution: Normal, Link: Normal. TMIG index: Tokyo Metropolitan Institute of Gerontology index of competence. IADL: instrumental activity of daily living. CI: confidence interval.

3.4. Effects of Nutritional Status, Self-Asssessed Chewing Ability, and IADL on Mortality

To assess the mortality rate at the 15-year follow up, nutritional status evaluated by the serum level of albumin, subscales of self-assessed chewing ability, and the IADL were analyzed using Cox's proportional hazard model. The results are presented in Table 3.

Table 3. Hazard ratios of nutritional status, self-assessed chewing ability, and IADL.

		Men		Women	
		Hazard Ratio (95 CI)	*p*-Value	Hazard Ratio (95 CI)	*p*-Value
Nutritional status, Self-assessed chewing ability, number of remaining teeth					
Serum Albumin (<3.7 g/dL/≥3.7 g/dL)		1.294 (0.634–2.641)	0.479	2.621 (1.184–5.803)	0.018
Self-assessed Chewing ability	Moderate hard and hard	1.144 (0.853–1.534)	0.368	1.164 (0.873–1.529)	0.300
	Slight hard	1.821 (1.082–3.049)	0.024	1.149 (0.681–1.946)	0.602
	Easy	1.661 (0.876–3.155)	0.120	0.718 (0.442–1.166)	0.180
Number of remaining teeth		1.028 (0.995–1.060)	0.094	0.966 (0.925–1.009)	0.119
IADL (TMIG Index)					
Self-management (≤4 points/>5 points)		1.212 (0.774–1.898)	0.401	1.548 (0.916–2.616)	0.103
Intellectual activity (≤2 points/>3 points)		2.033 (1.271–3.398)	0.043	1.391 (0.870–2.224)	0.168
Social role (≤2 points/>3 points)		1.569 (0.995–2.475)	0.053	1.345 (0.850–2.130)	0.206

TMIG index: The Tokyo Metropolitan Institute of Gerontology index of competence. CI: confidence interval.

For women, only serum albumin level was shown to have a statistically significant effect on mortality, and its hazard ratio was the highest. In contrast, for men, the self-assessed chewing ability of moderate hard food, and intercellular activity had statistically significant effects on mortality. The number of remaining teeth did not have a statistically significant effect. However, when classified as edentulous or dentate, the hazard ratio of edentulous was statistically significant in men (hazard ratio: 1.766, 95% CI; 1.119–2.788, $p = 0.015$). Additionally, hazard ratios of chewing ability were adjusted by health status evaluated by blood tests. Results were shown in Supplementary Table S10.

For men, adjusted hazard ratios of self-assessed chewing ability were statistically significant except for Creatinine.

The Kaplan–Meier analysis was used to calculate the survival rate. As self-assessed chewing ability is a contentious variable, the ability to chew three foods (konnyaku jelly, tubular roll of boiled fish paste, and steamed rice) was used as a dichotomous variable. The means and medians of the survival rate are shown in Supplementary Table S11. The survival curves of the statistically significant factors are shown in Figure 4.

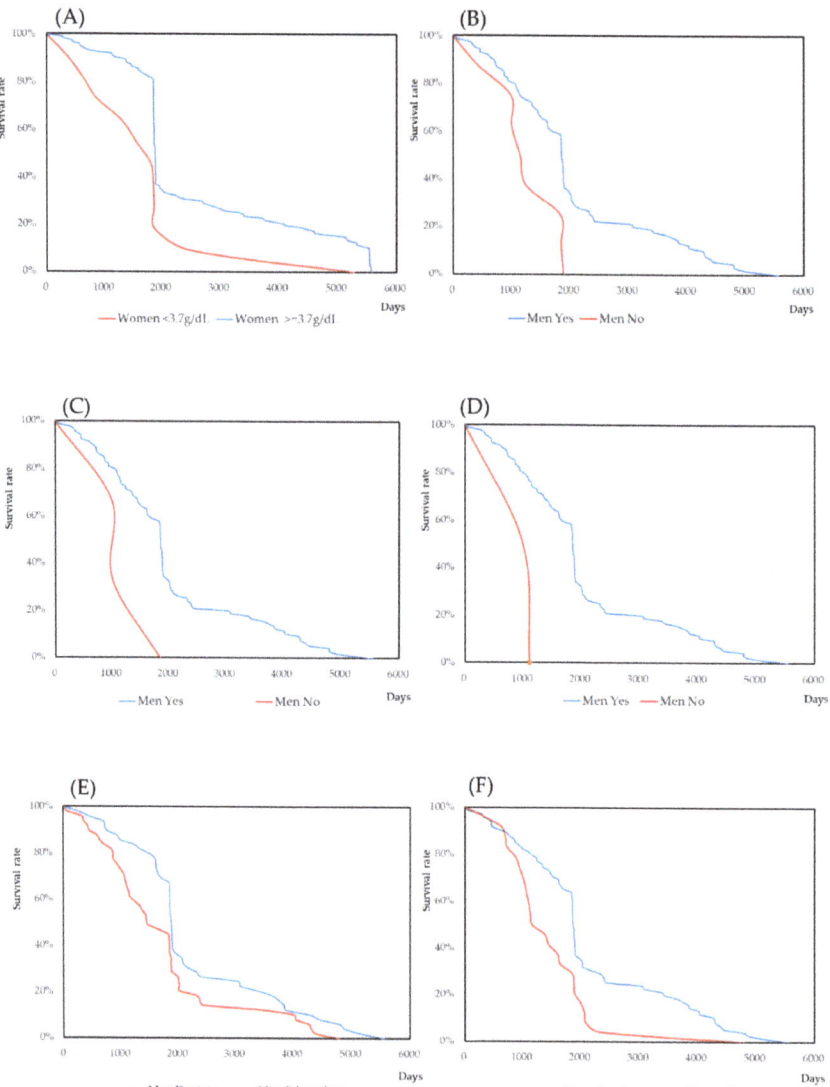

Figure 4. Survival curves of the significant factors for mortality. (**A**) Serum levels of albumin for women. (**B**) Ability to chew Konnyaku-jelly of men. (**C**) Ability to chew Tubular roll of boiled fish paste of men. (**D**) Ability to chew Steamed rice of men. (**E**) Edentulous. (**F**) Intellectual activity of men.

3.5. Overview of the Interactions Among Health-Related Factors

Finally, by using all health-related factors investigated in this study, multiple group structural equation modeling was conducted for men and women. The results are presented in Figure 5. Black lines indicated statistical significance for both men and women, blue lines indicate significance only in men, red lines indicate significance only in women, and orange lines indicated no significance for either men or women. Self-assessed chewing ability was not associated with serum albumin. ADLs were not associated with QOL.

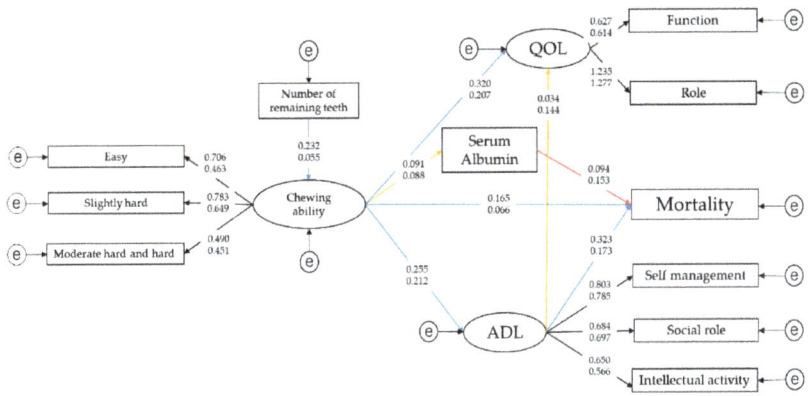

RMSEA 0.123 (90% CI: 0.114-0.131)

Figure 5. Overview of the interactions among health-related factors. Black lines indicated statistical significance for both men and women, blue lines indicate significance only in men, red lines indicate significance only in women, and orange lines indicated no significance for either men or women. e: Error variable. QOL: quality of live. ADL: activity of daily living. REMSEA: root-mean-square error of approximation.

4. Discussion

In this study, nutritional status, evaluated by the serum level of albumin, was associated with mortality in women. Self-assessed chewing ability was significantly associated with quality of life (QOL) and the instrumental activity of daily living (IADL) evaluated by the TIMG Index.

The subjects who participated in this study were functionally independent and could attend mass check-ups held at the local city hall or gymnasium. No subjects were hospitalized or living in a nursing home. According to the Kaplan–Meier analysis, their mean life expectancy was 91.28 years for men and 94.38 years for women (Supplementary Table S6). The subjects who participated in this study represented a healthy and long-living population. A previous report showed a large difference in mortality between participants and non-participants in health check-ups [51]. The results of this study may not applicable for hospitalized older adults or older adults residing in nursing homes.

Several studies have suggested that regular diet [52] and nutritional status [53–57] affect the QOL of community-dwelling older adults. Another study showed that chewing ability is significantly greater in subjects with high QOL scores. Dietary intake was not associated with QOL [58]. In this study, chewing ability was significantly associated with two dimensions of QOL. However, nutritional status, as evaluated by the serum level of albumin, and number of remaining teeth were not directly associated with QOL. As shown in Figure 3, the number of remaining teeth is a morphological background factor in oral function [59,60]. Therefore, the number of remaining teeth is not directly associated with QOL. Nutritional status was evaluated by the serum albumin level, which is one of the limitations of this study. A more precise evaluation of nutritional status or regular diet by a validated questionnaire may lead to more precise results. However, these tools were not available when the survey was conducted in 2002.

In this study, the self-assessed chewing ability was associated with three subscales of the TMIG index. The number of remaining teeth and the serum level of albumin were not associated with the IADL. A previous report showed that tooth loss is associated with future decline in higher-level functional capacity [61]. Tooth loss can be compensated for by prosthodontic treatment. In addition, the Japanese national insurance system covers most conventional prosthodontic treatments. Recently, the concept of functional teeth was introduced, and it could be used as a predictor of mortality instead of the number of remaining teeth [62]. One of the limitations of this study is that we did not have data on functional teeth. However, there were only three out of 196 (1.5%) edentulous subjects who did not use dentures.

Recently, the concept of frailty, including oral frailty, has been widely accepted [63–65]. Frailty has been evaluated by physical conditions that can be improved by nutritional interventions. For nutritional intervention studies, frail is a more optimal outcome variable than ADLs [66–70]. ADLs do not only describe limited physical conditions. They include other dimensions such as social function and intellectual activity [71]. A previous study showed that physical activity, social role, and mental health are associated with ADLs [41,43,72]. This may be one of the reasons why the serum level of albumin was not significantly associated with the ADL subscales.

Nutritional factors affect mortality in older adults [73]. In this study, malnutrition was evaluated by the serum level of albumin [74]. A low level of serum albumin is a well-known predictor of mortality in older persons in both the short and long term [74–80]. The results of this study are consistent with another report conducted in women; however, it was not applicable in men. Except for one subject, all women with less than the cut-off point of albumin died within the observational period. They died within 2000 days. In contrast, one man was alive after the observational period and he became a centenarian. When men and women were combined, the hazard ratio for the serum level of albumin was 1.979 (95% CI: 1.172–3.341, $p = 0.011$).

Self-assessed chewing ability was significantly correlated with QOL and mortality in men. The number of remaining teeth was not statistically significantly correlated with mortality. The subjective method for the evaluation of chewing ability requires a specific device, labor, and costs. Due to its ease of use and cost effectiveness, masticatory dysfunction has generally been assessed by self-assessment-specific questionnaires in epidemiological studies. Studies have shown that the mortality of older adults is influenced by the number of remaining teeth. However, they failed to show a dose–response relationship [81,82]. As mentioned for the QOL, this may be because the effects of tooth loss can be compensated for by the use of proper dentures. In this study, the number of remaining teeth did not directly influence mortality. However, for edentulous subjects, not using dentures was significantly high risk in men (Hazard ratio: 15.160 ($p = 0.019$)). Therefore, tooth loss should be used in combination with the use of dentures [83,84]. Therefore, the concept of functional teeth is reasonable [62]. However, complete denture wearers and subjects with all-natural teeth were treated as equivalent. Further study is necessary to apply the concept of functional teeth in epidemiological studies. The number of remaining teeth should be considered as one of the indicators of oral function. Mortality is a multifactorial issue, and some related factors cause either tooth loss or mortality. In particular, socioeconomic status and health literacy may be important factors in mortality. In this study, we could not obtain these data. It is one of the limitations of this study. However, the association of self-assessed chewing ability with mortality rather than the number of teeth was a reasonable result. Hazard ratio of self-assessed chewing ability for slight hard food was statistically significant for men. It was also significant adjusted by blood tests except for creatinine. Creatinine reflects the muscle activity. Self-assessed chewing ability may reflect the exercise in daily life. However, as shown in Figure 4, clear survival curves were obtained. Self-assessed chewing ability for slight hard food can be the indicator for the prediction of mortality.

There is a sex difference in mortality related to the number of remaining teeth [46,85–88]. Most studies have shown that tooth loss is a risk factor for mortality in men and not in women [85,87,88]. Other studies have shown contradictory results [46,86]. One report had statistically not significant between men and women [89]. Follow-up periods, the baseline number of remaining teeth, and statistical methods were different between studies. In addition, mortality is a multifactorial issue, and some related factors cause either tooth loss or mortality. Prevalence of noncommunicable diseases may be different between studies. Health care supply system varies from country to country. In addition, the prevalence of noncommunicable diseases may be different between men and women. It is impossible to reach a clear conclusion for the sex difference of mortality.

Figure 5 shows one of the models. The interactions between health-related factors are different between men and women. When planning a health promotion plan for older adults, different strategies may be necessary for men and women.

5. Conclusions

Self-assessed chewing ability was not associated with the serum level of albumin. In dental practice, recovering oral function is not enough for the health promotion of older adults. Additional nutritional instruction is indispensable. Health-related factors were found to interact with each other. However, the interactions were different for men and women. In terms of a health promotion plan for older adults, different strategies are necessary for men and women.

Supplementary Materials: The following are available online at http://www.mdpi.com/2072-6643/12/11/3315/s1, Figure S1. Diagram of the study design, Figure S2: Item response curve and item information curve of the 15 foods, Table S1: Results of blood tests for the subjects who participated in this study, Table S2: Descriptive statistics of the subscales of the SF 36, Table S3: Factor analysis for the subscales of the SF 36, Table S4: Frequency of items in the TMIG index for subjects who answered yes or able, Table S5: Frequency of scores of the TIMIG Index, Table S6: Factor analysis for the items in the TMIG index, Table S7: Three parameter logistic model of 15 foods, Table S8: Factor analysis for the 15 foods, Table S9: Correlations of number of remaining teeth, serum albumin level, and self-assessed chewing ability with subscales of the QOL, Table S10: Hazard ratios of self-assessed chewing ability of slight hard food adjusted by blood tests, Table S11: Means and medians of survival days.

Author Contributions: Y.N. planned the study design and management and analysis of the data and wrote the original draft. E.K., A.O., R.O., M.S., Y.T., C.T. and K.A. collected and managed the data. Y.N., H.D., T.S. and N.H. contributed to funding acquisition, planning the study design, and reviewing and editing the manuscript. All authors have read and agreed to the published version of the manuscript.

Funding: This study was supported by JSPS KAKENHI (grant numbers 17K12030, 20K10303), SECOM Science and Technology Foundation and an 8020 Research Grant for fiscal year 2017 from the 8020 Promotion Foundation (grant number 17-2-05). None of the funders played a role in the design of the study, data collection or analysis, interpretation of the results, or writing of the manuscript.

Conflicts of Interest: The authors state that they have no financial or nonfinancial conflicts of interest regarding this research.

References

1. Leonardi, M.; Chatterji, S.; Koskinen, S.; Mateos, A.J.L.; Haro, J.M.; Frisoni, G.; Frattura, L.; Martinuzzi, A.; Adamczyk, T.B.; Gmurek, M.; et al. Determinants of health and disability in ageing population: The COURAGE in Europe Project. *Clin. Psychol. Psychother.* **2014**, *21*, 193–198. [CrossRef]
2. Gómez, H.A.I.; Ayala, A.; García, R.M.P.; Blázquez, R.T.C.; Rodríguez, R.T.V.; Pérez, V.F.; Mayoralas, F.G.; Laso, R.A.; Larrañaga, C.A.; Forjaz, M.J. The WHO active ageing pillars and its association with survival: Findings from a population-based study in Spain. *Arch. Gerontol. Geriatr.* **2020**, *90*, 104114. [CrossRef]
3. Turner, H.Y.C.; Peel, N.M.; Hubbard, R.E. Health assets in older age: A systematic review. *BMJ Open.* **2017**, *7*, e013226. [CrossRef] [PubMed]
4. Kehoe, L.; Walton, J.; Flynn, A. Nutritional challenges for older adults in Europe: Current status and future directions. *Proc. Nutr. Soc.* **2019**, *78*, 221–233. [CrossRef]
5. Gabrovec, B.; Veninšek, G.; Samaniego, L.L.; Carriazo, A.M.; Antoniadou, E.; Jelenc, M. The role of nutrition in ageing: A narrative review from the perspective of the European joint action on frailty—ADVANTAGE JA. *Eur. J. Int. Med.* **2018**, *56*, 26–32. [CrossRef] [PubMed]

6. Lemacks, J.; Wells, B.A.; Ilich, J.Z.; Ralston, P.A. Interventions for improving nutrition and physical activity behaviors in adult African American populations: A systematic review, January 2000 through December 2011. *Prev. Chronic. Dis.* **2013**, *10*, E99. [CrossRef] [PubMed]
7. Raffaele, B.; Matarese, M.; Alvaro, R.; Marinis, D.M.G. Health-promotion theories in nutritional interventions for community-dwelling older adults: A systematic review. *Annali dell'Istituto Superiore di Sanità* **2017**, *53*, 146–151. [CrossRef] [PubMed]
8. Lyons, B.P. Nutrition education intervention with community-dwelling older adults: Research challenges and opportunities. *J. Community Health* **2014**, *39*, 810–818. [CrossRef] [PubMed]
9. Takayama, K.; Atagi, S.; Imamura, F.; Tanaka, H.; Minato, K.; Harada, T.; Katakami, N.; Yokoyama, T.; Yoshimori, K.; Takiguchi, Y.; et al. Quality of life and survival survey of cancer cachexia in advanced non-small cell lung cancer patients-Japan nutrition and QOL survey in patients with advanced non-small cell lung cancer study. *Support Care Cancer* **2016**, *24*, 3473–3480. [CrossRef]
10. Raynaud, K.; Seguy, D.; Rogosnitzky, M.; Saulnier, F.; Pruvot, F.R.; Zerbib, P. Conservative management of severe caustic injuries during acute phase leads to superior long-term nutritional and quality of life (QoL) outcome. *Langenbecks Arch. Surg.* **2016**, *401*, 81–87. [CrossRef]
11. Ha, L.; Hauge, T.; Spenning, A.B.; Iversen, P.O. Individual, nutritional support prevents undernutrition, increases muscle strength and improves QoL among elderly at nutritional risk hospitalized for acute stroke: A randomized, controlled trial. *Clin. Nutr.* **2010**, *29*, 567–573. [CrossRef] [PubMed]
12. Dent, E.; Visvanathan, R.; Piantadosi, C.; Chapman, I. Nutritional screening tools as predictors of mortality, functional decline, and move to higher level care in older people: A systematic review. *J. Nutr. Gerontol. Geriatr.* **2012**, *31*, 97–145. [CrossRef] [PubMed]
13. Kiesswetter, E.; Pohlhausen, S.; Uhlig, K.; Diekmann, R.; Lesser, S.; Uter, W.; Heseker, H.; Stehle, P.; Sieber, C.C.; Volkert, D. Prognostic differences of the Mini Nutritional Assessment short form and long form in relation to 1-year functional decline and mortality in community-dwelling older adults receiving home care. *J. Am. Geriatr. Soc.* **2014**, *62*, 512–517. [CrossRef]
14. Malafarina, V.; Reginster, J.Y.; Cabrerizo, S.; Bruyère, O.; Kanis, J.A.; Martinez, J.A.; Zulet, M.A. Nutritional status and nutritional treatment are related to outcomes and mortality in older adults with hip fracture. *Nutrients* **2018**, *10*, 555. [CrossRef] [PubMed]
15. Keller, U. Nutritional laboratory markers in malnutrition. *J. Clin. Med.* **2019**, *8*, 775. [CrossRef] [PubMed]
16. Copur, S.; Siriopol, D.; Afsar, B.; Comert, M.C.; Uzunkopru, G.; Sag, A.A.; Ortiz, A.; Covic, A.; van Raalte, D.H.; Cherney, D.Z.; et al. Serum glycated albumin predicts all-cause mortality in dialysis patients with diabetes mellitus: Meta-analysis and systematic review of a predictive biomarker. *Acta Diabetol.* **2020**, *30*. Online ahead of print. [CrossRef]
17. Sun, J.; Su, H.; Lou, Y.; Wang, M. Association between serum albumin level and all-cause mortality in patients with chronic kidney disease: A retrospective cohort study. *Am. J. Med. Sci.* **2020**. Online ahead of print. [CrossRef]
18. Akirov, A.; Gorshtein, A.; Adler-Cohen, C.; Steinmetz, T.; Shochat, T.; Shimon, I. Low serum albumin levels predict short- and long-term mortality risk in patients hospitalized to general surgery wards. *Intern. Med. J.* **2019**. Online ahead of print. [CrossRef]
19. Kendall, H.; Abreu, E.; Cheng, A.L. Serum albumin trend is a predictor of mortality in ICU patients with sepsis. *Biol. Res. Nurs.* **2019**, *21*, 237–244. [CrossRef]
20. Touma, E.; Bisharat, N. Trends in admission serum albumin and mortality in patients with hospital readmission. *Int. J. Clin. Pract.* **2019**, *73*, e13314. [CrossRef]
21. Wu, C.Y.; Hu, H.Y.; Huang, N.; Chou, Y.C.; Li, C.P.; Chou, Y.J. Albumin levels and cause-specific mortality in community-dwelling older adults. *Prev. Med.* **2018**, *112*, 145–151. [CrossRef] [PubMed]
22. Umeki, Y.; Adachi, H.; Enomoto, M.; Fukami, A.; Nakamura, S.; Nohara, Y.; Nakao, E.; Sakaue, A.; Tsuru, T.; Morikawa, N.; et al. Serum albumin and cerebro-cardiovascular mortality during a 15-year study in a community-based cohort in tanushimaru, a cohort of the seven countries study. *Intern. Med.* **2016**, *55*, 2917–2925. [CrossRef]
23. Tanaka, M.; Momosaki, R.; Wakabayashi, H.; Kikura, T.; Maeda, K. Relationship between nutritional status and improved ADL in individuals with cervical spinal cord injury in a convalescent rehabilitation ward. *Spinal Cord.* **2019**, *57*, 501–508. [CrossRef]

24. Pedersen, J.L.; Pedersen, P.U.; Damsgaard, E.M. Early nutritional follow-up after discharge prevents deterioration of ADL functions in malnourished, independent, geriatric patients who live alone—A randomized clinical trial. *J. Nutr. Health Aging* **2016**, *20*, 845–853. [CrossRef]
25. Nishioka, S.; Wakabayashi, H.; Momosaki, R. Nutritional status changes and activities of daily living after hip fracture in convalescent rehabilitation units: A retrospective observational cohort study from the Japan rehabilitation nutrition database. *J. Acad. Nutr. Diet.* **2018**, *118*, 1270–1276. [CrossRef]
26. Fueki, K.; Kimoto, K.; Ogawa, T.; Garrett, N.R. Effect of implant-supported or retained dentures on masticatory performance: A systematic review. *J. Prosthet. Dent.* **2007**, *98*, 470–477. [CrossRef]
27. Kumar, Y.; Chand, P.; Arora, V.; Singh, S.V.; Mishra, N.; Alvi, H.A.; Verma, U.P. Comparison of rehabilitating missing mandibular first molars with implant- or tooth-supported prostheses using masticatory efficiency and patient satisfaction outcomes. *J. Prosthodont.* **2017**, *26*, 376–380. [CrossRef]
28. Li, S.; Flint, A.; Pai, J.K.; Forman, J.P.; Hu, F.B.; Willett, W.C.; Rexrode, K.M.; Mukamal, K.J.; Rimm, E.B. Low carbohydrate diet from plant or animal sources and mortality among myocardial infarction survivors. *J. Am. Heart Assoc.* **2014**, *22*, e001169. [CrossRef] [PubMed]
29. Shirai, K. Ideal body mass index determined by mortality in Europe, and adequate high protein and low carbohydrate diet to maintain bodyweight. *J. Diabetes Investig.* **2011**, *30*, 421–422. [CrossRef]
30. Lagiou, P.; Sandin, S.; Weiderpass, E.; Lagiou, A.; Mucci, L.; Trichopoulos, D.; Adami, H.O. Low carbohydrate-high protein diet and mortality in a cohort of Swedish women. *J. Intern. Med.* **2007**, *261*, 366–374. [CrossRef]
31. Host, A.; McMahon, A.T.; Walton, K.; Charlton, K. Factors influencing food choice for independently living older people-A systematic literature review. *J. Nutr. Gerontol. Geriatr.* **2016**, *35*, 67–94. [CrossRef] [PubMed]
32. Nomura, Y.; Tsutsumi, I.; Nagasaki, M.; Tsuda, H.; Koga, F.; Kashima, N.; Uraguchi, M.; Okada, A.; Kakuta, E.; Hanada, N. Supplied food consistency and oral functions of institutionalized elderly. *Int. J. Dent.* **2020**, *2020*, 3463056. [CrossRef] [PubMed]
33. Fukuhara, S.; Bito, S.; Green, J.; Hsiao, A.; Kurokawa, K. Translation, adaptation, and validation of the SF-36 Health Survey for use in Japan. *J. Clin. Epidemiol.* **1998**, *51*, 1037–1044. [CrossRef]
34. Fukuhara, S.; Ware, J.J.E.; Kosinski, M.; Wada, S.; Gandek, B. Psychometric and clinical tests of validity of the Japanese SF-36 Health Survey. *J. Clin. Epidemiol.* **1998**, *51*, 1045–1053. [CrossRef]
35. Brazier, J.E.; Fukuhara, S.; Roberts, J.; Kharroubi, S.; Yamamoto, Y.; Ikeda, S.; Doherty, J.; Kurokawa, K. Estimating a preference-based index from the Japanese SF-36. *J. Clin. Epidemiol.* **2009**, *62*, 1323–1331. [CrossRef] [PubMed]
36. Koyano, W.; Shibata, H.; Nakazato, K.; Haga, H.; Suyama, Y. Measurement of competence: Reliability and validity of the TMIG Index of Competence. *Arch. Gerontol. Geriatr.* **1991**, *13*, 103–116. [CrossRef]
37. Nomura, Y.; Kakuta, E.; Okada, A.; Otsuka, R.; Shimada, M.; Tomizawa, Y.; Taguchi, C.; Arikawa, K.; Daikoku, H.; Sato, T.; et al. Effects of self-assessed chewing ability, tooth loss and serum albumin on mortality in 80-year-old individuals: A 20-year follow-up study. *BMC Oral. Health* **2020**, *20*, 122. [CrossRef]
38. Nomura, Y.; Kakuta, E.; Okada, A.; Otsuka, R.; Shimada, M.; Tomizawa, Y.; Taguchi, C.; Arikawa, K.; Daikoku, H.; Sato, T.; et al. Oral microbiome in four female centenarians. *Appl. Sci.* **2020**, *10*, 5312. [CrossRef]
39. Ishizaki, T.; Kai, I.; Kobayashi, Y.; Imanaka, Y. Functional transitions and active life expectancy for older Japanese living in a community. *Arch. Gerontol. Geriatr.* **2002**, *35*, 107–120. [CrossRef]
40. Kiyoshige, E.; Kabayama, M.; Gondo, Y.; Masui, Y.; Inagaki, H.; Ogawa, M.; Nakagawa, T.; Yasumoto, S.; Akasaka, H.; Sugimoto, K.; et al. Age group differences in association between IADL decline and depressive symptoms in community-dwelling elderly. *BMC Geriatr.* **2019**, *19*, 309. [CrossRef]
41. Komatsu, M.; Obayashi, K.; Tomioka, K.; Morikawa, M.; Jojima, N.; Okamoto, N.; Kurumatani, N.; Saeki, K. The interaction effect between physical and cultural leisure activities on the subsequent decline of instrumental ADL: The Fujiwara-kyo study. *Environ. Health Prev. Med.* **2019**, *24*, 71. [CrossRef]
42. Hama, Y.; Kubota, C.; Moriya, S.; Onda, R.; Watanabe, Y.; Minakuchi, S. Factors related to removable denture use in independent older people: A cross-sectional study. *J. Oral. Rehabil.* **2020**, *47*, 998–1006. [CrossRef]
43. Cho, S.; Park, S.; Takahashi, S.; Yoshiuchi, K.; Shephard, R.J.; Aoyagi, Y. Changes in and interactions between physical and mental health in older Japanese: The Nakanojo Study. *Gerontology* **2019**, *65*, 340–352. [CrossRef]
44. Okamoto, N.; Hisashige, A.; Tanaka, Y.; Kurumatani, N. Development of the Japanese 15D instrument of health-related quality of life: Verification of reliability and validity among elderly people. *PLoS ONE* **2013**, *8*, e61721. [CrossRef]

45. Kimura, M.; Moriyasu, A.; Kumagai, S.; Furuna, T.; Akita, S.; Kimura, S.; Suzuki, T. Community-based intervention to improve dietary habits and promote physical activity among older adults: A cluster randomized trial. *BMC Geriatr.* **2013**, *13*, 8. [CrossRef]
46. Ansai, T.; Takata, Y.; Soh, I.; Akifusa, S.; Sogame, A.; Shimada, N.; Yoshida, A.; Hamasaki, T.; Awano, S.; Fukuhara, M.; et al. Relationship between chewing ability and 4-year mortality in a cohort of 80-year-old Japanese people. *Oral. Dis.* **2007**, *13*, 214–219. [CrossRef]
47. Nomura, Y.; Kakuta, E.; Okada, A.; Yamamoto, Y.; Tomonari, H.; Hosoya, N.; Hanada, N.; Yoshida, N.; Takei, N. Prioritization of the skills to be mastered for the daily jobs of Japanese dental hygienists. *Int. J. Dent.* **2020**, *2020*, 4297646. [CrossRef]
48. Nomura, Y.; Matsuyama, T.; Fukai, K.; Okada, A.; Ida, M.; Yamauchi, N.; Hanamura, H.; Yabuki, Y.; Watanabe, K.; Sugawara, M.; et al. PRECEDE-PROCEED model based questionnaire and saliva tests for oral health checkup in adult. *J. Oral. Sci.* **2019**, *61*, 544–548. [CrossRef]
49. Nomura, Y.; Maung, K.; Khine, K.E.M.; Sint, K.M.; Lin, M.P.; Myint, W.M.K.; Aung, T.; Sogabe, K.; Otsuka, R.; Okada, A.; et al. Prevalence of dental caries in 5- and 6-year-old Myanmar children. *Int. J. Dent.* **2019**, *2019*, 5948379. [CrossRef]
50. Nomura, Y.; Ishii, Y.; Suzuki, S.; Morita, K.; Suzuki, A.; Suzuki, S.; Tanabe, J.; Ishiwata, Y.; Yamakawa, K.; Chiba, Y.; et al. Nutritional status and oral frailty: A community based study. *Nutrients* **2020**, *12*, E2886. [CrossRef]
51. Iwasa, H.; Yoshida, H.; Kim, H.; Yoshida, Y.; Kwon, J.; Sugiura, M.; Furuna, T.; Suzuki, T. A mortality comparison of participants and non-participants in a comprehensive health examination among elderly people living in an urban Japanese community. *Aging. Clin. Exp. Res.* **2007**, *19*, 240–245. [CrossRef]
52. Sun, W.; Aodeng, S.; Tanimoto, Y.; Watanabe, M.; Han, J.; Wang, B.; Yu, L.; Kono, K. Quality of life (QOL) of the community-dwelling elderly and associated factors: A population-based study in urban areas of China. *Arch. Gerontol. Geriatr.* **2015**, *60*, 311–316. [CrossRef]
53. Luger, E.; Haider, S.; Kapan, A.; Schindler, K.; Lackinger, C.; Dorner, T.E. Association between nutritional status and quality of life in (pre) frail community-dwelling older persons. *J. Frailty Aging* **2016**, *5*, 141–148.
54. Smoliner, C.; Norman, K.; Scheufele, R.; Hartig, W.; Pirlich, M.; Lochs, H. Effects of food fortification on nutritional and functional status in frail elderly nursing home residents at risk of malnutrition. *Nutrition* **2008**, *24*, 1139–1144. [CrossRef]
55. Gollub, E.A.; Weddle, D.O. Improvements in nutritional intake and quality of life among frail homebound older adults receiving home-delivered breakfast and lunch. *J. Am. Diet. Assoc.* **2004**, *104*, 1227–1235. [CrossRef]
56. Izawa, S.; Kuzuya, M.; Okada, K.; Enoki, H.; Koike, T.; Kanda, S.; Iguchi, A. The nutritional status of frail elderly with care needs according to the mini-nutritional assessment. *Clin. Nutr.* **2006**, *25*, 962–967. [CrossRef]
57. Haller, J. Vitamins for the elderly: Reducing disability and improving quality of life. *Aging* **1993**, *5*, 65–70.
58. Mori, K.; Kawano, Y.; Tada, Y.; Hida, A.; Nagasawa, N.; Inoue, K.; Kamioka, H.; Inoue, K.; Ozeki, T. Relationship of dietary intake and lifestyle factors to health-related quality of life in the community-dwelling elderly. *J. Nutr. Sci. Vitaminol.* **2010**, *56*, 364–371. [CrossRef]
59. Gotfredsen, K.; Walls, A.W. What dentition assures oral function? *Clin. Oral Implants Res.* **2007**, *18*, 34–45. [CrossRef]
60. Sierpińska, T.; Gołębiewska, M.; Długosz, J.W. The relationship between masticatory efficiency and the state of dentition at patients with non rehabilitated partial lost of teeth. *Adv. Med. Sci.* **2006**, *51*, 196–199.
61. Sato, Y.; Aida, J.; Kondo, K.; Tsuboya, T.; Watt, R.G.; Yamamoto, T.; Koyama, S.; Matsuyama, Y.; Osaka, K. Tooth loss and decline in functional capacity: A prospective cohort study from the Japan gerontological evaluation study. *J. Am. Geriatr. Soc.* **2016**, *64*, 2336–2342. [CrossRef]
62. Maekawa, K.; Ikeuchi, T.; Shinkai, S.; Hirano, H.; Ryu, M.; Tamaki, K.; Yatani, H.; Kuboki, T.; Kimura-Ono, A.; Kikutani, T.; et al. Number of functional teeth more strongly predicts all-cause mortality than number of present teeth in Japanese older adults. *Geriatr. Gerontol. Int.* **2020**, *20*, 607–614. [CrossRef]
63. Xue, Q.L.; Roche, K.B.; Varadhan, R.; Zhou, J.; Fried, L.P. Initial manifestations of frailty criteria and the development of frailty phenotype in the Women's Health and Aging Study II. *J. Gerontol. A Biol. Sci. Med. Sci.* **2008**, *63*, 984–990. [CrossRef]

64. Signore, D.S.; Roubenoff, R. Physical frailty and sarcopenia (PF&S): A point of view from the industry. *Aging Clin. Exp. Res.* **2017**, *29*, 69–74. [CrossRef]
65. Tanaka, T.; Takahashi, K.; Hirano, H.; Kikutani, T.; Watanabe, Y.; Ohara, Y.; Furuya, H.; Tetsuo, T.; Akishita, M.; Iijima, K. Oral frailty as a risk factor for physical frailty and mortality in community-dwelling elderly. *J. Gerontol. A Biol. Sci. Med. Sci.* **2018**, *73*, 1661–1667. [CrossRef]
66. Avgerinou, C.; Bhanu, C.; Walters, K.; Croker, H.; Tuijt, R.; Rea, J.; Hopkins, J.; Barr, M.; Kharicha, K.K. Supporting nutrition in frail older people: A qualitative study exploring views of primary care and community health professionals. *Br. J. Gen. Pract.* **2020**, *70*, e138–e145. [CrossRef]
67. Tomata, Y.; Watanabe, T.; Sugiyama, K.; Zhang, S.; Sugawara, Y.; Tsuji, I. Effects of a community-based program for oral health and nutrition on cost-effectiveness by preventing disability in Japanese frail elderly: A quasi-experimental study using propensity score matching. *J. Am. Med. Dir. Assoc.* **2017**, *18*, 678–685. [CrossRef]
68. Orlandoni, P.; Peladic, J.N.; Spazzafumo, L.; Venturini, C.; Cola, C.; Sparvoli, D.; Giorgini, N.; Basile, R.; Fagnani, D. Utility of video consultation to improve the outcomes of home enteral nutrition in a population of frail older patients. *Geriatr. Gerontol. Int.* **2016**, *16*, 762–767. [CrossRef]
69. Hirakawa, Y.; Kimata, T.; Uemura, K. Current challenges in home nutrition services for frail older adults in Japan-A qualitative research study from the point of view of care managers. *Healthcare* **2013**, *1*, 53–63. [CrossRef]
70. Suffian, M.N.I.; Adznam, S.N.; Saad, A.H.; Chan, Y.M.; Ibrahim, Z.; Omar, N.; Murat, M.F. Frailty Intervention through Nutrition Education and Exercise (FINE). A health promotion intervention to prevent frailty and improve frailty status among pre-frail elderly-A study protocol of a cluster randomized controlled trial. *Nutrients* **2020**, *12*, E2758. [CrossRef]
71. Fujiwara, Y.; Shinkai, S.; Kumagai, S.; Amano, H.; Yoshida, Y.; Yoshida, H.; Kim, H.; Suzuki, T.; Ishizaki, T.; Haga, H.; et al. Longitudinal changes in higher-level functional capacity of an older population living in a Japanese urban community. *Arch. Gerontol. Geriatr.* **2003**, *36*, 141–153. [CrossRef]
72. Cappelli, M.; Bordonali, A.; Giannotti, C.; Montecucco, F.; Nencioni, A.; Odetti, P.; Monacelli, F. Social vulnerability underlying disability amongst older adults: A systematic review. *Eur. J. Clin. Investig.* **2020**, *50*, e13239. [CrossRef]
73. Shibata, H. Nutritional factors on longevity and quality of life in Japan. *J. Nutr. Health Aging* **2001**, *5*, 97–102.
74. Don, B.R.; Kaysen, G. Serum albumin: Relationship to inflammation and nutrition. *Semin. Dial.* **2004**, *17*, 432–437. [CrossRef]
75. Okamura, T.; Hayakawa, T.; Hozawa, A.; Kadowaki, T.; Murakami, Y.; Kita, Y.; Abbott, R.D.; Okayama, A.; Ueshima, H. Lower levels of serum albumin and total cholesterol associated with decline in activities of daily living and excess mortality in a 12-year cohort study of elderly Japanese. *J. Am. Geriatr. Soc.* **2008**, *56*, 529–535. [CrossRef]
76. Takata, Y.; Ansai, T.; Soh, I.; Awano, S.; Sonoki, K.; Akifusa, S.; Kagiyama, S.; Hamasaki, T.; Torisu, T.; Yoshida, A.; et al. Serum albumin levels as an independent predictor of 4-year mortality in a community-dwelling 80-year-old population. *Aging Clin. Exp. Res.* **2010**, *22*, 31–35. [CrossRef]
77. Takata, Y.; Ansai, T.; Yoshihara, A.; Miyazaki, H. Serum albumin (SA) levels and 10-year mortality in a community-dwelling 70-year-old population. *Arch. Gerontol. Geriatr.* **2012**, *54*, 39–43. [CrossRef]
78. Goldwasser, P.; Feldman, J. Association of serum albumin and mortality risk. *J. Clin. Epidemiol.* **1997**, *50*, 693–703. [CrossRef]
79. Sahyoun, N.R.; Jacques, P.F.; Dallal, G.; Russell, R.M. Use of albumin as a predictor of mortality in community dwelling and institutionalized elderly populations. *J. Clin. Epidemiol.* **1996**, *49*, 981–988. [CrossRef]
80. Cohen, K.H.; Connor, B.E.L.; Edelstein, S.L. Albumin levels as a predictor of mortality in the healthy elderly. *J. Clin. Epidemiol.* **1992**, *45*, 207–212. [CrossRef]
81. Nakanishi, N.; Hino, Y.; Ida, O.; Fukuda, H.; Shinsho, F.; Tatara, K. Associations between self-assessed masticatory disability and health of community-residing elderly people. *Community Dent Oral. Epidemiol.* **1999**, *27*, 366–371. [CrossRef] [PubMed]
82. Nakanishi, N.; Fukuda, H.; Takatorige, T.; Tatara, K. Relationship between self-assessed masticatory disability and 9-year mortality in a cohort of community-residing elderly people. *J. Am. Geriatr. Soc.* **2005**, *53*, 54–58. [CrossRef]

83. Fukai, K.; Takiguchi, T.; Ando, Y.; Aoyama, H.; Miyakawa, Y.; Ito, G.; Inoue, M.; Sasaki, H. Mortality rates of community-residing adults with and without dentures. *Geriatr. Gerontol. Int.* **2008**, *8*, 152–159. [CrossRef] [PubMed]
84. Appollonio, I.; Carabellese, C.; Frattola, A.; Trabucchi, M. Dental status, quality of life, and mortality in an older community population: A multivariate approach. *J. Am. Geriatr. Soc.* **1997**, *45*, 1315–1323. [CrossRef] [PubMed]
85. Morita, I.; Nakagaki, H.; Kato, K.; Murakami, T.; Tsuboi, S.; Hayashizaki, J.; Toyama, A.; Hashimoto, M.; Simozato, T.; Morishita, N.; et al. Relationship between survival rates and numbers of natural teeth in an elderly Japanese population. *Gerodontology* **2006**, *23*, 214–218. [CrossRef] [PubMed]
86. Osterberg, T.; Carlsson, G.E.; Sundh, V.; Steen, B. Number of teeth—A predictor of mortality in the elderly? A population study in three Nordic localities. *Acta Odontol. Scand.* **2007**, *65*, 335–340. [CrossRef]
87. Hämäläinen, P.; Meurman, J.H.; Keskinen, M.; Heikkinen, E. Relationship between dental health and 10-year mortality in a cohort of community-dwelling elderly people. *Eur. J. Oral. Sci.* **2003**, *111*, 291–296. [CrossRef] [PubMed]
88. Osterberg, T.; Carlsson, G.E.; Sundh, V.; Mellström, D. Number of teeth–a predictor of mortality in 70-year-old subjects. *Community Dent Oral. Epidemiol.* **2008**, *36*, 258–268. [CrossRef]
89. Hirotomi, T.; Yoshihara, A.; Ogawa, H.; Miyazaki, H. Number of teeth and 5-year mortality in an elderly population. *Community Dent Oral. Epidemiol.* **2015**, *43*, 226–231. [CrossRef]

Publisher's Note: MDPI stays neutral with regard to jurisdictional claims in published maps and institutional affiliations.

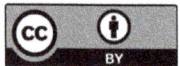

© 2020 by the authors. Licensee MDPI, Basel, Switzerland. This article is an open access article distributed under the terms and conditions of the Creative Commons Attribution (CC BY) license (http://creativecommons.org/licenses/by/4.0/).

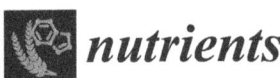

Article

Effect of Training-Detraining Phases of Multicomponent Exercises and BCAA Supplementation on Inflammatory Markers and Albumin Levels in Frail Older Persons

Adriana Caldo-Silva [1,2,*], Guilherme Eustáquio Furtado [2,3,*], Matheus Uba Chupel [2], André L. L. Bachi [4,5], Marcelo P. de Barros [6], Rafael Neves [1], Emanuele Marzetti [7,8], Alain Massart [1,2] and Ana Maria Teixeira [1,2]

1. University of Coimbra, Faculty of Sports Sciences and Physical Education—(FCDEF-UC), 3040-248 Coimbra, Portugal; rsneves.prof@gmail.com (R.N.); alainmassart@fcdef.uc.pt (A.M.); ateixeira@fcdef.uc.pt (A.M.T.)
2. Research Centre for Sport and Physical Activity, CIDAF-FCDEF-UC, 3040-248 Coimbra, Portugal; matheusuba@hotmail.com
3. Health Sciences Research Unit: Nursing (UICISAE), Nursing School of Coimbra (ESEnfC), 3000-232 Coimbra, Portugal
4. Department of Otorhinolaryngology, ENT Lab, Federal University of São Paulo (UNIFESP), São Paulo 04025-002, Brazil; allbachi77@gmail.com
5. Post-Graduation Program in Health Sciences, Santo Amaro University (UNISA), São Paulo 04829-300, Brazil
6. Institute of Physical Activity Sciences and Sports (ICAFE), Interdisciplinary Program in Health Sciences, Cruzeiro do Sul University, São Paulo 01506-000, Brazil; marcelo.barros@cruzeirodosul.edu.br
7. Fondazione Policlinico Universitario "Agostino Gemelli" IRCCS, 00168 Rome, Italy; emanuele.marzetti@policlinicogemelli.it
8. Università Cattolica del Sacro Cuore, 00168 Rome, Italy
* Correspondence: dricaldo@gmail.com (A.C.-S.); guilhermefurtado@esenfc.pt (G.E.F.)

Abstract: Nowadays, it is accepted that the regular practice of exercise and branched-chain amino acids supplementation (BCAAs) can benefit the immune responses in older persons, prevent the occurrence of physical frailty (PF), cognitive decline, and aging-related comorbidities. However, the impact of their combination (as non-pharmacological interventions) in albumin and the inflammatory markers is not fully understood. Therefore, we investigated the effect of a 40-week multifactorial intervention [MIP, multicomponent exercise (ME) associated or not with BCAAs] on plasma levels of inflammatory markers and albumin in frail older persons ($\geq$75 years old) living at residential care homes (RCH). This study consisted of a prospective, naturalistic, controlled clinical trial with four arms of multifactorial and experimental (interventions-wahshout-interventions) design. The intervention groups were ME + BCAAs ($n = 8$), ME ($n = 7$), BCAAs ($n = 7$), and control group ($n = 13$). Lower limb muscle-strength, cognitive profile, and PF tests were concomitantly evaluated with plasma levels of albumin, anti- and pro-inflammatory cytokines [Interleukin-10 (IL-10) and Tumor Necrosis Factor-alpha (TNF-α) respectively], TNF-α/IL-10 ratio, and myeloperoxidase (MPO) activity at four different time-points: Baseline (T1), after 16 weeks of multifactorial intervention (T2), then after a subsequent 8 weeks washout period (T3) and finally, after an additional 16 weeks of multifactorial intervention (T4). Improvement of cognitive profile and muscle strength-related albumin levels, as well as reduction in the TNF-α levels were found particularly in ME plus BCAAs group. No significant variations were observed over time for TNF-α/IL-10 ratio or MPO activity. Overall, the study showed that MIP triggered slight alterations in the inflammatory and physical function of the frail older participants, which could provide independence and higher quality of life for this population.

Keywords: inflammaging; cognitive impairment; cytokines; protein intake; physical frailty

---

Citation: Caldo-Silva, A.; Furtado, G.E.; Chupel, M.U.; Bachi, A.L.L.; de Barros, M.P.; Neves, R.; Marzetti, E.; Massart, A.; Teixeira, A.M. Effect of Training-Detraining Phases of Multicomponent Exercises and BCAA Supplementation on Inflammatory Markers and Albumin Levels in Frail Older Persons. *Nutrients* 2021, 13, 1106. https://doi.org/10.3390/nu13041106

Academic Editors: Christiano Capurso and Catherine Féart

Received: 28 February 2021
Accepted: 21 March 2021
Published: 28 March 2021

Publisher's Note: MDPI stays neutral with regard to jurisdictional claims in published maps and institutional affiliations.

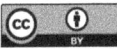

Copyright: © 2021 by the authors. Licensee MDPI, Basel, Switzerland. This article is an open access article distributed under the terms and conditions of the Creative Commons Attribution (CC BY) license (https://creativecommons.org/licenses/by/4.0/).

1. Introduction

Aging is characterized as a natural degenerative process strongly linked to diminished immune efficiency, and also to enhanced inflammatory responses, and thus, to higher risks of infections in older persons [1]. The sedentary lifestyle, per se, is one of the most important contributors to age-related illness, whereas regular physical exercises (rPE)—based on hormesis principles—could chronically slow down the aging immune/inflammatory dysfunctions [2]. In this sense, reduction of systemic levels of interleukin-10 (IL-10), a classical anti-inflammatory cytokine, with elevation on Tumor Necrosis Factor-alpha (TNF-α) levels are associated with aging [3]. Although the participation in rPE programs does not stop the progression of aging [4], staying in moderate rPE programs can help making the aging process more rewarding, with lower incidence of premature chronic diseases [5]. In addition to the comorbidities outcomes, both aging and the sedentary behavior may speed up the loss of mobility and functional autonomy [6], reducing the quality of life [7], and also increasing the susceptibility to physical frailty (PF) and cognitive decline [8].

The age-related PF syndrome is defined by loss of muscle mass (and sarcopenia), by low physical activity levels, and often accompanied by low protein intake [9]. Cognitive decline, in turn, is characterized by confusion and progressive loss of memory and neuromotor skills [10]. However, these two outcomes reveal biological and phenotypic similarities, which is the reason leading to the current scientific interest in investigating populations affected by these disorders [11]. In this sense, rPE could also provide protection against both PF and cognitive decline in very old people [12], with most of these benefits related, at least in part, to changes that occur in the immune system [13]. Recent findings have shown that multicomponent exercise (ME) interventions, those that include different types of endurance, muscle strength, and balance exercises in the same session, appear to have a superior effect on cognitively and physically frail older persons [14,15].

Participation of older persons in rPE ameliorates not only antigen recognition, but also immune responsiveness in general, as some evidence has shown that increased levels of physical activity using exercise routines can even extend the protection provided by the influenza vaccine in older persons [16], as well as a regulation of systemic inflammatory status [17]. Apart from the modulating effects of rPE, nutritional habits also play an important role in determining immune and inflammatory efficiency, especially in older persons [2]. In fact, malnutrition in older population is a serious concern for health systems around the world, since it increases the risk of comorbidities occurrence with subsequent higher health care costs [7,8]. Indeed, nutritional supplementation with vitamins, antioxidants, and protein components (including isolated amino acids) have already demonstrated positive results against PF, cognitive impairment, sarcopenia and other age-related disorders [18].

Supplementation with BCAA, in the absence of branched-chain aminotransferase (BCAT) activity in the liver implies that a dietary supply of BCCAs would ensure an almost intact passage through the liver directly to the muscle tissue, which seems to be advantagous to restrain sarcopenia and frailty [19]. Supplementation with BCAA, especially in association with regular exercises, was demonstrated to improve muscle strength and cognitive functions in the older population, which are safe and low-cost strategies to circumvent the general limitations imposed by the aging process [20–22].

Among several pro/anti-inflammatory biomarkers used in the context of exercise and nutrition sciences [23], myeloperoxidase (MPO) stands out as a valid marker largely released by activated neutrophils, with potent pro-oxidative/pro-inflammatory actions 24 [24]. MPO activity also appears as a biomarker that was strongly associated with frailty and risk of mortality in a study conducted in a large community-dwelling frail octogenarians and nonagenarians [25]. Recently, a similar intervention demonstrated the slight reduction of serum MPO activity triggered by the combination of Taurine and ME in older persons [26]. Instead, albumin concentrations are currently used for the assessment of the nutritional status of an individual, and low albumin concentrations have been associated with increased mortality after correlation for age, body mass index (BMI), gender, and several chronic comorbidities [27]. In this sense, multifatorial interventions programs

(MIP, exercise plus protein suplmentattion) that target to maintain (or even increase) albuminemia in older persons could characterize an important strategy to diminish the harmful effects of aging and its comorbidities [28].

Therefore, the aim of this work was to evaluate the effect of a 40-week MIPon plasma/serum pro- and anti-inflammatory markers of the immune system in older persons living in residential care homes (RCH). Furthermore, we hypothesized that ME plus BCAAs may have an impact on the systemic albumin levels, inflammatory variables, cognitive profile, and physical function of the participants.

2. Materials and Methods

2.1. Preliminary Procedures and Ethics

This is a prospective, naturalistic, controlled clinical trial (treatment vs care). All subjects volunteered to participate in the exercise classes or the supplementation programs. Consent forms were signed by the institution's directors, the participants and their legal representatives before testing and intervention. This study was approved by the Ethical Committee of Faculty of Sport Sciences and Physical Education, University of Coimbra (reference number: CE/FCDEFUC/00282018), respecting the Portuguese Resolution (Art.°4th; Law no. 12/2005, 1st series) on ethics in human research and the Helsinki's Declaration. This study was properly registered with clinicaltrials.gov register NCT04376463.

2.2. Participants Elegibility

Study participants were selected through a non-probabilistic trial (plus controlled sampling) living in public and private RCH. The eligible criteria for the participants in this study were, at the time of first screening: (i) Participants had to be 70 years old or more; (ii) physically frail and pre-frail; (iii) clinically stable with their drug therapy updated; (iv) being able to perform the Time Up and Go test in ≤ 50 s that indicate severe mobility independence [29]; (v) not participating in other structured rPE; (vi) not presenting any type of health condition or use medication that might prevent the functional self-sufficiency test performance or attention impairment (such as severe cardiopathy, hypertension, uncontrolled asthmatic bronchitis or severe musculoskeletal conditions); (vii) not presenting mental disorders or hearing/visual impairment that could prevent the evaluations and activities proposed, according to the institutional medical staff; (viii) not presenting morbid obesity (BMI ≥ 40). At the end of the recruitment process, 80 older persons entered the enrollment phase.

2.3. Participants Allocation

All the participants were selected through a non-probabilistic trial (plus controlled sampling) based on the geographical area of Coimbra, Portugal, living in public and private residential care homes (RCH) or frequenting day centres in the local community. From the 80 participants initially screened, 50 eligible participants were allocated in their respective intervention groups. However, for the specific reasons highlighted in Figure 1, only 35 participants (age = 83 ± 3 years-old) completed the 40 weeks multifactorial intervention, divided in the following groups: ME ($n = 7$), ME + BCAA ($n = 8$), BCAA ($n = 7$), and the no-regular exercise/no-supplementation control group (CG, $n = 13$). All the procedures were performed according to the Consolidated Standards of Reporting Trials (CONSORT) guidelines [30].

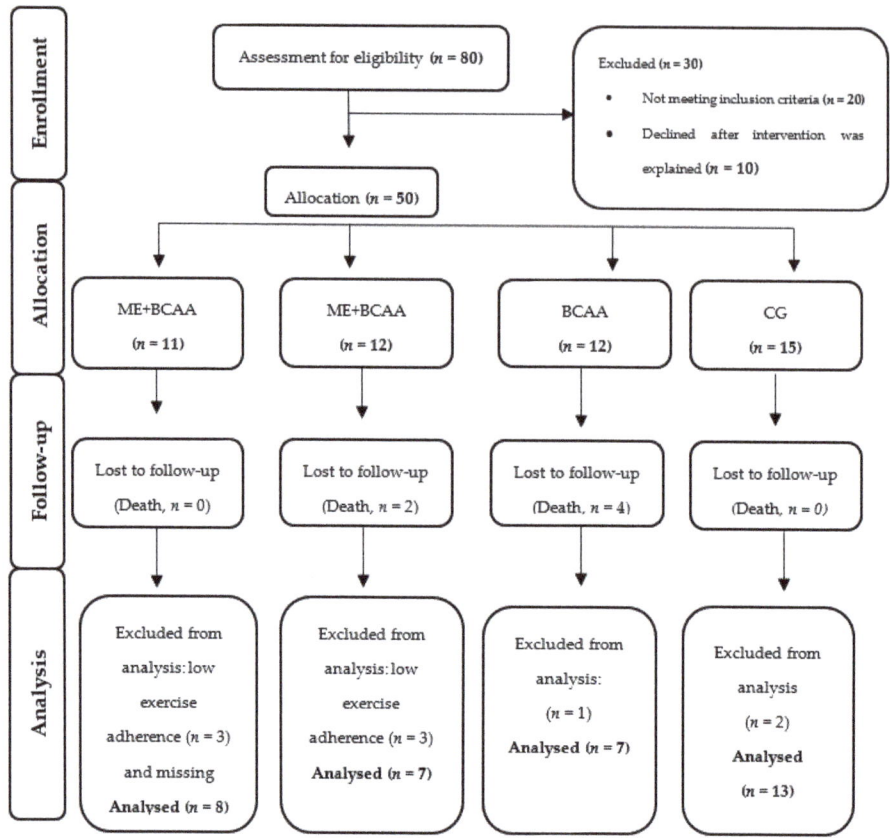

Figure 1. CONSORT Flowchart of study participants [30]. ME + BCAA, Multicomponent Exercise + Branched Chain Amino Acid; ME, Multicomponent Exercise; BCAA, Branched Chain Amino Acid; CG, Control Group.

2.4. Experimental Design

This study is a four-phase prospective, naturalistic, controlled clinical trial with four arms of MIP experimental design (ME + BCAAs, BCAAs, ME, and CG). In the first phase, a baseline data collection (T1) was done followed by 16 weeks of MIP. The second phase consisted of a second data collection (T2) followed by an 8 week washout phase. Phase 3 consisted of a third data collection, followed by the resumption of the MIP for a period of 16 weeks. The last data collection took place after the 16 weeks of intervention (T4) (Figure 2).

3. Outcome Measures

All the assessments were performed in the morning, between 10 and 11:45 a.m. One session was used to apply a short test battery to measure biosocial, global health status, cognition profile, nutritional, physical, and physical frailty status. In the second consecutive day, blood samples were collected and stored at −80 °C until further analysis.

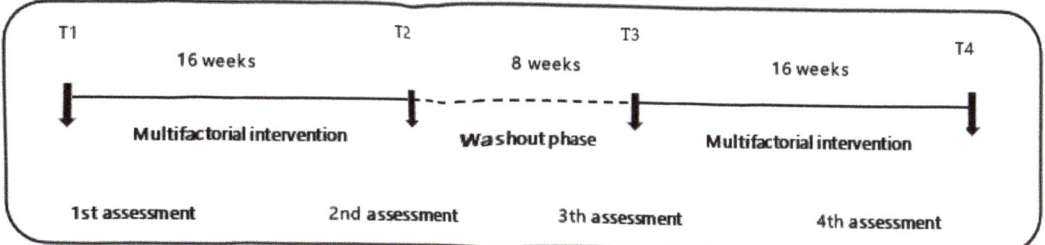

Figure 2. Chronological order of multifactorial interventions study design. T1 to T2 (elastic-band exercise, 16 weeks, 8 weeks), T2 to T3 (wash-out), T3 to T4 (multicomponent exercise, 16 weeks).

3.1. Physical Frailty Index

The phenotype of Fried's physical frailty index was used [9]. Weight loss was assessed by a self-report of unintentional weight loss of 4 kg or more in the last 6 months. Self-reported exhaustion was evaluated by a negative concordance of question number 7 and 20 of the Center of Epidemiologic Studies for Depression scale [31]. Hand-grip strength was assessed in kilograms by a hand-held (HGT) dynamometer (Lafayette 78,010, Sagamore, United States). The best result of the two trials was used for scoring purposes. Participants who were unable to perform the HGT and those in the lowest 20% were categorized as positive [32]. The cutoff reference values for HGT of ≥ 29 kg for male and ≥ 17 kg for female were adopted. Slowness was measured by the "15 feet (4.6 m) walking test". Based on the cutoff values of Fried's study population, the times of ≥ 7 s for males and ≥ 6 s for females were adopted for positive scores of slowness. The best time of the two trials was used for the final scoring. Low physical activity (PA) levels were assessed by the International PA Questionnaire short version (IPAQ-SV) [33]. There are three levels of PA suggested for classification: Inactive, minimally active, and highly active. Participants classified as inactive had a positive score for this PF component. A positive evaluation in one or two criteria classified the participants as pre-frail, in three or more criteria as frail, and as non-frail when the subject scored none of the five PF indicators. The prevalence of PF was calculated to generate a frailty total score, as well as the presence of each of the five criteria of the Fried's model (0 to 5 points). In this study, participants classified as frail (3 or more points) and pre-frail (2 points) were included.

3.2. Nutritional Assessment

Daily diet at the RCH was prescribed by a registered nutritionist and was provided for all the participants without any change or interference of the research staff. On the basis of the information provided, the diet was analyzed using specific tools (photographic quantification of portions, food table) for the Portuguese population [34–36]. Due to the relationship between the frailty status and severe decrease of muscle mass (or sarcopenia) which had already been demonstrated in several studies, the objective of this nutritional assessment was to characterize the protein consumption of the participants. In addition, the Mini Nutritional Assessment (MNA) questionnaire was applied [37,38]. This consists of 18 questions that present a maximum score of 30 points, and classifies the participants as malnourished (≤ 17 points), at risk of malnutrition ($17 < MNA < 23.5$ points), and as having a normal nutritional status (MNA > 23.5 points).

3.3. Lower Limb Muscle-Strength Test

The Five-Times-Sit-to-Stand-Test (5TSS test) was applied. This test assesses the functional strength of the lower limbs, transition movements, balance, and risk of falling. The participant is instructed to stand as quickly as possible five times, without stopping in the middle. In addition, the participant should be encouraged to keep his arms crossed over his chest. The instructor must count the time with a stopwatch and must count each position out loud so that the participant remains oriented. The test is stopped when the participant reaches the orthostatic position at the 5th repetition [29].

3.4. Clinical and Health Status

The Charlson comorbidity index (CCI) was calculated based on the registry of individual comorbidities combined with age and gender, to account for a final score [39]. The anthropometric assessment included body mass (kg) and stature (m). Body mass was determined using a portable scale (Seca®, model 770, Berlin, Germany) with a precision of 0.1 kg, whereas stature was determined using a portable stadiometer (Seca Body meter®, model 208, Berlin, Germany) with a precision of 0.1 cm. Body mass index (BMI) was calculated according to the formula (BMI = body mass/stature^2). The standardized procedures described in previous studies were followed [40].

3.5. Cognitive Profile

The Portuguese version of the Mini Mental State Examination (MMSE) was used [41]. The MMSE is a 30-point scale instrument that evaluates five domains of cognition: Orientation, immediate recall, attention and calculation, delayed recall, and language. This scale classifies individuals by progressive cognitive skills: (0–9 points) severe cognitive impairment; (10–18 points) moderate cognitive impairment; (19–24 points) mild cognitive impairment; and (25–30 points) normal cognitive profile [42].

3.6. Biochemical Analysis

Non-fasting blood collection was done in the morning (between 10:00 a.m. and 11:00 a.m.). Blood samples were collected by venipuncture, after 15 min of individual rest in an isolated and quiet room, at the four time-points of the study assessment. The participants were asked to avoid alcohol and caffeine intake on the previous day of blood collection, and also to maintain their sleep habits during the previous night. After centrifugation at 3000 rpm at 4 °C during 15 min, plasma and serum samples were aliquoted into Eppendorf tubes and stored at −80 °C until used for the determination of interleukin-10 (IL-10), tumour necrosis factor alpha (TNF-α), myeloperoxidase activity (MPO), and total albumin concentrations. The ELISA (Thermo Fisher, Gloucester, UK) intra-assay coefficients of variability were 4.1% for IL-10 and 3.0% for TNF-α.

3.7. Full Characterization of the MIP

3.7.1. Oral BCAAs

The BCAAs power mixture was composed of L-leucine (Leu), L-isoleucine (Ile), and L-valine (Val) in the proportion of 2:1:1 (MyProtein®, Cheshire, UK), accounting for 20 kcal per portion, comprising 5 grams (g) of supplement: 1.85 g Leu, 0.93 g Ile, and 0.93 g Val. The unflavored supplement was used as to not induce ingestion preferences for specific flavors. The BCCAs were diluted in 200 mL of water and given immediately after the exercise sessions to the participants in the ME + BCAAs and BCAAs groups [43]. The supplement dose was fixed at 0.21 g total BCAAs/kg/session, with individual portion sachets, administered in the morning, between 09:00 and 11:30 a.m. [44]. We opted to exclude maltodextrin or the carnosine-based placebo here, since the carbohydrate ingestion could mask the effort perception and cognitive indexes in our older persons volunteers, compared to the amino acid supplementation [45]. In addtion, carnosine, as well as other β-alanine derivatives, were shown to affect cognitive functions, including the perception of wellness, mood, and depression indexes [46]. Therefore, we decided to split BCAA-supplemented (ME + BCAAs and BCAAs) and BCAAs-absent groups (ME and CG) according to the proximity between the residential care homes (RCH), where the ME programs were effectively applied. No communication was reported between volunteers from the BCAA-supplemented and no-BCAA supplemented groups in our study.

3.7.2. Washout Period (Oral BCAAs)

In this phase, the participants endured a cessation period of 8 weeks, when supplementation of the ME + BCAAs and BCAAs groups was suspended in order to verify whether the supposed benefits of BCAAs were maintained or lost [21].

3.7.3. Exercise Intervention (Phase 1)

The exercise program was divided in two interventions of 16 weeks each, separated by an 8-week detraining (washout) period. Exercise sessions were offered twice a week, with an interval of 36 h for adequate physiological recovery and rest. The exercise protocol respected the guidelines of exercise prescription for older persons and the guidelines of exercise periodization by the American College of Sports Medicine (ACSM) [47,48]. The program started with an adaptation period of 2 weeks, in which seven different exercises were performed using elastic bands (TheraBand®, Hygenic Corporation, Akron, OH, USA). The participants were closely supervised for two initial sessions aiming for equipment familiarization and adjustments to the Rating Perceived Exertion (RPE OMNI) scale [49]. During these familiarization sessions, the participants learned the correct technique of the exercises, and selected the proper color, length, and grip width of the elastic bands. The exercise intensity was indirectly calculated using the Karvonen's formula to predict the target heart rate (HR), with HR_{max} being calculated by an adjusted formula for older persons [50].

$$HR = ((HR_{max} - \text{resting HR}) \times \%\text{Intensity}) + \text{resting HR} \quad (1)$$

After the adaptation period, the exercise program was progressively intensified by increments in both the number of exercises (from 8 to 10 exercises during the rest of the exercise intervention) and the proposed physical effort, imposed by different intensity color bands, according to the OMNI table [49]. The elastic-band exercises applied in the Phase 1 period are shown in Table 1. For safety reasons, the exercise programs were also monitored using heart rate monitors (Polar M200; Polar Electro Oy, Kempele, Finland). Additionally, intensity was measured through the specific rating perceived exertion (RPE) scales for each exercise program [51]. The RPE used is an arbitrary scale ranging from 0 to 10 points, with identical intervals and with reference to the quality of effort: (0) Nothing at all; (1) very weak; (2) weak; (3) moderate; (4) somewhat strong; (5–6) strong; (7–9) very strong; (10) very, very strong (almost maximal).

Table 1. Example of elastic-band exercise sessions applied in phase 1.

Warm-Up				5 min	PSE 1–3	Progression	Weeks	Intensity (Color)
Exercises (8–10)	Sets	Repetitions	Cadence	Interval	PSE	2×10	2	Yellow
Front squat	2–3	10–20	2:3	30–45 s	4 to 6	3×20	2	Yellow
Chair unilateral hip flexion	2–3	10–20	2:3	30–45 s	4 to 6	3×10	2	Red
Chair Bench over row (with flexion)	2–3	10–20	2:3	30–45 s	4 to 6	3×20	2	Red
Chest Press (stand and/or chair)	2–3	10–20	2:3	30–45 s	4 to 6	3×10	2	Green
Standing (or chair) reverse fly	2–3	10–20	2:3	30–45 s	4 to 6	3×20	2	Green
Shoulder Press/twist arm position	2–3	10–20	2:3	30–45 s	4 to 6	3×15	2	Blue
Chair (or stand) frontal total raiser	2–3	10–20	2:3	30–45 s	4 to 6	$3\text{–}4 \times 10^{-15}$	2	Blue
Biceps arm curl (stand and/or chair)	2–3	10–20	2:3	30–45 s	4 to 6			
Chair Overhead triceps extension	2–3	10–20	2:3	30–45 s	4 to 6			
Cooling down				5 min	PSE 1–2			

Notes: PSE—Perception subjective effort.

3.7.4. Washout (ME Detraining)

In this phase, the participants endured a detraining period of 8 weeks, when the ME programs were suspended. The aim was to check if the physiological adaptations acquired during the first phase of ME were maintained or if an 8-week interruption was able to revert the possible effects on immune changes [52].

3.7.5. Exercise Retraining Protocol

The phase 3 (exercise retraining) protocol was also based on the resistant TheraBand (TheraBand®, Hygenic Corporation, Akron, OH, USA) elastic bands (Table 2), but included walking, steps, and balance exercises (sometimes with dumbbells and ankle/wrist weights) to compose a multicomponent exercise program for an identical 16-week period (twice a week, on alternate days, also totalizing 32 sessions). The multicomponent program (Table 2) was described by Furtado et al. [53]. The phase 3 program aimed to reproduce most of the daily activities of the older persons in this study [54].

Table 2. Example of multicomponent exercise sessions applied in phase 2.

Exercises (8–10)	Sets	Repetitions	Cadence	Interval	PSE
Front squat	2–3	10–20	2:3	30–45 s	4 to 6
Chair unilateral hip flexion	2–3	10–20	2:3	30–45 s	4 to 6
Chair Bench over row (with flexion)	2–3	10–20	2:3	30–45 s	4 to 6
Chest Press (stand and/or chair)	2–3	10–20	2:3	30–45 s	4 to 6
Standing (or chair) reverse fly	2–3	10–20	2:3	30–45 s	4 to 6
Shoulder Press/twist arm front position	2–3	10–20	2:3	30–45 s	4 to 6
Chair (or stand) frontal total raiser	2–3	10–20	2:3	30–45 s	4 to 6
Biceps arm curl (stand and/or chair)	2–3	10–20	2:3	30–45 s	4 to 6
Chair Overhead triceps extension	2–3	10–20	2:3	30–45 s	4 to 6
Circuit Training					
Walking around the room	2–3	3 min		30–45 s	4 to 6
Balance/agility exercise	2–3	3 min		30–45 s	4 to 6

Notes: PSE—Perception subjective effort.

3.8. Statistical Analysis

The descriptive statistics for each group, at the baseline and follow-up evaluations, were reported as the mean plus standard deviation (M ± SD), except when mentioned otherwise. All the variables were checked for the normally residual distribution and values were logarithmically transformed when appropriate. One-way Analysis of Variance ANOVA was used to determine baseline differences between the four groups in all the parameters. Effects of time, group, and time x group interactions were assessed through repeated measures ANOVA and Bonferroni post-hoc for multiple comparisons. Additionally, univariate analysis was performed using the paired t-test for comparisons during the first phase of interventions (T1 vs. T2). All statistical analyses were performed using the SPSS 21 (SPSS Inc., Chicago, IL, USA), and the level of significance was set at $p < 0.05$.

4. Results

The dynamics of the MIP groups and drop-outs are presented in detail in Figure 1. From the 50 (100%) participants initially selected, only 35 participants (70%) completed the intervention. This is an expected experimental loss, as reported by several previous studies [55]. None of the dropouts left the intervention due to injuries or adverse responses. Reported deaths were due to acute events triggered by chronic clinical conditions. Table 3 shows the characterization of participants by MIP groups at the baseline, including nutritional, cognitive, frailty, anthropometric, and body composition status. No statistically significant differences in all the variables appeared, expect for time in residential care and nutritional status assessed by MNA ($p < 0.05$). However, all the groups were within the well-nourished category.

Table 3. Characterization of participants by intervention groups at baseline.

Variables	ME + BCAA (n = 8) M ± SD	ME (n = 7) M ± SD	BCAA (n = 7) M ± SD	CG (n = 13) M ± SD	p-Value
Age (years)	80 ± 6.1	86.7 ± 4	84.2 ± 5.8	83.1 ± 5.4	0.139
Time in residential care (years)	3.6 ± 1	4.7 ± 1.4	4.5 ± 1.1	5 ± 1	0.06
MNA (0–30 pts)	25.5 ± 2.2	24 ± 2.7	21.7 ± 2.8	24.7 ± 1.8	0.02
BMI (kg/m^2)	28.53 ± 5.1	28.7 ± 5.6	25.8 ± 3.1	30.2 ± 3.7	0.23
Stature (cm)	158 ± 0.05	150 ± 0.06	161 ± 0.12	155 ± 011	0.16
Comorbidity index (0–10 pts)	4.87 ± 1.12	5.28 ± 0.95	5.42 ± 1.1	4.92 ± 1.2	0.71
Schooling time (years)	4 ± 0	4 ± 0	4 ± 0	4 ± 0	0.99
Cognitive profile (0–30 pts)	26.00 (3.11)	21.00 (3.78)	20.85 (2.79)	21.69 (2.89)	0.00
Physical Frailty index (0–5 pts)	2.00 (0.53)	2.71 (1.1)	3.00 (0.57)	2.16 (0.71)	0.40
Daily Individual Protein (gr/kg/day)	1.42 ± 0.28	1.83 ± 0.44	1.48 ± 0.22	1.60 ± 0.23	0.159
BCAAs (per person/gr/week)	30.3 ± 6.0	n.d.	28.4 ± 5.0	n.d.	

Notes: BMI: Body mass index; MNA: Mini nutritional assessment; M ± SD: Mean (standard and deviation); pts: Points; Kg/m^2: Kilograms; cm: Centimeters; One-way ANOVA was used to compare groups, except for the Comorbidity index (Fisher Exact Test). BCAA Branched Chain Amino Acids.

4.1. Biochemical Analysis

Table 4 shows the results for IL-10, TNF-α and TNF-α/IL-10 ratio, MPO, albumin, 5TSS-Test, as well as Fried (score) and MMSE. Concerning the IL-10 levels, a classical anti-inflammatory cytokine, not only no effects of time ($p = 0.690$) or time vs. experimental groups were found (CG, BCAAs, ME, and ME + BCAAs), F(degrees of freedom-df:9, 51) = 1.567, $p = 150$), but also Bonferroni post-hoc comparisons did not result in significant variations between time vs. groups ($p > 0.05$). Regarding the TNF-α levels, although we did not observe any interference of time on these pro-inflammatory cytokine levels ($p > 0.05$, Table 4), repeated ANOVA analyses revealed significant interactions between time vs. groups: F(df: 6.758, 47.303) = 2.524, $p = 0.029$. In addition, Bonferroni post-hoc comparisons showed not only higher TNF-α values in the ME + BCAAs group between T2 and T3 ($p = 0.01$), but also a significant decrease of TNF-α was observed between T3 and T4 within the same experimental group (ME + BCAAs, $p < 0.01$). The TNF-α values were unchanged in all other experimental groups. Regarding the TNF-α/IL-10 ratios, no significant variations were observed over time ($p = 0.703$) or within the interactions (time vs. group, $p = 0.638$).

Concerning MPO activity, Table 4 shows that this biomarker was not influenced by time (T1, T2, T3, and T4), except for a slight tendency regarding interactions (time vs. group): F(df: 9, 48) = 2.010, $p = 0.059$. Particularly, the Bonferroni post-hoc comparisons showed that the BCAAs group presented higher MPO activity after re-supplementation (T4) than the values found in the T2 time-point (after the first 16 weeks of the supplementation period, $p = 0.026$). No significant alterations in the MPO activity were observed in other comparisons between groups.

In terms of serum albumin (Table 4), a statistically significant difference in the effect of time was found (F(df: 1949; 46,784) = 3.841, $p = 0.02$), but no other (time vs. group) significant difference was detected between the albumin levels ($p = 0.219$). The pairwise comparison using Bonferroni post-hoc showed a decrease of albumin levels in the BCAAs group in the T3 time-point (after the washout period, $p = 0.04$) as compared to the values found in T1, whereas no other significant variations were observed in the other groups ($p > 0.05$).

4.2. Five-Times-Sit-to-Stand-Test (5TSS test)

Table 4 shows no effect of time ($p = 0.841$) or interactions (time vs. group, $p = 0.846$) on the time elapsed to perform the 5TSS test. However, post-hoc adjustments showed that the ME + BCAAs and BCAAs groups presented a significant reduction of the time elapsed to perform this test at time-points T2, T3, and T4 ($p = 0.009$, $p = 0.014$, and $p = 0.024$, respectively).

Table 4. Statistical analysis comparison of four time-points moments of multifactorial intervention for biochemical, cognitive profile, physical frailty index, and functional fitness test.

Biomarker/Variables	Groups	T1 M ± SD	T2 M ± SD	T3 M ± SD	T4 M ± SD	Effect	F	Overall p
IL-10 (µg/mL)	ME + BCAA	10.36 (6.96)	12.0 (6.53)	15.99 (7.98)	11.52 (7.56)	Time	0.491	0.690
	ME	8.68 (7.68)	12.25 (12.35)	4.16 (3.39)	10.53 (5.82)			
	BCAA	7.71 (2.54)	9.24 (4.15)	13.83 (6.94)	9.85 (10.89)	Time*group	1.567	0.150
	CG	16.10 (7.4)	12.21 (2.81)	12.74 (7.36)	20.45 (5.42)			
TNF-α (pg/mL)	ME + BCAA	62.44 (53.65)	71.42 (38.06)	112.86 (62.51)	57.37 (31.18)	Time	1.552	0.210
	ME	41.78 (54.08)	45.83 (21.07)	24.92 (15.60)	54.05 (29.19)			
	BCAA	32.65 (15.74)	37.18 (26.91)	62.93 (35.77)	60.02 (55.42)	Time*group	2.524	0.015
	CG	44.46 (41.72)	44.81 (37.16)	41.78 (37.86)	57.01 (44.15)			
TNF-α/IL-10 ratio (pg/mL)	ME + BCAA	6.24 (4.46)	7.47 (4.09)	6.96 (1.63)	6.10 (3.25)	Time	0.472	0.703
	ME	4.43 (1.99)	9.06 (10.46)	8.64 (7.36)	5.70 (3.27)			
	BCAA	5.44 (3.39)	3.85 (1.84)	5.45 (1.54)	11.19 (9.77)	Time*group	0.777	0.638
	CG	4.10 (1.27)	5.37 (1.56)	4.56 (1.80)	4.41 (0.38)			
MPO (µg/mL)	ME + BCAA	5653.91 (1106.71)	5871.97 (1159.09)	4843.50 (1221.63)	5196.53 (591.62)	Time	1.191	0.323
	ME	5935.71 (1315.33)	5252.76 (1084.06)	4685.42 (1043.31)	4512.34 (794.61)			
	BCAA	5139.04 (909.07)	4069.64 (1009.10)	5416.47 (1539.50)	5575.80 (1181.43)	Time*group	2.010	0.059
	CG	4623.56 (699.03)	4593.56 (1310.34)	4655.42 (815.10)	4327.39 (863.95)			
Albumin (g/dL)	ME + BCAA	3.60 (0.39)	3.63 (0.61)	3.82 (0.54)	3.75 (0.63)	Time	3.841	0.013
	ME	3.73 (0.61)	4.12 (0.74)	3.57 (0.43)	4.13 (0.22)			
	BCAA	3.77 (0.39)	3.61 (0.40)	1.56 (2.15)	2.83 (1.60)	Time*group	1.446	0.185
	CG	3.75 (0.72)	3.60 (0.35)	2.59 (1.85)	2.96 (1.69)			
5TSS test (s)	ME + BCAA	21.87 (3.64)	18.71 (3.59)	20.66 (4.98)	17.54 (4.4)	Time	0.165	0.841
	ME	26.69 (12.98)	28.02 (11.28)	26.08 (10.46)	27.56 (12.24)			
	BCAA	36.54 (14.14)	36.24 (13.39)	36.74 (11.89)	35.76 (17.28)	Time*group	0.436	0.846
	CG	24.58 (8.99)	24.76 (9.0)	23.66 (9.30)	25.17 (9.75)			
Physical Frailty (index)	ME + BCAA	2.00 (0.53)	1.50 (0.53)	2.12 (0.99)	2.00 (0.53)	Time	2.702	0.05
	ME	2.71 (1.1)	2.57 (1.13)	2.14 (0.69)	2.00 (0.81)			
	BCAA	3.00 (0.57)	2.14 (0.37)	2.28 (1.25)	2.71 (0.48)	Time*group	3.799	0.00
	CG	2.16 (0.71)	2.25 (0.75)	2.66 (0.49)	3.16 (0.71)			
MMSE (0–30 points)	ME + BCAA	26.00 (3.11)	26.37 (2.44)	26.00 (2.87)	24.37 (3.58)	Time	4.262	0.13
	ME	21.00 (3.78)	22.42 (2.99)	21.00 (4.65)	20.00 (3.91)			
	BCAA	20.85 (2.79)	19.42 (4.07)	20.71 (4.02)	19.57 (3.64)	Time*group	1.214	0.305
	CG	21.69 (2.89)	23.92 (3.47)	23.23 (3.83)	21.76 (2.94)			

Notes: M ± SD: Mean (standard and deviation); ME: Multicomponent exercise; BCAA: Branched-chain amino acids; IL: Interleukin; TNF-α: Tumor Necrosis Factor-alpha; MPO: Myeloperoxidase; MMSE: Mini Mental State Exam; 5TSS test: Five-Times-Sit-to-Stand-Test; T1 to T2 (elastic-band exercise, 16 weeks, 8 weeks), T2 to T3 (wash-out), T3 to T4 (multicomponent exercise, 16 weeks). * time versus group interactions. Statistically significant differences are denoted in bold.

4.3. Cognitive Assessment

The results obtained in the cognitive profile (Table 4), show that, at baseline (T1), 65.7% of the participants (n = 23) scored below the 24-point threshold in the MMSE test, indicating that a significant fraction of participants was within the mild/moderate cognitive impairment classification. In addition, at the same time-point (T1), significant differences were found for the cognitive score between the ME + BCAAs group and the other groups ($p < 0.05$). An effect of time (F(df: 3, 93) = 4.262, $p = 0.007$), but not interaction (time vs. group, $p = 0.296$), was observed for the MMSE results. The cognitive MMSE scores increased in the control group between T1 and T2 but decreased subsequently in T3 and T4 ($p = 0.008$). No significant alterations were observed in the other groups. At baseline, 45.7% of the participants were classified as frail and 54.3% as pre-frail.

5. Discussion

This study evaluated the effects of exercise and BCAAs on biomarkers of immunity, total albumin, and the cognitive profile of institutionalized older persons. The main findings were that ME showed more proemint result, particullary with BCAA in the improve cognitive profile and muscle strength-related albumin levels in plasma and diminish the frailty status. Moreover, exercise induced slight changes on the pro-inflammatory marker TNF-α.

Albumin levels tend to decrease with age, and this effect seems to imply an increased risk of complications and higher rate of mortality, morbidity, and disabilities such as sarcopenia and frailty [56]. Despite the key participation of albumin on the pH balance and ionic homeostasis in blood, most of the free fatty acid (and some other lipids) transport in the bloodstream is also performed by serum albumin [57]. Not surprisingly, the age-related impaired albuminemia and elevated serum anion gap are known to be associated with hypertension, low cardiorespiratory fitness, and decreased renal function, which are common morbidities of advanced aged people [58]. Therefore, interventions that aim to sustain (or even increase) albuminemia in older persons could represent an important strategy to mitigate the harmful effects of aging and its comorbidities. In this respect, some studies have already shown that BCAAs apparently increases albumin levels in older persons suffering from malnutrition [59].

Our results showed that the serum albumin levels were efficiently sustained or even augmented, in exercising participants (both ME and ME + BCAAs groups) during the first 16 weeks of intervention (phase 1). However, the withdrawal of BCAAs during the washout period (phase 2) quickly decreased those albumin levels, especially in the BCAAs group. The prominent effect of exercise on albumin levels was evident since its levels in both ME and ME + BCAAs groups were fully restored after the phase 3 period (T3 to T4 time-points), whereas only partial recoveries were observed in albumin levels in the BCAAs group at the same time-point. Low serum albumin levels were shown to be the most relevant biomarkers associated with poor physical strength in the older persons [60].

It is broadly accepted that the regular practice of exercise training imposes metabolic, endocrine/physiological, immune, and cognitive adaptations that, among many benefits, can increase skeletal muscle mass and strength, thus, circumventing the deleterious effects of sarcopenia in older persons [61].

The chronic exercise-mediated adjustments on insulin/glucagon balance, thyroid, and steroid hormones, such as testosterone, cortisol, and estrogens, can also be involved in the enhancement of hepatic and protein muscle metabolism (proteolysis, proteogenesis, and protein turnover), with clear consequences on the circulating amino acid levels (e.g., glutamine and alanine), blood pH and electrolyte balance (hydric/ionic homeostasis), and renal functions [62].

However, it was reported that the putative effect of amino acid/protein supplementation in older women could be masked by sufficient daily protein intake, as we attested in all institutionalized participants in this study [63]. Thus, the proper mechanism behind this effect still needs to be fully understood for this special population. In fact, to our knowledge, this is the first study to show the potential of physical exercise associated or not with BCAAs supplementation to maintain serum albumin levels in older persons living in RCH.

Contrarily to the albumin results, the monitored inflammatory markers (IL-10, TNF-α, and MPO) did not show significant alterations over time. Apparently, we can putatively suggest, that the physical exercise intensities reached in the sessions, as well as the BCAAs supplementation effect compared to the daily protein intake in this population, were not sufficient to induce a significant impact on the inflammatory status in the participants in this study. Other interventions with older persons have been able to show a strong anti-inflammatory effect of exercise training, but it seems that these results were observed for intervention periods longer than 16 weeks [43,44].

Interestingly, even though an increase in the levels of the pro-inflammatory cytokine TNF-α was observed in the ME + BCAAs group from T1 to T2 and T3, this finding was accompanied by a proportional increase of the anti-inflammatory cytokine IL-10, since the TNF-α/IL-10 ratio was not different in this group over time. Moreover, at the end of the intervention, TNF-α levels significantly decreased in this group. In accordance with the literature, IL-10 is a key anti-inflammatory cytokine that acts by inhibiting systemic inflammation mediated by TNF-α [64].

Concomitantly, BCAAs alone did not induce alterations in both IL-10 and TNF-α levels. These results differ slightly from what is observed in the literature regarding this type of intervention on inflammatory status [65]. Based on the literature, there is a close interaction between the inflammatory status and aging, and in this respect, it is widely accepted that older persons, especially sedentary people, present a chronic, systemic, sterile low-grade inflammation associated with aging, a phenomenon named inflammaging [66]. It is highlighted that inflammaging plays an important role in the loss of lean mass, which leads to sarcopenia and frailty, as well as increases the risk of the development of diseases and comorbidities, such as cognitive decline, atherosclerosis, insulin resistance, etc. [67].

Despite the fact that literature defines the ability to induce an anti-inflammatory change as a hallmark of physical exercise, in general, our results did not corroborate this fact. It is paramount to mention that some factors could putatively influence the lack of significant results in the inflammatory analysis. Firstly, the occurrence of inflammaging and pathophysiological disturbances in our participants could be crucial for the response magnitude observed during the interventions here. Second, the low level of physical activity of our participants before the interventions could mitigate the benefits that would be achieved with the physical exercise sessions and, consequently, limit physiological adaptation. These factors, associated with polypharmacy, a high rate of comorbidities, and the small sample size that finished the study, may determine the lack of significant effects observed.

There is a consensus in the literature that physical exercise sessions stimulate the release of cytokines, such as IL-6, IL-10, and TNF-α, in response to contracting skeletal muscles, which are responsible not only for tissue restoration and energy metabolism, but also for the adjustment of the systemic inflammatory status [68]. As appealing as these effects are, physical exercise training also improves human antioxidant defenses as observed in several studies which may also justify the use of exercise interventions to counteract the progression of oxidative-related diseases [69].

There are solid pieces of evidence that the loss of muscle strength and power in the lower limbs, which is characterized by a decline of up to 50% in overall muscle strength from the age of 30 to 80 years [52,53] is associated with an increased incidence of falls.

Particularly, physical exercise training improves body composition, muscle strength, metabolic parameters, bone health, and functionality as well as reduces the risk of mortality, chronic diseases, cognitive deterioration, falls, and depression [70]. Here, we observed that only the ME + BCAAs group presented an improved physical performance in the 5TSS test. Neither ME or BCAAs alone were sufficient to mediate improvements in lower body strength. Only the combination of exercise and supplementation did so. This result was achieved probably due to multiple factors, from physiological to cognitive positive effects that were not directly assessed by the applied methodology here. According to the literature, the 5TSS test is an important performance test that invokes physical skills and abilities that could have been particularly developed during phase 3 of this study. The phase 3 of our study included walking activities, steps, and balance exercises, which mimic the participants' regular daily life activities.

It is important to point out that strength exercise training has been proposed as one of the most effective methodologies, presenting best results in bringing back safety in performing the common tasks of daily life, focusing on the optimization of neuromuscular function for better benefits [71].

Multicomponent programs combine aerobic and strength exercises, including other physical skills, such as balance and flexibility [54], in order to optimize the functional capacity of frail older persons [72], as well as to maintain their independence to perform basic activities of daily living [73]. Concerning supplementation, it was reported that branched-chain amino acids, particularly L-leucine, showed significant results in inducing hypertrophy in older persons and improving their functional capacity [58,59].

Taking into account that cognitive impairment is one of the main factors that cause morbidity and high health costs worldwide [74], our results show that physical exercise training, in association or not with BCAAs, was able to maintain the cognitive scores of the participants and could have important practical applications. Considering the population enrolled here (pre-frail and frail octogenarians) and the trend for the natural decline of their cognitive functions, the maintenance of those cognitive scores by exercise is, per se, a remarkable achievement. The literature supports the positive effect of BCAAs in older persons, to improve their mood state [75], the perception of fatigue, and their performance in a mental task [76], which are abilities that were not evaluated here. Leucine is important since it activates the mammalian target of rapamycin complex 1 (mTORC1) and the downstream phosphorylation of p70S6 kinase and 4E (eIF4E)-binding protein 1 (4E-BP1) and related signaling pathways [77]. The aging muscle is less responsive to lower doses of amino acids when compared to the young muscle and may require higher quantities of protein to acutely stimulate equivalent muscle protein synthesis [78]. Nevertheless, the dose and duration of BCAAs proposed here did not affect the cognition scores in our participants.

Study Limitation and Perspectives for Future Researchers

The entire study was conducted with human octogenarians and, given the difficulty to control several influencing factors in this type of population, this study had the additional merit of causing a minimal impact on their daily routines at the residential care homes. In addition, our results here represent real-world data reflecting the reality at residential care homes. We screened participants with disabilities and comorbidities that, although expecting high rate of dropouts and low motivational issues, we could accomplish the proposed goals with a reasonable number of participants. The execution of a controlled study over 40 weeks with such a particular population also introduces other limitations. We suggest that the use of other methods of exercise training, such as the use of playful activities (dance and music sessions) might elevate the adherence of this population to the program.

6. Conclusions

This study showed that multicompetent exercise training, with minor effect of BCAAs, triggered alterations in the inflammatory status and physical profiles of older persons, while helping maintain cognitive levels. Taken together, the achieved results, could help increase autonomy and efficiency in the performance of daily activities. Unlike other studies, our results showed that supplementation with BCAA did not induce substantial changes in health-related parameters at older ages. It is possible that the heterogeneity and limited sample size might have limited the statistical relevance of our results. Despite a slight and transient variation over time observed in some inflammatory and cognitive parameters, it is possible that the results here were influenced by the comorbidity status of each group.

Author Contributions: A.C.-S. drafted the paper; G.E.F. worked on the methodology of the study aspects of RCT; R.N. helped with data acquisition; M.U.C. statically analyzed the data; A.M.T., A.M. and E.M. developed the study proposal, revised the manuscript critically, and suggested additional statistical analyses; A.M.T. coordinated the research study and, together with M.P.d.B. and A.L.L.B., revised the manuscript critically. All authors have read and agreed to the published version of the manuscript.

Funding: Portuguese Foundation for Science and Technology—CIDAF (UID/DTP/0413/2020). BCAA supplement provided free of cost by MyProtein®, Cheshire, UK.

Institutional Review Board Statement: This study was conducted according to the guidelines of the and approved by the University of Coimbra, Faculty of Sport Sciences and Physical Education Ethical Committee (reference number: CE/FCDEFUC/00282018), https://clinicaltrials.gov/ct2/show/NCT04376463 (accessed on 5 May 2020).

Informed Consent Statement: Informed consent was obtained from all subjects involved in the study.

Data Availability Statement: The data presented in this study are available on request from the corresponding author. Data supporting the reported results is the property of CIDAF, Faculty of Sport Sciences and Physical Education, University of Coimbra, Coimbra, Portugal.

Acknowledgments: We would like to thank the RCH for accepting to participate in this study. Thanks to the Pedro Alexandre Ferreira Filipe nurse for volunteering with the data collection and Ana Vieira-Pedrosa and Rafael Rodrigues for helping with the data collection. The authors would like to thank Jonatas Bussador do Amaral for his assistance in the graphical abstract. The authors M.P.B. and A.L.L.B. are fellows of the Brazilian National Council for Scientific and Technology Development (CNPq; M.P.B.: PQ-2 #305818/2018-0; A.L.L.B.: PQ-2 #307674/2017-7, Brazil).

Conflicts of Interest: The authors declare that there are no conflict of interest.

References

1. Aiello, A.; Farzaneh, F.; Candore, G.; Caruso, C.; Davinelli, S.; Gambino, C.M.; Ligotti, M.E.; Zareian, N.; Accardi, G. Immunosenescence and its hallmarks: How to oppose aging strategically? A review of potential options for therapeutic intervention. *Front. Immunol.* **2019**, *10*, 1–19. [CrossRef]
2. Duggal, N.A.; Niemiro, G.; Harridge, S.D.; Simpson, R.J.; Lord, J.M. Can physical activity ameliorate immunosenescence and thereby reduce age-related multi-morbidity? *Nat. Rev. Immunol.* **2019**, *19*, 563–572. [CrossRef] [PubMed]
3. Amirato, G.R.; Borges, J.O.; Marques, D.L.; Santos, J.M.B.; Santos, C.A.F.; Andrade, M.S.; Furtado, G.E.; Rossi, M.; Luis, L.N.; Zambonatto, R.F.; et al. L-glutamine supplementation enhances strength and power of knee muscles and improves glycemia control and plasma redox balance in exercising elderly women. *Nutrients* **2021**, *13*, 1025. [CrossRef]
4. Chodzko-Zajko, W.; Schwingel, A. Successful Aging: The Role of Physical Activity. *Am. J. Lifestyle Med.* **2008**, *3*, 20–28. [CrossRef]
5. Bauman, A.; Merom, D.; Bull, F.C.; Buchner, D.M.; Fiatarone Singh, M.A. Updating the Evidence for Physical Activity: Summative Reviews of the Epidemiological Evidence, Prevalence, and Interventions to Promote "active Aging". *Gerontologist* **2016**, *56*, S268–S280. [CrossRef]
6. Sherrington, C.; Fairhall, N.; Kirkham, C.; Clemson, L.; Howard, K.; Vogler, C.; Close, J.C.; Moseley, A.M.; Cameron, I.D.; Mak, J.; et al. Exercise and fall prevention self-management to reduce mobility-related disability and falls after fall-related lower limb fracture in older people: Protocol for the RESTORE (Recovery Exercises and Stepping on after Fracture) randomised controlled trial. *BMC Geriatr.* **2016**, *16*, 34. [CrossRef] [PubMed]
7. Cavalcante, P.A.M.; Doro, M.R.; Suzuki, F.S.; Rica, R.L.; Serra, A.J.; Pontes Junior, F.L.; Evangelista, A.L.; Figueira Junior, A.J.; Baker, J.S.; Bocalini, D.S. Functional Fitness and Self-Reported Quality of Life of Older Women Diagnosed with Knee Osteoarthrosis: A Cross-Sectional Case Control Study. *J. Aging Res.* **2015**, *2015*, 841985. [CrossRef]
8. Covinsky, K.E.; Eng, C.; Lui, L.-Y.; Sands, L.P.; Yaffe, K. The last 2 years of life: Functional trajectories of frail older people. *J. Am. Geriatr. Soc.* **2003**, *51*, 492–498. [CrossRef]
9. Fried, L.P.; Tangen, C.M.; Walston, J.; Newman, A.B.; Hirsch, C.; Gottdiener, J.; Seeman, T.; Tracy, R.; Kop, W.J.; Burke, G.; et al. Frailty in Older Adults: Evidence for a Phenotype. *J. Gerontol. Ser. A Biol. Sci. Med. Sci.* **2001**, *56*, M146–M157. [CrossRef]
10. Rodakowski, J.; Saghafi, E.S.; Butters, M.A.; Skidmore, E.R. Nonpharmacological Interventions in Adults with MCI and Early dementia. *Mol. Asp. Med.* **2015**, 38–53. [CrossRef]
11. Ruan, Q.; Yu, Z.; Chen, M.; Bao, Z.; Li, J.; He, W. Cognitive frailty, a novel target for the prevention of elderly dependency. *Ageing Res. Rev.* **2015**, *20*, 1–10. [CrossRef]
12. Higueras-Fresnillo, S.; Cabanas-Sánchez, V.; Lopez-Garcia, E.; Esteban-Cornejo, I.; Banegas, J.R.; Sadarangani, K.P.; Rodríguez-Artalejo, F.; Martinez-Gomez, D. Physical Activity and Association Between Frailty and All-Cause and Cardiovascular Mortality in Older Adults: Population-Based Prospective Cohort Study. *J. Am. Geriatr. Soc.* **2018**, *66*, 2097–2103. [CrossRef]
13. Gleeson, M.; Bishop, N.C.; Stensel, D.J.; Lindley, M.R.; Mastana, S.S.; Nimmo, M.A. The anti-inflammatory effects of exercise: Mechanisms and implications for the prevention and treatment of disease. *Nat. Rev. Immunol.* **2011**, *11*, 607–615. [CrossRef]
14. Tarazona-Santabalbina, F.J.; Gómez-Cabrera, M.C.; Pérez-Ros, P.; Martínez-Arnau, F.M.; Cabo, H.; Tsaparas, K.; Salvador-Pascual, A.; Rodriguez-Mañas, L.; Viña, J. A Multicomponent Exercise Intervention that Reverses Frailty and Improves Cognition, Emotion, and Social Networking in the Community-Dwelling Frail Elderly: A Randomized Clinical Trial. *J. Am. Med. Dir. Assoc.* **2016**, *17*, 426–433. [CrossRef]
15. Theou, O.; Stathokostas, L.; Roland, K.P.; Jakobi, J.M.; Patterson, C.; Vandervoort, A.A.; Jones, G.R. The effectiveness of exercise interventions for the management of frailty: A systematic review. *J. Aging Res.* **2011**, *2011*, 569194. [CrossRef]
16. Woods, J.A.; Keylock, K.T.; Lowder, T.; Vieira, V.J.; Zelkovich, W.; Dumich, S.; Colantuano, K.; Lyons, K.; Leifheit, K.; Cook, M.; et al. Cardiovascular exercise training extends influenza vaccine seroprotection in sedentary older adults: The immune function intervention trial. *J. Am. Geriatr. Soc.* **2009**, *57*, 2183–2191. [CrossRef]
17. Paixão, V.; Almeida, E.B.; Amaral, J.B.; Roseira, T.; Monteiro, F.R.; Foster, R.; Sperandio, A.; Rossi, M.; Amirato, G.R.; Santos, C.A.F.; et al. Elderly Subjects Supplemented with L-Glutamine Shows an Improvement of Mucosal Immunity in the Upper Airways in Response to Influenza Virus Vaccination. *Vaccines* **2021**, *9*, 107. [CrossRef]

18. Abizanda, P.; Sinclair, A.; Barcons, N.; Lizán, L.; Rodríguez-Mañas, L. Costs of Malnutrition in Institutionalized and Community-Dwelling Older Adults: A Systematic Review. *J. Am. Med. Dir. Assoc.* **2016**, *17*, 17–23. [CrossRef]
19. Goates, S.; Du, K.; Braunschweig, C.A.; Arensberg, M.B. Economic burden of disease-associated malnutrition at the state level. *PLoS ONE* **2016**, *11*, 1–15. [CrossRef]
20. Artaza-Artabe, I.; Sáez-López, P.; Sánchez-Hernández, N.; Fernández-Gutierrez, N.; Malafarina, V. The relationship between nutrition and frailty: Effects of protein intake, nutritional supplementation, vitamin D and exercise on muscle metabolism in the elderly. A systematic review. *Maturitas* **2016**, *93*, 89–99. [CrossRef] [PubMed]
21. Ikeda, T.; Aizawa, J.; Nagasawa, H.; Gomi, I.; Kugota, H.; Nanjo, K.; Jinno, T.; Masuda, T.; Morita, S. Effects and feasibility of exercise therapy combined with branched-chain amino acid supplementation on muscle strengthening in frail and pre-frail elderly people requiring long-term care: A crossover trial. *Appl. Physiol. Nutr. Metab.* **2016**, *41*, 438–445. [CrossRef] [PubMed]
22. Ikeda, T.; Matsunaga, Y.; Kanbara, M.; Kamono, A.; Masuda, T.; Watanabe, M.; Nakanishi, R.; Jinno, T. Effect of exercise therapy combined with branched-chain amino acid supplementation on muscle strength in elderly women after total hip arthroplasty: A randomized controlled trial. *Asia Pac. J. Clin. Nutr.* **2019**, *28*, 720–726. [CrossRef] [PubMed]
23. Giannopoulou, I.; Fernhall, B.; Carhart, R.; Weinstock, R.S.; Baynard, T.; Figueroa, A.; Kanaley, J.A. Effects of diet and/or exercise on the adipocytokine and inflammatory cytokine levels of postmenopausal women with type 2 diabetes. *Metabolism* **2005**, *54*, 866–875. [CrossRef]
24. Loria, V.; Dato, I.; Graziani, F.; Biasucci, L.M. Myeloperoxidase: A new biomarker of inflammation in ischemic heart disease and acute coronary syndromes. *Mediat. Inflamm.* **2008**, *2008*. [CrossRef] [PubMed]
25. Giovannini, S.; Onder, G.; Leeuwenburgh, C.; Carter, C.; Marzetti, E.; Russo, A.; Capoluongo, E.; Pahor, M.; Bernabei, R.; Landi, F. Myeloperoxidase levels and mortality in frail community-living elderly individuals. *J. Gerontol. Ser. A Biol. Sci. Med. Sci.* **2010**, *65 A*, 369–376. [CrossRef]
26. Chupel, M.U.; Minuzzi, L.G.; Furtado, G.E.; Santos, M.L.; Ferreira, J.P.; Filaire, E.; Teixeira, A.M. Taurine supplementation reduces myeloperoxidase and matrix—Metalloproteinase—9 levels and improves the effects of exercise in cognition and physical fitness in older women. *Amino Acids* **2021**, 1–13. [CrossRef]
27. Alcorta, M.D.; Alvarez, P.C.; Cabetas, R.N.; Martín, M.A.; Valero, M.; Candela, C.G. The importance of serum albumin determination method to classify patients based on nutritional status. *Clin. Nutr. ESPEN* **2018**, *25*, 110–113. [CrossRef]
28. Abizanda, P.; López, M.D.; García, V.P.; de Estrella, J.D.; da Silva, G.Á.; Vilardell, N.B.; Torres, K.A. Effects of an Oral Nutritional Supplementation Plus Physical Exercise Intervention on the Physical Function, Nutritional Status, and Quality of Life in Frail Institutionalized Older Adults: The ACTIVNES Study. *J. Am. Med. Dir. Assoc.* **2015**, *1*, 439.e9–439.e16. [CrossRef]
29. Guralnik, J.M.; Ferrucci, L.; Simonsick, E.M.; Salive, M.E.; Wallace, R.B. A short physical performance battery Assessing Lower Extremety Function: Association with self reported disability and prediction of mortality and nursing home admission. *J. Gerontol.* **1994**, *49*, M85–M94. [CrossRef]
30. Begg, M.; Eastwood, E.; Horton, R.; Moher, M.; Ingram, O.; Pitkin, R.; Drummond, R.; Schulz, K.; Simel, D.; Stroup, D. Improving the Quality of Reporting of Randomized Controlled Trials The CONSORT Statement. *JAMA* **1996**, *J276*, 637–639. [CrossRef]
31. Gonçalves, B.; Fagulha, T.; Ferreira, A.; Reis, N. Depressive symptoms and pain complaints as predictors of later development of depression in Portuguese middle-aged women. *Health Care Women Int.* **2014**, *35*, 1228–1244. [CrossRef] [PubMed]
32. Syddall, H.; Cooper, C.; Martin, F.; Briggs, R.; Aihie Sayer, A. Is grip strength a useful single marker of frailty? *Age Ageing* **2003**, *32*, 650–656. [CrossRef]
33. Campaniço Validade Simultânea do Questionário. Internacional de Actividade Física Através da Medição Objectiva da Actividade Física por Actigrafia Proporcional. 2016. Available online: http://hdl.handle.net/10400.5/11866 (accessed on 1 March 2021).
34. Torres, D.; Oliveira, A.; Severo, M.; Alarcão, V.; Guiomar, S.; Mota, J.; Teixeira, P.; Rodrigues, S.; Vilela, S.; Oliveira, L.; et al. Inquérito Alimentar Nacional e de Atividade Física. *Inq. Aliment. Nac. Ativ. Fís. IAN-AF 2015–2016* **2016**, *53*, 1689–1699.
35. Goios, A. Pesos e Porções de Alimentos (2a Edição). In *Pesos e Porções de Alimentos (2ª Edição)*; U. Porto Press: Porto, Portugal, 2016; ISBN 9789897461033.
36. INSA. Tabela da Composição de Alimentos. 2006. Available online: http://www2.insa.pt/sites/INSA/Portugues/AreasCientificas/AlimentNutricao/AplicacoesOnline/TabelaAlimentos/Paginas/TabelaAlimentos.aspx (accessed on 2 March 2021).
37. Vellas, B.; Guigoz, Y.; Garry, P.J.; Nourhashemi, F.; Bennahum, D.; Lauque, S.; Albarede, J.L.; Vellas, B. The Mini Nutritional Assessment (MNA) for grading the nutritional state of elderly patients: Presentation of the MNA, history and validation. *Nestle Nutr. Workshop Ser. Clin. Perform. Programme* **1999**, *1*, 3–11. [CrossRef]
38. Loureiro, M.H.V.S. Validação do "Mini-Nutricional Assessement" em Idosos. Available online: https://estudogeral.uc.pt/handle/10316/10439 (accessed on 1 March 2021).
39. Charlson, M.; Szatrowski, T.P.; Peterson, J.; Gold, J. Validation of a combined comorbidity index. *J. Clin. Epidemiol.* **1994**, *47*, 1245–1251. [CrossRef]
40. Lohman, T.G.; Roche, A.F.; Martorell, R. *Lohman Anthropometric Standardization Reference Manual*; Human Kinetics Books: Champaign, IL, USA, 1992.
41. Morgado, J.; Rocha, C.S.; Maruta, C.; Guerreiro, M.; Martins, I.P. Novos valores normativos do mini-mental state examination. *Sinapse* **2009**, *9*, 2009.
42. Folstein Mini-mental State. A grading the cognitive state of patients for the clinician. *J. Psychiatr Res.* **1975**, *12*, 189–198. [CrossRef]

43. Ispoglou, T.; White, H.; Preston, T.; McElhone, S.; McKenna, J.; Hind, K. Double-blind, placebo-controlled pilot trial of L-Leucine-enriched amino-acid mixtures on body composition and physical performance in men and women aged 65-75 years. *Eur. J. Clin. Nutr.* **2016**, *70*, 182–188. [CrossRef]
44. Negro Perna, S.; Spadaccini, D.; Castelli, L.; Calanni, L.; Barbero, M.; Cescon, C.; Rondanelli, M. D´antonaEffects of 12 Weeks of Essential Amino Acids (EAA)-Based Multi-Ingredient Nutritional Supplementation on Muscle Mass, Muscle Strength, Muscle Power and Fatigue in Healthy Elderly Subjects: A Randomized Controlled Double-Blind Study. *J. Nutr. Health Aging* **2019**, *23*, 414–424. [CrossRef]
45. Honka, X.M.J.; Bucci, M.; Andersson, J.; Huovinen, V.; Guzzardi, M.A.; Sandboge, S.; Savisto, N.; Salonen, M.K.; Badeau, R.M.; Parkkola, R.; et al. Resistance training enhances insulin suppression of endogenous glucose production in elderly women. *J. Appl. Physiol.* **2016**, *120*, 633–639. [CrossRef] [PubMed]
46. Solis, M.Y.; Cooper, S.; Hobson, R.M.; Artioli, G.G.; Otaduy, M.C.; Roschel, H.; Robertson, J.; Martin, D.; Painelli, V.S.; Harris, R.C.; et al. Effects of beta-alanine supplementation on brain homocarnosine/carnosine signal and cognitive function: An exploratory study. *PLoS ONE* **2015**, *10*, 1–16. [CrossRef] [PubMed]
47. Nelson, M.E.; Rejeski, W.J.; Blair, S.N.; Duncan, P.W.; Judge, J.O.; King, A.C.; Macera, C.A.; Castaneda-Sceppa, C. Physical activity and public health in older adults: Recommendation from the American College of Sports Medicine and the American Heart Association. *Med. Sci. Sports Exerc.* **2007**, *39*, 1435–1445. [CrossRef] [PubMed]
48. de Souto Barreto, P.; Morley, J.E.; Chodzko-Zajko, W.; Pitkala, K.H.; Weening-Dijksterhuis, E.; Rodriguez-Mañas, L.; Barbagallo, M.; Rosendahl, E.; Sinclair, A.; Landi, F.; et al. Recommendations on Physical Activity and Exercise for Older Adults Living in Long-Term Care Facilities: A Taskforce Report. *J. Am. Med. Dir. Assoc.* **2016**, *17*, 381–392. [CrossRef] [PubMed]
49. Colado, J.C.; Pedrosa, F.M.; Juesas, A.; Gargallo, P.; Carrasco, J.J.; Flandez, J.; Chupel, M.U.; Teixeira, A.M.; Naclerio, F. Concurrent validation of the OMNI-Resistance Exercise Scale of perceived exertion with elastic bands in the elderly. *Exp. Gerontol.* **2018**, *103*, 11–16. [CrossRef]
50. Tanaka, H.; Monahan, K.D.; Seals, D.R. Age-predicted maximal heart rate revisited. *J. Am. Coll. Cardiol.* **2001**, *37*, 153–156. [CrossRef]
51. Borg, G.A. Psychophysical Bases of Perception Exertion. *Med. Sci. Sports Exerc.* **1982**, *14*, 377–381. [CrossRef]
52. Sakugawa, R.L.; Moura, B.M.; Orssatto, L.B.d.R.; Bezerra, E.d.S.; Cadore, E.L.; Diefenthaeler, F. Effects of resistance training, detraining, and retraining on strength and functional capacity in elderly. *Aging Clin. Exp. Res.* **2019**, *31*, 31–39. [CrossRef]
53. Furtado, G.E.; Carvalho, H.M.; Loureiro, M.; Patrício, M.; Uba-Chupel, M.; Colado, J.C.J.C.; Hogervorst, E.; Ferreira, J.P.J.P.; Teixeira, A.M. Chair-based exercise programs in institutionalized older women: Salivary steroid hormones, disabilities and frailty changes. *Exp. Gerontol.* **2020**, *130*, 110790. [CrossRef]
54. Baker, M.K.; Atlantis, E.; Fiatarone Singh, M.A. Multi-modal exercise programs for older adults. *Age Ageing* **2007**, *36*, 375–381. [CrossRef]
55. Rivera-Torres, S.; Fahey, T.D.; Rivera, M.A. Adherence to Exercise Programs in Older Adults: Informative Report. *Gerontol. Geriatr. Med.* **2019**, *5*, 233372141882360. [CrossRef]
56. Vandewoude, M.F.J.; Alish, C.J.; Sauer, A.C.; Hegazi, R.A. Malnutrition-sarcopenia syndrome: Is this the future of nutrition screening and assessment for older adults? *J. Aging Res.* **2012**, *2012*. [CrossRef] [PubMed]
57. Pilgeram, L. Control of fibrinogen biosynthesis: Role of the FFA/Albumin ratio. *Cardiovasc. Eng.* **2010**, *10*, 78–83. [CrossRef]
58. Ahn, S.Y.; Ryu, J.; Baek, S.H.; Han, J.W.; Lee, J.H.; Ahn, S.; Kim, K.I.; Chin, H.J.; Na, K.Y.; Chae, D.W.; et al. Serum anion gap is predictive of mortality in an elderly population. *Exp. Gerontol.* **2014**, *50*, 122–127. [CrossRef]
59. Hiroshige, K.; Sonta, T.; Suda, T.; Kanegae, K.; Ohtani, A. Oral supplementation of branched-chain amino acid improves nutritional status in elderly patients on chronic haemodialysis. *Nephrol. Dial. Transplant.* **2001**, *16*, 1856–1862. [CrossRef]
60. Barbalho, S.M.; Flato, U.A.P.; Tofano, R.J.; Goulart, R.d.A.; Guiguer, E.L.; Detregiachi, C.R.P.; Buchaim, D.V.; Araújo, A.C.; Buchain, R.L.; Reina, F.T.R.; et al. Physical exercise and myokines: Relationships with sarcopenia and cardiovascular complications. *Int. J. Mol. Sci.* **2020**, *21*, 3607. [CrossRef]
61. Pedrero-Chamizo, R.; Albers, U.; Palacios, G.; Pietrzik, K.; Meléndez, A.; González-Gross, M. Health risk, functional markers and cognitive status in institutionalized older adults: A longitudinal study. *Int. J. Environ. Res. Public Health* **2020**, *17*, 7303. [CrossRef] [PubMed]
62. Starling, R.D.; Ades, P.A.; Poehlman, E.T. Physical activity, protein intake, and appendicular skeletal muscle mass in older men. *Am. J. Clin. Nutr.* **1999**, *70*, 91–96. [CrossRef]
63. Zhu, K.; Kerr, D.A.; Meng, X.; Devine, A.; Solah, V.; Binns, C.W.; Prince, R.L. Two-year whey protein supplementation did not enhance muscle mass and physical function in well-nourished healthy older postmenopausal women. *J. Nutr.* **2015**, *145*, 2520–2526. [CrossRef]
64. Saraiva, M.; O'Garra, A. The regulation of IL-10 production by immune cells. *Nat. Rev. Immunol.* **2010**, *10*, 170–181. [CrossRef] [PubMed]
65. Ohno, T.; Tanaka, Y.; Sugauchi, F.; Orito, E.; Hasegawa, I.; Nukaya, H.; Kato, A.; Matunaga, S.; Endo, M.; Tanaka, Y.; et al. Suppressive effect of oral administration of branched-chain amino acid granules on oxidative stress and inflammation in HCV-positive patients with liver cirrhosis. *Hepatol. Res.* **2008**, *38*, 683–688. [CrossRef]

66. Franceschi, C.; Capri, M.; Monti, D.; Giunta, S.; Olivieri, F.; Sevini, F.; Panourgia, M.P.; Invidia, L.; Celani, L.; Scurti, M.; et al. Inflammaging and anti-inflammaging: A systemic perspective on aging and longevity emerged from studies in humans. *Mech. Ageing Dev.* **2007**, *128*, 92–105. [CrossRef] [PubMed]
67. Liu, Y.Z.; Wang, Y.X.; Jiang, C.L. Inflammation: The common pathway of stress-related diseases. *Front. Hum. Neurosci.* **2017**, *11*, 1–11. [CrossRef]
68. Pedersen, B.K.; Febbraio, M.A. Muscles, exercise and obesity: Skeletal muscle as a secretory organ. *Nat. Rev. Endocrinol.* **2012**, *8*, 457–465. [CrossRef] [PubMed]
69. Simioni, C.; Zauli, G.; Martelli, A.; Vitale, M.; Sacchetti, G.; Gonelli, A.; Neri, L. Oxidative stress: Role of physical exercise and antioxidant nutraceuticals in adulthood and aging. *Oncotarget* **2018**, *9*, 17181–17198. [CrossRef] [PubMed]
70. Beard, J.R.; Officer, A.M.; Cassels, A.K. WHO World Report on Ageing And HeAltH. *Gerontologist* **2016**, *56*, S163–S166. [CrossRef]
71. Cadore, E.L.; Casas-Herrero, A.; Zambom-Ferraresi, F.; Idoate, F.; Millor, N.; Gómez, M.; Rodriguez-Mañas, L.; Izquierdo, M. Multicomponent exercises including muscle power training enhance muscle mass, power output, and functional outcomes in institutionalized frail nonagenarians. *Age (Omaha)* **2014**, *36*, 773–785. [CrossRef]
72. Villareal, D.T.; Smith, G.I.; Sinacore, D.R.; Shah, K.; Mittendorfer, B. Regular Multicomponent Exercise Increases Physical Fitness and Muscle Protein Anabolism in Frail, Obese, Older Adults. *Obesity* **2011**, *19*, 312–318. [CrossRef]
73. Casas-Herrero, A.; Anton-Rodrigo, I.; Zambom-Ferraresi, F.; Sáez De Asteasu, M.L.; Martinez-Velilla, N.; Elexpuru-Estomba, J.; Marin-Epelde, I.; Ramon-Espinoza, F.; Petidier-Torregrosa, R.; Sanchez-Sanchez, J.L.; et al. Effect of a multicomponent exercise programme (VIVIFRAIL) on functional capacity in frail community elders with cognitive decline: Study protocol for a randomized multicentre control trial. *Trials* **2019**, *20*, 1–12. [CrossRef]
74. Alzheimer's Association. 2020 Alzheimer's disease facts and figures. *Alzheimer's Dement.* **2020**, *16*, 391–460. [CrossRef]
75. Gariballa, S.; Forster, S. Effects of dietary supplements on depressive symptoms in older patients: A randomised double-blind placebo-controlled trial. *Clin. Nutr.* **2007**, *26*, 545–551. [CrossRef]
76. Fernstrom, J.D. Large neutral amino acids: Dietary effects on brain neurochemistry and function. *Amino Acids* **2013**, *45*, 419–430. [CrossRef] [PubMed]
77. Neishabouri, H.; Hutson, S.; Davoodi, J. Chronic activation of mTOR complex 1 by branched chain amino acids and organ hypertrophy. *Amino Acids* **2015**, *47*, 1167–1182. [CrossRef] [PubMed]
78. Ko Wu, S.; Wang, S.; Chang, Y.; Chang, C.; Kuan, T.; Chuang, H.; Chang, C.; Chou, W.; Wu, C. Effects of enriched branched-chain amino acid supplementation on sarcopenia. *Aging (Albany N. Y.)* **2020**, *12*, 15091–15103. [CrossRef]

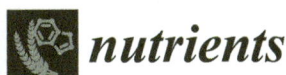

Article

The Dietary Inflammatory Index Is Associated with Low Muscle Mass and Low Muscle Function in Older Australians

Marlene Gojanovic [1,*], Kara L. Holloway-Kew [1], Natalie K. Hyde [1], Mohammadreza Mohebbi [2], Nitin Shivappa [3,4], James R. Hebert [3,4], Adrienne O'Neil [1] and Julie A. Pasco [1,5,6]

[1] IMPACT Institute for Mental and Physical Health and Clinical Translation, Deakin University, Geelong, Victoria 3220, Australia; k.holloway@deakin.edu.au (K.L.H.-K.); natalie.hyde@deakin.edu.au (N.K.H.); adrienne.oneil@deakin.edu.au (A.O.); julie.pasco@deakin.edu.au (J.A.P.)
[2] Biostatistics Unit, Faculty of Health, Deakin University, Geelong, Victoria 3220, Australia; m.mohebbi@deakin.edu.au
[3] Cancer Prevention and Control Program and Department of Epidemiology and Biostatistics, Arnold School of Public Health, University of South Carolina, Columbia, SC 29208, USA; shivappa@email.sc.edu (N.S.); jhebert@mailbox.sc.edu (J.R.H.)
[4] Department of Nutrition, Connecting Health Innovations LLC, Columbia, SC 29201, USA
[5] Department of Medicine-Western Health, University of Melbourne, St Albans, Victoria 3021, Australia
[6] University Hospital Geelong, Barwon Health, Geelong, Victoria 3220, Australia
* Correspondence: mgojanovic@icloud.com

Abstract: Age-associated chronic, low grade systemic inflammation has been recognised as an important contributing factor in the development of sarcopenia; importantly, diet may regulate this process. This cross-sectional study examined the association of diet-related inflammation with components of sarcopenia. Participants (n = 809) aged 60–95 years from the Geelong Osteoporosis Study were studied. Body composition was measured by dual energy X-ray absorptiometry. In this study, low appendicular lean mass (ALM/height^2, kg/m^2) was defined as T-score < −1 and low muscle function as Timed-Up-and-Go >10 s over 3 m (TUG > 10). Dietary inflammatory index (DII®) scores, based on specific foods and nutrients, were computed using dietary data collected from a food frequency questionnaire. Associations between DII scores and low muscle mass and low muscle function, alone and combined, were determined using linear and logistic regression. After adjusting for covariates, higher DII score was associated with lower ALM/height^2 (β −0.05, standard error (SE) 0.02, p = 0.028), and higher natural log-transformed (ln) (TUG) (β 0.02, standard error 0.01, p = 0.035) and higher likelihood for these components combined (odds ratio 1.33, 95% confidence interval 1.05 to 1.69, p = 0.015). A pro-inflammatory diet, as indicated by higher DII score, is associated with lower muscle mass, poorer muscle function and increased likelihood for the combination of low muscle mass and low muscle function. Further studies investigating whether anti-inflammatory dietary interventions could reduce the risk of sarcopenia are needed.

Keywords: aged; dietary inflammatory index; dietary patterns; frailty; inflammation; muscle function; muscle mass; sarcopenia

Citation: Gojanovic, M.; Holloway-Kew, K.L.; Hyde, N.K.; Mohebbi, M.; Shivappa, N.; Hebert, J.R.; O'Neil, A.; Pasco, J.A. The Dietary Inflammatory Index Is Associated with Low Muscle Mass and Low Muscle Function in Older Australians. *Nutrients* 2021, 13, 1166. https://doi.org/10.3390/nu13041166

Academic Editors: Cristiano Capurso, Catherine Féart and Louise Deldicque

Received: 1 March 2021
Accepted: 29 March 2021
Published: 1 April 2021

Publisher's Note: MDPI stays neutral with regard to jurisdictional claims in published maps and institutional affiliations.

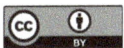

Copyright: © 2021 by the authors. Licensee MDPI, Basel, Switzerland. This article is an open access article distributed under the terms and conditions of the Creative Commons Attribution (CC BY) license (https://creativecommons.org/licenses/by/4.0/).

1. Introduction

Sarcopenia, the loss of muscle mass and function with age, is an important underlying cause of physical disability and frailty, leading to increased risk of falls and fractures, nursing home admission, hospitalisation, decreased quality of life and mortality [1–3]. Sarcopenia is common in older adults with an estimated prevalence of 5% to 13% in adults aged 60 to 70 years and 11% to 50% in adults over 80 years of age [4]. In Australia, sarcopenia prevalence has been estimated to be 2.9% for men and 5.9% for women aged 60 to 96 years [5]. The large variability in prevalence is related to the populations studied, different methods used to assess muscle mass, muscle strength and physical performance, and criteria used to define sarcopenia [6,7]. With the ageing of populations, the overall prevalence and number of individuals with sarcopenia is expected to increase. This will present an ever-increasing greater burden on the health care system; making it ever more important to identify novel modifiable risk factors for the prevention and treatment of sarcopenia [8].

Age-associated chronic, low grade systemic inflammation, termed "inflammaging", has been recognised as an important contributing factor in the development of sarcopenia [9–11]. It has been proposed that inflammaging is caused by increased oxidative stress or reduced immune function (immunosenescence) [11]. While the mechanisms are not yet fully understood, there is consensus that inflammaging is accompanied by increased levels of pro-inflammatory cytokines, mainly tumour necrosis factor-alpha (TNF-α) and interleukin-6 (IL-6), and the acute phase protein, C-reactive protein (CRP) [11,12]. More recently, study findings have suggested that inflammaging may stimulate muscle wasting and loss of muscle quality [9,12]. Thus, chronic inflammation may be implicated in the development and progression of sarcopenia.

Importantly, diet may be involved in this process. Specific nutrients, foods and dietary patterns have been associated with biomarkers of inflammation; yet the role of inflammation in the diet as a whole has not been properly investigated [13]. Single nutrient analysis is limited by the high correlation and interactions between many nutrients that make it difficult to distinguish between individual and combined effects [14]. Dietary pattern analysis has emerged as a new, more holistic approach to examine relationships between diet and health outcomes [15]. The dietary inflammatory index (DII®) is a validated tool that quantifies the inflammatory potential of nutrients and foods in the context of a dietary pattern [16]. The DII has been used to investigate the association of an inflammatory dietary pattern with various health outcomes associated with ageing, including cardiovascular disease [17], risk of fracture [18], frailty [19,20], and cancer [21]. However, few studies have examined the association of DII scores in relation to sarcopenia and its components [22–25]. We propose that chronic inflammation is a contributor to sarcopenia and that the inflammatory potential of the diet has a regulatory role on chronic inflammation and thus, sarcopenia.

The overall objective of this study was to examine associations between the inflammatory potential of diet and the components of sarcopenia in men and women aged 60 years and over. Specifically, we aimed to evaluate associations between DII score and (1) lean mass (as a surrogate measure of muscle mass), (2) muscle function and (3) a combination of these two as a representation of sarcopenia.

2. Materials and Methods

2.1. Study Design

In this population-based study, participants were men and women from the Geelong Osteoporosis Study (GOS). The GOS is an age-stratified sample of men and women aged 20 to 96 years randomly selected from electoral rolls for the Barwon Health Statistical Division in south-eastern Australia. Details of study design, participation and retention have been described elsewhere [26]. The participants were assessed at baseline and have participated in follow-up assessments every few years. Cross-sectional data from two different timepoints, baseline for men (2001–2006) and 15-year for women (2011–2014), were used in this study due to availability of comparable data for the exposure, outcomes and covariates.

The study protocol was approved by the Barwon Health Human Research Ethics Committee. All participants provided written informed consent.

2.2. Participants

Individuals aged 60 years and over were included in this analysis, but were excluded if (1) their weight exceeded the limit of the dual energy X-ray absorptiometry (DXA) scanners ($\geq$120 kg), (2) a limb was affected by a prosthesis, plates or screws or had been amputated, (3) a full body scan, and/or a Timed-Up-and-Go (TUG) test was not performed, (4) a food frequency questionnaire (FFQ) was not completed or (5) excessively high or low daily nutritional energy intakes were reported on the FFQ (i.e., <3360 or >16,800 kJ/day for men and <2100 or >14,700 kJ/day for women) [27].

2.3. Outcome Measures

2.3.1. Muscle Mass and Muscle Function

As a surrogate for skeletal muscle mass, lean mass was measured by whole body DXA, which is the preferred method for assessing body composition in a research setting [28]. Appendicular lean mass (ALM, kg) was calculated as the sum of the lean mass measurements for arms and legs, expressed relative to height squared (ALM/height^2, kg/m^2).

A Lunar DPX-L (Lunar; Madison, WI, USA) was used to scan the first 544 men at baseline until an upgrade to a GE-Prodigy (Prodigy; GE Lunar, Madison, WI, USA). Cross-calibration was performed on 40 subjects aged 21 to 82 years to ensure comparability of the DXA scanners; no differences were detected in lumbar spine or femoral neck bone mineral density [26]. All scans for the women at 15-year assessment were performed on the GE Lunar Prodigy. The DXA scanner was calibrated three times per week with an anthropometric phantom (Hologic) to preserve the repeatability and accuracy of measures. Muscle function was assessed using a timed "Up-and-Go" (TUG) test, which measures the time taken to rise from a seated position in a chair with no arm rests, walk 3 metres, turn around, walk back and sit down [29].

In this study, a combination of low muscle mass and low muscle function was used as a representation of sarcopenia [28]. Low muscle mass was defined as ALM/height^2 < 7.87 kg/m^2 for men and <6.07 kg/m^2 for women (equal to T-score <−1) [30]. Cut points for ALM/height^2 were calculated using DXA from a sample of 374 men and 308 women aged 20–39 years from the GOS [30]. As suggested by the European Working Group on Sarcopenia in Older People (EWGSOP), low muscle function can be defined either as low muscle strength or low physical performance [28]. In this study, low muscle function was defined as TUG > 10 s for 3 metres [29]; the TUG is a recognised assessment tool for physical performance [28,31]. Measures of handgrip strength, used to assess low muscle strength, were not available for the recently updated definition of sarcopenia (EWGSOP2) [31].

2.3.2. Exposure: Dietary Inflammatory Index (DII)

Dietary data were collected using the Dietary Questionnaire for Epidemiological Studies (DQES version 2), an FFQ created by Cancer Council Victoria, which was completed by participants at each assessment phase [32]. In this study, the baseline timepoint was used to assess diet from the FFQ for men and the 15-year timepoint for women. The FFQ DQES was designed for use in epidemiological studies and has been validated for the Australian population [33,34]; it captures usual eating habits over the past 12 months covering five types of dietary intake, incorporating 80 items: (1) cereal foods, sweets and snacks, (2) dairy products, meats and fish, (3) fruit, (4) vegetables, and (5) alcoholic beverages on a ten-point frequency scale. Portion sizes are based on dietary data collected on older Australian residents (mean age 61 years), which matches the sample used in our analyses [32]. Analysis of questionnaires for assessment of dietary intakes was undertaken by the Nutritional Assessment Office, Cancer Council Victoria. The output of the FFQ analysis provided estimated intakes of macronutrients and a range of micronutrients which were used to compute DII scores for all participants.

The DII is based upon up to 45 food parameters which have been scored based on reported pro-inflammatory or anti-inflammatory effects on specific inflammatory markers (IL-1β, IL-4, IL-6, IL-10, TNF-α, and CRP) using 1943 peer-reviewed articles published through to December 2010. Details of the development of the DII have been reported elsewhere [16,35] and validation work using inflammatory biomarkers are also available [35–39]. Briefly, the scoring algorithm uses a global reference database (food consumption from eleven populations globally) and food parameter-specific inflammatory effect scores to create an overall DII score for an individual. The DII scores individuals' diets on a continuum from strongly anti-inflammatory (−8.87) to strongly pro-inflammatory (+7.98).

To calculate DII scores for the participants in this study, dietary intake data were used to calculate an individuals' intake of food parameters which were then compared to the global reference database. A Z-score for each of the food parameters for each participant was calculated based on the global mean and standard deviation; this was achieved by subtracting the global mean from the amount reported and dividing this value by the standard deviation. The Z-scores were converted to a proportion to minimise the effects of outliers ("right-skewing"). The standardised dietary intake data (proportion) was centred by doubling and subtracting 1 and then multiplied by the inflammatory effect score of each food parameter and summed to obtain an overall DII score for every participant in the study. In this study, a total of 22 of 45 food parameters were available from the FFQ for computing the overall DII scores. These included energy, carbohydrate, protein, total fat, fibre, cholesterol, saturated fat, monounsaturated fat, polyunsaturated fat, omega-3 fatty acids, omega-6 fatty acids, niacin, thiamine, riboflavin, iron, magnesium, zinc, vitamin C, vitamin E, folic acid, beta-carotene and alcohol.

2.4. Covariates

Data on age, sex, body fat percentage, height and mobility were collected at all assessment phases. Barefoot standing height (±0.1 cm) was measured using a wall-mounted stadiometer [26]. Measurements of body fat percentage were obtained from whole body DXA scans. Mobility was self-reported and divided into seven categories ranging from "very active" to "bedfast". For these analyses, two categories of mobility were considered; sedentary (included "sedentary", "limited", "inactive", "chair or bedridden" and "bedfast") and active (included "very active" and "active").

2.5. Statistical Analyses

All statistical tests were performed using Minitab 17 (Minitab, LLC, State College, PA, USA). The DII was analysed as a continuous variable. Kolmogorov–Smirnov test was used to investigate normality of the data. Independent sample t test was used to compare continuous characteristics between sex or other dichotomised factors. If necessary, a non-parametric Mann–Whitney U test was used for this purpose, and a Chi-square test was used for categorical variables. The natural log-transformation was used to normalise TUG scores (used to assess muscle function), which were positively skewed.

Separate linear regression models were used to examine the association between DII and muscle mass and muscle function. A logistic regression model was used to examine the association between DII score and these components combined. Bivariable regression models with no adjustment for participant characteristics were presented (model 1), followed by multivariable regression models that accounted for age (years), sex (male/female) and body fat percentage (%) (model 2). Further adjustments were made for mobility (active/inactive) for ALM/height^2, and height (m) for ln (TUG). Interaction between co-variables were tested and retained in the final model (model 3) if the interaction term was statistically significant ($p < 0.05$). To test for interaction terms, DII was dichotomised according to the median. Daily nutritional energy intake was not included in the multivariable models as a covariate because energy is already included as a constituent of the DII [36]. Results are presented as standardised beta coefficient (β) and standard error (SE), or as an odds ratio (OR) and 95% confidence interval (95% CI).

3. Results

3.1. Participants

Out of a total of 2389 individuals (1540 men at baseline and 849 women who participated in the 15-year assessment), 1071 (694 men and 377 women) were ≥60 years. Of these, 262 (163 men and 99 women) were excluded from this analysis because they met one or more of the exclusion criteria: 9 weighed ≥120 kg, 98 were affected by lower limb prostheses, plates or screws, 2 were unilaterally affected by a lower limb amputation, 98 did not provide a full body scan, 112 did not perform a TUG test, 66 did not complete an FFQ, and 20 reported excessively high or low daily FFQ-derived energy intakes. Thus, analyses included data from 809 individuals (531 men and 278 women).

3.2. Characteristics of Participants in the Study Sample

Key characteristics are described pooled and by sex in Table 1. Participants' ages ranged from 60 to 95 years, with 34% identified as female. The DII scores for the sample ranged from −2.7 to 2.5. Median DII scores for women were 0.8 (interquartile range: −0.2 to 1.5) and 0.4 (interquartile range: −0.4 to 1.2) for men. Compared with men, women had higher TUG and DII scores ($p = 0.02$ and $p = 0.003$, respectively), lower ALM/height^2 and reported lower levels of mobility ($p < 0.001$ and $p = 0.001$, respectively). No differences were detected in proportions of men and women with low muscle mass and low muscle function combined (8.6% vs. 10.9%, $p = 0.31$).

Table 1. Key Characteristics of the Participants; Data are Shown for All, and According to Sex.

Characteristics	Total (n = 809)	Females (n = 278)	Males (n = 531)	p Value
DII score	0.6 (−0.3, 1.3)	0.8 (−0.2, 1.5)	0.4 (−0.4, 1.2)	0.003
Age (yr)	66.4 (72.4, 78.8)	70.6 (65.0, 75.3)	74.0 (67.0, 81.3)	<0.001
Height (cm)	167.9 ± 8.7	159.9 ± 6.0	172.1 ± 6.6	<0.001
Weight (kg)	78.2 ± 13.7	73.5 ± 14.6	80.6 ± 12.5	<0.001
BMI (kg/m^2)	27.7 ± 4.5	28.8 ± 5.6	27.2 ± 3.8	<0.001
Body fat (%)	32.0 ± 10.1	42.1 ± 8.0	26.7 ± 6.4	<0.001
ALM/h^2 (kg/m^2)	7.7 ± 1.1	6.6 ± 0.8	8.2 ± 0.9	<0.001
TUG (s)	8.9 (7.6, 10.3)	9.1 (7.8, 10.8)	8.6 (7.6, 10.1)	0.02
Mobility level (active) *	533 (66.2)	161 (58.8)	372 (70.0)	0.001
ALM/h^2 cutpoint (below) †	257 (31.8)	74 (26.6)	183 (34.5)	0.02
TUG >10 s (yes)	183 (22.6)	76 (27.3)	107 (20.1)	0.02
Low ALM/h^2 and TUG > 10 s (yes)	82 (10.1)	24 (8.6)	58 (10.9)	0.31

DII, dietary inflammatory index; ALM/h^2, appendicular lean mass/height^2; TUG, Timed-Up-and-Go. Data are presented as mean ± standard deviation, median (interquartile range) or n (%). Comparison of characteristics between male and female participants was performed using independent sample t test with parametric continuous variables, Mann–Whitney U test with non-parametric continuous variables, and Chi-square test with categorical variables. * Missing values: 4 for mobility level. † ALM/height^2 cutpoints: <7.87 kg/m^2 for men, <6.07 kg/m^2 for women.

Table 2 shows the total daily energy intake and nutrient intake of participants which was used to calculate DII scores. Calcium intake was similar between men and women; however, men had higher intakes of energy, protein, carbohydrate, fats and alcohol ($p < 0.001$ for all).

3.3. Dietary Inflammatory Index and Muscle Mass and Muscle Function

Table 3 shows the results of linear and logistic regression modelling for the association between DII and low muscle mass and low muscle function, alone and combined. A negative association was observed between DII and ALM/height^2 in the unadjusted model ($\beta = -0.13$, SE = 0.04 for model 1). This association persisted after adjustment for age, sex and body fat percentage ($\beta = -0.05$, SE = 0.02 for model 2) and for the interaction of age and sex ($\beta = -0.05$, SE = 0.02 for model 3). Repeating the statistical analysis with model 2 but including mobility as a covariate did not change the association ($\beta = -0.05$, SE = 0.02).

Table 2. Total Daily Energy and Nutrient Intake of Participants; Data is Shown for All, and According to Sex.

Nutrient	Total (n = 809)		Females (n = 278)		Males (n = 531)		p Value
	Median	IQR	Median	IQR	Median	IQR	
Energy (kJ)	6927.9	(5593.3, 8632.0)	5991.5	(4784.0, 7438.5)	7353.2	(6195.3, 9230.9)	<0.001
Protein (g)	78.2	(63.0, 96.4)	70.0	(55.1, 88.5)	83.1	(67.6, 100.0)	<0.001
Carbohydrate (g)	186.7	(146.7, 234.6)	154.0	(119.8, 194.2)	205.0	(164.0, 251.1)	<0.001
Total fat (g)	66.8	(51.0, 85.4)	57.5	(45.4, 72.5)	71.3	(56.4, 92.3)	<0.001
Saturated fats (g)	26.4	(19.6, 34.6)	23.4	(17.7, 30.5)	28.1	(21.0, 36.4)	<0.001
Polyunsaturated fatty acids (g)	10.6	(7.2, 14.9)	8.7	(6.1, 12.1)	12.1	(8.3, 16.2)	<0.001
Monounsaturated fatty acids (g)	23.2	(17.6, 30.1)	20.1	(15.4, 25.5)	24.6	(19.2, 32.0)	<0.001
Sugar (g)	86.4	(67.3, 111.8)	74.1	(55.1, 95.4)	93.3	(74.0, 120.8)	<0.001
Starch (g)	97.4	(73.0, 126.2)	78.8	(60.2, 99.8)	109.3	(85.0, 138.6)	<0.001
Fibre (g)	20.5	(16.4, 26.3)	18.8	(14.6, 23.4)	21.5	(16.9, 27.8)	<0.001
Alcohol (g)	5.6	(0.3, 21.9)	2.1	(0.0, 12.7)	10.1	(0.9, 26.7)	<0.001
Beta-carotene (µg)	2358.2	(1680.8, 3323.5)	2246.8	(1624.0, 3089.6)	2440.9	(1710.6, 3539.8)	0.02
Calcium (mg)	849.0	(672.3, 1061.7)	848.8	(648.6, 1113.3)	849.1	(683.0, 1047.1)	0.67
Cholesterol (mg)	239.2	(182.0, 316.3)	221.8	(167.5, 297.9)	249.6	(190.1, 322.0)	0.001
Folate (µg)	255.0	(197.9, 321.1)	227.3	(185.7, 291.7)	271.2	(214.8, 335.6)	<0.001
Iron (mg)	11.7	(9.0, 14.7)	10.3	(7.7, 13.3)	12.4	(9.6, 16.0)	<0.001
Magnesium (mg)	270.2	(217.3, 336.3)	247.8	(197.0, 310.4)	282.6	(227.6, 346.2)	<0.001
Niacin (mg)	33.7	(26.7, 42.1)	30.4	(22.8, 37.9)	35.9	(28.5, 44.4)	<0.001
Phosphorus (mg)	1393.7	(1100.6, 1708.0)	1281.7	(1025.5, 1616.7)	1440.1	(1150.8, 1732.3)	0.001
Potassium (mg)	2684.6	(2196.3, 3270.8)	2451.4	(1979.5, 3015.7)	2830.4	(2300.8, 3379.9)	<0.001
Retinol (µg)	965.8	(609.7, 966.7)	686.7	(532.0, 858.4)	810.4	(641.3, 1020.1)	<0.001
Riboflavin (mg)	2.1	(1.7, 2.7)	2.0	(1.6, 2.5)	2.2	(1.7, 2.8)	0.002
Sodium (mg)	2163.1	(1688.1, 2767.2)	1840.5	(1459.1, 2306.2)	2317.1	(1875.9, 2976.4)	<0.001
Thiamine (mg)	1.4	(1.1, 1.8)	1.2	(1.0, 1.5)	1.5	(1.2, 2.0)	<0.001
Vitamin C (mg)	102.1	(71.6, 148.5)	92.1	(67.8, 125.7)	107.0	(75.7, 160.6)	0.001
Vitamin E (mg)	5.9	(4.6, 7.6)	5.4	(4.0, 7.0)	6.2	(4.8, 8.0)	<0.001
Zinc (mg)	10.2	(8.1, 12.8)	9.1	(7.1, 11.6)	10.7	(8.8, 13.1)	<0.001

IQR, interquartile range. Comparison of daily dietary intakes between females and males was performed using Mann–Whitney U test.

A positive association between DII score and ln (TUG) was observed in the unadjusted model (β = 0.03, SE = 0.01 for model 1). This association remained significant after adjustment for age, sex and body fat percentage (β = 0.02, SE = 0.01 for model 2) and for the interaction of age and sex (β = 0.02, SE = 0.01 for model 3). Repeating the statistical analysis with model 2 but including height as a covariate did not change the association (β = 0.01, SE = 0.01).

Each one-unit increase in DII was positively associated with a 33% increase in combined low ALM/h^2 plus TUG > 10 s in the unadjusted and adjusted logistic model (OR 1.34, 95% CI 1.08 to 1.67 for model 1; OR 1.33, 95% CI 1.05 to 1.69 for model 2). There were no significant interactions found between covariates.

Table 3. Linear and Logistic Regression Results for the Association between DII Score and Low Muscle Mass and Low Muscle Function, Alone and Combined, for All Participants, Geelong Osteoporosis Study (GOS), 2001 to 2014.

Outcome Variable	Model 1 *			Model 2 †			Model 3 ‡		
	β	SE	p Value	β	SE	p Value	β	SE	p Value
ALM/h^2 (kg/m^2)	−0.13	0.04	<0.001	−0.05	0.02	0.036	−0.05	0.02	0.028
ln(TUG) (s)	0.03	0.01	<0.001	0.02	0.01	0.028	0.02	0.01	0.035
	OR	95% CI	p Value	OR	95% CI	p Value			
Low ALM/h^2 and TUG > 10 s (yes)	1.34	1.08, 1.67	0.007	1.33	1.05, 1.69	0.015			

β, standardised beta coefficient; SE, standard error; ALM/h^2, appendicular lean mass/height^2; ln(TUG), natural log-transformed Timed-Up-and-Go; OR, odds ratio; CI, confidence interval. Standardised beta coefficients and standard errors and odds ratios and confidence intervals are for DII scores. * Model 1: unadjusted. † Model 2: adjusted for age, sex and body fat percentage. ‡ Model 3: adjusted for co-variables in model 2 as well as sex*age interaction term.

4. Discussion

In this cross-sectional study, higher DII score, indicating a more pro-inflammatory diet, was associated with lower muscle mass, poorer muscle function and higher likelihood for the combination of low muscle mass and low muscle function. The sex*age interaction term identified that the relationship between DII and ALM/height^2 and ln (TUG) was different between men and women and that the size of this difference increased with increasing age.

In this study, higher DII score (indicating a more pro-inflammatory diet) was associated with lower ALM/height^2, indicating lower muscle mass. Other studies examining the relationship between DII and muscle mass have reported similar results. In a prospective longitudinal study of 1098 individuals aged 50 to 79 years from the Tasmanian Older Adult Cohort Study (TASOAC), inverse associations were shown between energy-adjusted DII scores and appendicular lean mass in men but not in women after controlling for age and percent body fat (semi-adjusted model) [24]. Findings from a study of 466 Chinese boys and girls aged 6 to 9 years reported that DII score was inversely associated with relative appendicular skeletal muscle mass (ASM/height^2) [40]. In a longitudinal study with 494 female participants aged 21 to 89 years from the GOS, while the DII was not predictive of skeletal muscle index (ALM/height^2) significance increased with adjustment; thus, suggesting a higher DII score was associated with increases in skeletal muscle index [23]. Together, these findings highlight the potential role for overall diet quality based on the inflammatory potential of diet in the maintenance of skeletal muscle mass across the life course.

Other studies that have looked at anti-inflammatory dietary patterns like the Mediterranean diet and muscle mass have produced differing results [41,42]. In a cross-sectional study of women aged 18 to 79 years from the Twins UK study, higher adherence to a Mediterranean diet was associated with higher FFM% (fat-free mass/weight × 100) after adjustment for age, physical activity, smoking, energy and protein intake and misreporting; specifically, FFM% was 1.0% higher in the highest quartile (Q4) compared to the lowest quartile (Q1) [41]. In contrast, in a study conducted in Iran among community-dwelling men and women with an average age of 66 years, no differences in mean muscle mass were detected in the higher tertiles of a Mediterranean dietary pattern compared with the lower tertiles; although the direction of the association was as expected (i.e., lower adherence to a Mediterranean dietary pattern was associated with lower muscle mass) [42]. These inconsistencies may be due to a range of factors including insufficient sample size, the use of samples with different age ranges (e.g., some including both pre and postmenopausal women), different ranges of the DII scores and the different settings.

Another finding of our study was that higher DII score is associated with higher ln (TUG). Handgrip strength, a clinical marker of poor mobility, and gait speed can also be used to assess low muscle function for the diagnosis of sarcopenia [28]. Several studies have explored these measures, but results have been inconsistent. In a cohort study of 1948 individuals aged 60 years or older from the Seniors-ENRICA study, higher DII score was associated with slow gait speed, as a low score in the Short Physical Performance Battery (SPPB) test [20], which is somewhat comparable to our study findings. In a study of 321 individuals aged 70 to 85 years, low gait speed and low grip strength were positively associated with higher DII scores [43]. Furthermore, in a cross-sectional study of 78 frail individuals aged 65 years or older from South Korea, a higher SPPB score was associated with lower levels of TNF-α, suggesting that improving muscle function may lower levels of inflammation [44]. Conversely, no significant associations have been observed between DII and gait speed or handgrip strength in other studies [22,24,40]. The inconsistency of results could be due to different methods used to assess muscle function, age-group differences and limited DII score ranges. More research is therefore required to determine the effects of dietary inflammation on muscle function in older adults.

The final component considered in this study was a combination of low muscle mass and low muscle function as a representation of sarcopenia. We found that higher DII score was associated with a higher likelihood for these components combined. Our findings are in agreement with a cross-sectional study of 300 individuals aged 55 years or older from Iran by Bagheri et al. [22], who found that those in the top tertile of DII had higher odds of sarcopenia than those in the bottom tertile. In a study of 1344 postmenopausal Korean women aged 50 years or older, a pro-inflammatory diet, as determined by DII score over the median, was associated with increased odds for sarcopenic obesity. However, this result was attenuated and did not reach statistical significance after adjustment for age, family income, regular exercise, education status, smoking and female hormone supplements [25]. Interestingly, a pro-inflammatory diet was associated with increased odds for osteosarcopenic obesity in the adjusted model [25]. However, a direct comparison between these results and ours is made difficult by several factors; sarcopenic obesity is a distinct condition [31], two different criteria were used to define sarcopenia (low muscle mass and function vs. low muscle mass alone) and muscle mass was adjusted for body size in different ways (ALM/height^2 vs. ASM/weight %). Cut-off values also differ because of ethnicity, body size, lifestyles and culture between European and Asian populations [45], and there is no consensus about which method is best for adjusting for body size [31].

To date, evidence that a pro-inflammatory diet is associated with sarcopenia has been limited. Previous studies have mainly focused on the association of "healthy eating", high fruit and vegetable intake, and Mediterranean anti-inflammatory dietary patterns with sarcopenia [42,46–49]. Our findings support those observed by Hashemi et al. [42] who found that a Mediterranean dietary pattern was associated with lower odds for EWGSOP-defined sarcopenia among community-dwelling men and women with an average age of 66 years. Given that the inflammatory potential of the Mediterranean diet is comparable to a DII score of −3.96, indicating a strong anti-inflammatory potential, in a similar way, these results are consistent with our study findings [50]. In contrast, Chan, Leung and Woo [47] found no association between Mediterranean Diet Score (MDS) and the Asian Working Group for Sarcopenia (AWGS)-defined sarcopenia in a prospective cohort study of community-dwelling Chinese men and women aged 65 years and older. The absence of associations may be due to the differences in the Chinese diet compared to the traditional Mediterranean diet. Additionally, cut points for muscle mass were lower (<7.0 kg/m^2 for men and <5.4 kg/m^2 for women) than those used in this study, which may have affected the case ascertainment of sarcopenia.

Consistent with the findings of this study, other studies have suggested that a pro-inflammatory diet, as measured by the DII, is associated with increased hip fracture risk and frailty, which are associated with loss of muscle mass and/or function [18,19,51,52]. Research indicates that chronic low-grade inflammation plays a role in the development of sarcopenia, and that diet plays a role in the regulation of chronic inflammation, supporting the findings of this study that the inflammatory potential of the diet may be a modifiable risk factor for sarcopenia [9,13,53].

There were several strengths to this study. The secondary analysis of existing data from the GOS allowed for access to a large data set. Not only was this efficient but the random sampling method used in the GOS strengthened the external validity of this study by achieving a sample that was representative of the underlying population [26]. Objective measures were used to assess muscle mass and muscle function. Furthermore, a systematic approach was adopted for addressing confounding and effect modification with adjustment for a number of variables. The validity of the Cancer Council Victoria FFQ has been assessed against weighed food records in Australian men and women ranging from 31 to 75 years [33] and in young to middle-aged women [34] with good agreement; thus, confirming that the FFQ used was a valid tool in the assessment of dietary intake in our study sample of Australian men and women.

Despite its strengths, our study had several limitations. The primary limitation of cross-sectional studies is the inability to account for temporality, and as a result, causality cannot be established. Reliance on long-term memory for some self-reported data may have affected the accuracy of dietary and lifestyle self-reported data, resulting in recall bias and increased random measurements error [54,55]. Despite using objective measures to confirm some self-reported data, biases may still exist. As well, the presence of selection bias due to non-response and attrition rates cannot be excluded. Additionally, the fact that data were pooled from different study periods for men and women may have introduced bias. Data also may have been affected by the exclusion criteria; as a consequence, the study findings may not be applicable to individuals who weigh $\geq$120 kg or who are affected by lower limb prostheses, plates or screws. The original definition of sarcopenia by EWGSOP focussed on the detection of low muscle mass. More recent definitions have turned attention to low muscle strength as the primary diagnostic criterion of sarcopenia [31,56]. In the absence of muscle strength measures in this data set, we have not adopted the latest version of the definition. Furthermore, the absence of data on 23 parameters may have limited the range of DII scores, which appear to be somewhat narrower than other studies [57]. This may have contributed to the narrow effective range of the DII score, which is about half of that normally observed in other studies that typically range from about -5 to $+5$ [57]. Increasing the effective range of the independent variable often increases magnitude of the observed effect [58]. Therefore, our results actually may underestimate the relationship between DII score and the combined low muscle mass and low muscle function components.

5. Conclusions

A pro-inflammatory diet, as indicated by higher DII score, is associated with lower muscle mass, poorer muscle function and increased likelihood for the combination of low muscle mass and low muscle function among older Australian men and women. These results support the notion that a pro-inflammatory diet negatively affects muscle mass and muscle function and exacerbates the risk of developing sarcopenia. Future studies could consider the relationship between DII and the sarcopenia trajectory and investigate whether anti-inflammatory dietary interventions could reduce the risk of sarcopenia.

Author Contributions: Conceptualisation, M.G., K.L.H.-K., N.K.H. and J.A.P.; methodology, M.G., K.L.H.-K., N.K.H., M.M., N.S., J.R.H. and J.A.P.; software, N.S. and J.R.H.; validation, M.G., M.M., N.S., J.R.H. and J.A.P.; formal analysis, M.G., M.M., N.S., J.R.H. and J.A.P.; investigation, M.G., K.L.H.-K., N.S., J.R.H. and A.O.; resources, N.S., J.R.H. and J.A.P.; data curation, J.A.P.; writing—original draft preparation, M.G.; writing—review and editing, M.G., K.L.H.-K., N.K.H., M.M., N.S., J.R.H., A.O. and J.A.P.; visualisation, M.G.; supervision, J.A.P.; project administration, J.A.P.; funding acquisition, J.A.P. All authors have read and agreed to the published version of the manuscript.

Funding: The Geelong Osteoporosis Study was funded by the National Health and Medical Research Council (NHMRC) Australia, grant numbers 251638, 628582 and 299831.

Institutional Review Board Statement: The study was conducted according to the guidelines of the Declaration of Helsinki, and approved by the Barwon Health Human Research Ethics Committee (projects 92/01 and 00/56).

Informed Consent Statement: Informed consent was obtained from all subjects involved in the study.

Data Availability Statement: The data that support the findings of this study are available from the corresponding author upon reasonable request.

Acknowledgments: The authors thank G. Giles of the Cancer Epidemiology Centre of The Cancer Council Victoria for permission to use the Dietary Questionnaire for Epidemiological Studies (Version 2), Melbourne: The Cancer Council Victoria, Australia, 1996.

Conflicts of Interest: K.L.H.-K. was supported by an Alfred Deakin Postdoctoral Research Fellowship. She has received funding from the Prolia BCGP Competitive Grant Program and Amgen Investigator Sponsored Studies Grant. N.K.H. was supported by a Dean's Research Postdoctoral Fellowship (Deakin University). A.O. is supported by a Future Leader Fellowship (#101160) from the Heart Foundation Australia and Wilson Foundation. She has received research funding from National Health and Medical Research Council (NHMRC) Australia, Australian Research Council, University of Melbourne, Deakin University, Sanofi, Meat and Livestock Australia and Woolworths Limited and Honoraria from Novartis. The Food and Mood Centre with which A.O. is affiliated has received funding from the Fernwood Foundation, the A2 Milk Company and Be Fit Foods. J.A.P. has received funding from the NHMRC, the Medical Research Future Fund (MRFF) Australia, Barwon Health, Deakin University, Amgen, The BUPA Foundation, Osteoporosis Australia, Australian and New Zealand Bone and Mineral Society, the Geelong Community Foundation, the Western Alliance and the Norman Beischer Foundation. J.R.H. owns controlling interest in Connecting Health Innovations LLC (CHI), a company that has licensed the right to his invention of the dietary inflammatory index (DII®) from the University of South Carolina in order to develop computer and smart phone applications for patient counselling and dietary intervention in clinical settings. N.S. is an employee of CHI. The subject matter of this paper will not have any direct bearing on that work, nor has that activity exerted any influence on this project. The funders had no role in the design of the study; in the collection, analyses, or interpretation of data; in the writing of the manuscript, or in the decision to publish the results.

References

1. Beaudart, C.; Rizzoli, R.; Bruyère, O.; Reginster, J.-Y.; Biver, E. Sarcopenia: Burden and challenges for public health. *Arch. Public Health* **2014**, *72*, 45. [CrossRef] [PubMed]
2. Pasco, J.A.; Mohebbi, M.; Holloway, K.L.; Brennan-Olsen, S.L.; Hyde, N.K.; Kotowicz, M.A. Musculoskeletal decline and mortality: Prospective data from the Geelong Osteoporosis Study. *J. Cachexia Sarcopenia Muscle* **2017**, *8*, 482–489. [CrossRef] [PubMed]
3. Pasco, J.A.; Sui, S.X.; Tembo, M.C.; Holloway Kew, K.L.; Rufus, P.G.; Kotowicz, M.A. Sarcopenic obesity and falls in the elderly. *J. Gerontol. Geriatr. Res.* **2018**, *7*, 2–5. [CrossRef]
4. Von Haehling, S.; Morley, J.E.; Anker, S.D. An overview of sarcopenia: Facts and numbers on prevalence and clinical impact. *J. Cachexia Sarcopenia Muscle* **2010**, *1*, 129–133. [CrossRef]
5. Sui, S.X.; Holloway-Kew, K.L.; Hyde, N.K.; Williams, L.J.; Tembo, M.C.; Leach, S.; Pasco, J.A. Definition-specific prevalence estimates for sarcopenia in an Australian population: The Geelong Osteoporosis Study. *JCSM Clin. Rep.* **2020**, *5*, 89–98.
6. Morley, J.E.; Anker, S.D.; von Haehling, S. Prevalence, incidence, and clinical impact of sarcopenia: Facts, numbers, and epidemiology-update 2014. *J. Cachexia Sarcopenia Muscle* **2014**, *5*, 253–259. [CrossRef]
7. Pasco, J.A. Age-related changes in muscle and bone. In *Osteosarcopenia: Bone, Muscle and Fat Interactions*; Duque, G., Ed.; Springer: Berlin/Heidelberg, Germany, 2019; pp. 45–71.
8. Ethgen, O.; Beaudart, C.; Buckinx, F.; Bruyere, O.; Reginster, J.-Y. The future prevalence of sarcopenia in Europe: A claim for public health action. *Calcif. Tissue Int.* **2017**, *100*, 229–234. [CrossRef]
9. Bano, G.; Trevisan, C.; Carraro, S.; Solmi, M.; Luchini, C.; Stubbs, B.; Manzato, E.; Sergi, G.; Veronese, N. Inflammation and sarcopenia: A systematic review and meta-analysis. *Maturitas* **2017**, *96*, 10–15. [CrossRef]
10. Pérez-Baos, S.; Prieto-Potin, I.; Román-Blas, J.A.; Sánchez-Pernaute, O.; Largo, R.; Herrero-Beaumont, G. Mediators and patterns of muscle loss in chronic systemic inflammation. *Front. Physiol.* **2018**, *9*, 409. [CrossRef]
11. Xia, S.; Zhang, X.; Zheng, S.; Khanabdali, R.; Kalionis, B.; Wu, J.; Wan, W.; Tai, X. An update on inflamm-aging: Mechanisms, prevention, and treatment. *J. Immunol. Res.* **2016**, *2016*, 12. [CrossRef]
12. Ogawa, S.; Yakabe, M.; Akishita, M. Age-related sarcopenia and its pathophysiological bases. *Inflamm. Regen.* **2016**, *36*, 17. [CrossRef]
13. Barbaresko, J.; Koch, M.; Schulze, M.B.; Nöthlings, U. Dietary pattern analysis and biomarkers of low-grade inflammation: A systematic literature review. *Nutr. Rev.* **2013**, *71*, 511–527. [CrossRef]
14. Calder, P.C.; Ahluwalia, N.; Brouns, F.; Buetler, T.; Clement, K.; Cunningham, K.; Esposito, K.; Jönsson, L.S.; Kolb, H.; Lansink, M.; et al. Dietary factors and low-grade inflammation in relation to overweight and obesity. *Br. J. Nutr.* **2011**, *106*, S5–S78. [CrossRef]
15. Hu, F.B. Dietary pattern analysis: A new direction in nutritional epidemiology. *Curr. Opin. Lipidol.* **2002**, *13*, 3–9. [CrossRef]
16. Shivappa, N.; Steck, S.E.; Hurley, T.G.; Hussey, J.R.; Hébert, J.R. Designing and developing a literature-derived, population-based dietary inflammatory index. *Public Health Nutr.* **2014**, *17*, 1689–1696. [CrossRef]

17. O'Neil, A.; Shivappa, N.; Jacka, F.N.; Kotowicz, M.A.; Kibbey, K.; Hebert, J.R.; Pasco, J.A. Pro-inflammatory dietary intake as a risk factor for CVD in men: A 5-year longitudinal study. *Br. J. Nutr.* **2015**, *114*, 2074–2082. [CrossRef]
18. Orchard, T.; Yildiz, V.; Steck, S.E.; Hébert, J.R.; Ma, Y.; Cauley, J.A.; Li, W.; Mossavar-Rahmani, Y.; Johnson, K.C.; Sattari, M.; et al. Dietary inflammatory index, bone mineral density and risk of fracture in postmenopausal women: Results from the Women's Health Initiative. *J. Bone Miner. Res.* **2017**, *32*, 1136–1146. [CrossRef]
19. Shivappa, N.; Stubbs, B.; Hébert, J.R.; Cesari, M.; Schofield, P.; Soysal, P.; Maggi, S.; Veronese, N. The relationship between the dietary inflammatory index and incident frailty: A longitudinal cohort study. *J. Am. Med. Dir. Assoc.* **2018**, *19*, 77–82. [CrossRef]
20. Laclaustra, M.; Rodriguez-Artalejo, F.; Guallar-Castillon, P.; Banegas, J.R.; Graciani, A.; Garcia-Esquinas, E.; Lopez-Garcia, E. The inflammatory potential of diet is related to incident frailty and slow walking in older adults. *Clin. Nutr.* **2020**, *39*, 185–191. [CrossRef]
21. Sardo Molmenti, C.L.; Steck, S.E.; Thomson, C.A.; Hibler, E.A.; Yang, J.; Shivappa, N.; Greenlee, H.; Wirth, M.D.; Neugut, A.I.; Jacobs, E.T.; et al. Dietary inflammatory index and risk of colorectal adenoma recurrence: A pooled analysis. *Nutr. Cancer* **2017**, *69*, 238–247. [CrossRef]
22. Bagheri, A.; Soltani, S.; Hashemi, R.; Heshmat, R.; Motlagh, A.D.; Esmaillzadeh, A. Inflammatory potential of the diet and risk of sarcopenia and its components. *Nutr. J.* **2020**, *19*, 129. [CrossRef] [PubMed]
23. Davis, J.A.; Mohebbi, M.; Collier, F.; Loughman, A.; Shivappa, N.; Hébert, J.R.; Pasco, J.A.; Jacka, F.N. Diet quality and a traditional dietary pattern predict lean mass in Australian women: Longitudinal data from the Geelong Osteoporosis Study. *Prev. Med. Rep.* **2021**, *21*. [CrossRef]
24. Cervo, M.M.; Shivappa, N.; Hebert, J.R.; Oddy, W.H.; Winzenberg, T.; Balogun, S.; Wu, F.; Ebeling, P.; Aitken, D.; Jones, G.; et al. Longitudinal associations between dietary inflammatory index and musculoskeletal health in community-dwelling older adults. *Clin. Nutr.* **2020**, *39*, 516–523. [CrossRef] [PubMed]
25. Park, S.; Na, W.; Sohn, C. Relationship between osteosarcopenic obesity and dietary inflammatory index in postmenopausal women: 2009 to 2011 Korea National Health and Nutrition Examination Surveys. *J. Clin. Biochem. Nutr.* **2018**, *63*, 211–216. [CrossRef] [PubMed]
26. Pasco, J.A.; Nicholson, G.C.; Kotowicz, M.A. Cohort profile: Geelong Osteoporosis Study. *Int. J. Epidemiol.* **2012**, *41*, 1565–1575. [CrossRef] [PubMed]
27. Willett, W. *Nutritional Epidemiology*; Oxford University Press: New York, NY, USA, 2013. [CrossRef]
28. Cruz-Jentoft, A.J.; Baeyens, J.P.; Bauer, J.M.; Boirie, Y.; Cederholm, T.; Landi, F.; Martin, F.C.; Michel, J.-P.; Rolland, Y.; Schneider, S.M.; et al. Sarcopenia: European consensus on definition and diagnosis: Report of the European Working Group on Sarcopenia in Older People. *Age Ageing* **2010**, *39*, 412–423. [CrossRef] [PubMed]
29. Podsiadlo, D.; Richardson, S. The timed "Up & Go": A test of basic functional mobility for frail elderly persons. *J. Am. Geriatr. Soc.* **1991**, *39*, 142–148.
30. Gould, H.; Brennan, S.L.; Kotowicz, M.A.; Nicholson, G.C.; Pasco, J.A. Total and appendicular lean mass reference ranges for Australian men and women: The Geelong Osteoporosis Study. *Calcif. Tissue Int.* **2014**, *94*, 363–372. [CrossRef]
31. Cruz-Jentoft, A.J.; Bahat, G.; Bauer, J.; Boirie, Y.; Bruyère, O.; Cederholm, T.; Cooper, C.; Landi, F.; Rolland, Y.; Sayer, A.A.; et al. Sarcopenia: Revised European consensus on definition and diagnosis. *Age Ageing* **2019**, *48*, 16–31. [CrossRef]
32. Giles, C.G.; Ireland, P.D. *Dietary Questionnaire for Epidemiological Studies (Version 2)*; The Cancer Council Victoria: Melbourne, Australia, 1996.
33. Xinying, P.X.; Noakes, M.; Keogh, J. Can a food frequency questionnaire be used to capture dietary intake data in a 4 week clinical intervention trial? *Asia Pac. J. Clin. Nutr.* **2004**, *13*, 318–323. [CrossRef]
34. Hodge, A.; Patterson, A.J.; Brown, W.J.; Ireland, P.; Giles, G. The Anti Cancer Council of Victoria FFQ: Relative validity of nutrient intakes compared with weighed food records in young to middle-aged women in a study of iron supplementation. *Aust. N. Z. J. Public Health* **2000**, *24*, 576–583. [CrossRef]
35. Shivappa, N.; Steck, S.E.; Hurley, T.G.; Hussey, J.R.; Ma, Y.; Ockene, I.S.; Tabung, F.; Hébert, J.R. A population-based dietary inflammatory index predicts levels of C-reactive protein in the Seasonal Variation of Blood Cholesterol Study (SEASONS). *Public Health Nutr.* **2014**, *17*, 1825–1833. [CrossRef]
36. Tabung, F.K.; Steck, S.E.; Zhang, J.; Ma, Y.; Liese, A.D.; Agalliu, I.; Hingle, M.; Hou, L.; Hurley, T.G.; Jiao, L.; et al. Construct validation of the dietary inflammatory index among postmenopausal women. *Ann. Epidemiol.* **2015**, *25*, 398–405. [CrossRef]
37. Shivappa, N.; Hébert, J.R.; Rietzschel, E.R.; De Buyzere, M.L.; Langlois, M.; Debruyne, E.; Marcos, A.; Huybrechts, I. Associations between dietary inflammatory index and inflammatory markers in the Asklepios Study. *Br. J. Nutr.* **2015**, *113*, 665–671. [CrossRef]
38. Wirth, M.D.; Shivappa, N.; Davis, L.; Hurley, T.G.; Ortaglia, A.; Drayton, R.; Blair, S.N.; Hébert, J.R. Construct validation of the dietary inflammatory index among African Americans. *J. Nutr. Health Aging* **2017**, *21*, 487–491. [CrossRef]
39. Kotemori, A.; Sawada, N.; Iwasaki, M.; Yamaji, T.; Shivappa, N.; Hebert, J.R.; Ishihara, J.; Inoue, M.; Tsugane, S. Validating the dietary inflammatory index using inflammatory biomarkers in a Japanese population: A cross-sectional study of the JPHC-FFQ validation study. *Nutrition* **2020**, *69*, 110569. [CrossRef]
40. Amakye, W.K.; Zhang, Z.; Wei, Y.; Shivappa, N.; Hebert, J.R.; Wang, J.; Su, Y.; Mao, L. The relationship between dietary inflammatory index (DII) and muscle mass and strength in Chinese children aged 6–9 years. *Asia Pac. J. Clin. Nutr.* **2018**, *27*, 1315–1324. [CrossRef]

41. Kelaiditi, E.; Jennings, A.; Steves, C.J.; Skinner, J.; Cassidy, A.; MacGregor, A.J.; Welch, A.A. Measurements of skeletal muscle mass and power are positively related to a Mediterranean dietary pattern in women. *Osteoporos. Int.* **2016**, *27*, 3251–3260. [CrossRef]
42. Hashemi, R.; Motlagh, A.D.; Heshmat, R.; Esmaillzadeh, A.; Payab, M.; Yousefinia, M.; Siassi, F.; Pasalar, P.; Baygi, F. Diet and its relationship to sarcopenia in community dwelling iranian elderly: A cross sectional study. *Nutrition* **2015**, *31*, 97–104. [CrossRef]
43. Kim, D.; Park, Y. Association between the dietary inflammatory index and risk of frailty in older individuals with poor nutritional status. *Nutrients* **2018**, *10*, 1363. [CrossRef]
44. Kim, D.Y.; Kim, C.-O.; Lim, H. Quality of diet and level of physical performance related to inflammatory markers in community-dwelling frail, elderly people. *Nutrition* **2017**, *38*, 48–53. [CrossRef]
45. Chen, L.K.; Liu, L.K.; Woo, J.; Assantachai, P.; Auyeung, T.W.; Bahyah, K.S.; Chou, M.Y.; Chen, L.Y.; Hsu, P.S.; Krairit, O.; et al. Sarcopenia in Asia: Consensus report of the Asian Working Group for Sarcopenia. *J. Am. Med. Dir. Assoc.* **2014**, *15*, 95–101. [CrossRef]
46. Fanelli Kuczmarski, M.; Mason, M.A.; Beydoun, M.A.; Allegro, D.; Zonderman, A.B.; Evans, M.K. Dietary patterns and sarcopenia in an urban African American and white population in the United States. *J. Nutr. Gerontol. Geriatr.* **2013**, *32*, 291–316. [CrossRef]
47. Chan, R.; Leung, J.; Woo, J. A prospective cohort study to examine the association between dietary patterns and sarcopenia in Chinese community-dwelling older people in Hong Kong. *J. Am. Med. Dir. Assoc.* **2016**, *17*, 336–342. [CrossRef]
48. Kim, J.; Lee, Y.; Kye, S.; Chung, Y.S.; Kim, K.M. Association of vegetables and fruits consumption with sarcopenia in older adults: The Fourth Korea National Health and Nutrition Examination Survey. *Age Ageing* **2015**, *44*, 96–102. [CrossRef] [PubMed]
49. Granic, A.; Mendonça, N.; Sayer, A.A.; Hill, T.R.; Davies, K.; Siervo, M.; Mathers, J.C.; Jagger, C. Effects of dietary patterns and low protein intake on sarcopenia risk in the very old: The Newcastle 85+ study. *Clin. Nutr.* **2020**, *39*, 166–173. [CrossRef]
50. Steck, S.; Shivappa, N.; Tabung, F.; Harmon, B.; Wirth, M.; Hurley, T.; Hebert, J. The dietary inflammatory index: A new tool for assessing diet quality based on inflammatory potential. *Digest* **2014**, *49*, 1–9.
51. Zhang, Z.; Cao, W.; Shivappa, N.; Hebert, J.R.; Li, B.; He, J.; Tang, X.; Liang, Y.; Chen, Y. Association between diet inflammatory index and osteoporotic hip fracture in elderly Chinese population. *J. Am. Med. Dir. Assoc.* **2017**, *18*, 671–677. [CrossRef]
52. Resciniti, N.V.; Lohman, M.C.; Wirth, M.D.; Shivappa, N.; Hebert, J.R. Dietary inflammatory index, pre-frailty and frailty among older US adults: Evidence from the National Health and Nutrition Examination Survey, 2007-2014. *J. Nutr. Health Aging* **2019**, *23*, 323–329. [CrossRef]
53. Galland, L. Diet and inflammation. *Nutr. Clin. Pract.* **2010**, *25*, 634–640. [CrossRef]
54. Hébert, J.R.; Hurley, T.G.; Steck, S.E.; Miller, D.R.; Tabung, F.K.; Peterson, K.E.; Kushi, L.H.; Frongillo, E.A. Considering the value of dietary assessment data in informing nutrition-related health policy. *Adv. Nutr.* **2014**, *5*, 447–455. [CrossRef] [PubMed]
55. Adamson, A.J.; Collerton, J.; Davies, K.; Foster, E.; Jagger, C.; Stamp, E.; Mathers, J.C.; Kirkwood, T. Nutrition in advanced age: Dietary assessment in the Newcastle 85+ study. *Eur. J. Nutr.* **2009**, *63*, S6–S18. [CrossRef] [PubMed]
56. Bhasin, S.; Travison, T.G.; Manini, T.M.; Patel, S.; Pencina, K.M.; Fielding, R.A.; Magaziner, J.M.; Newman, A.B.; Kiel, D.P.; Cooper, C.; et al. Sarcopenia Definition: The Position Statements of the Sarcopenia Definition and Outcomes Consortium. *J. Am. Geriatr. Soc.* **2020**, *68*, 1410–1418. [CrossRef] [PubMed]
57. Hébert, J.R.; Shivappa, N.; Wirth, M.D.; Hussey, J.R.; Hurley, T.G. Perspective: The dietary inflammatory index (DII)—Lessons learned, improvements made, and future directions. *Adv. Nutr.* **2019**, *10*, 185–195. [CrossRef]
58. Wynder, E.L.; Hebert, J.R. Homogeneity in nutritional exposure: An impediment in cancer epidemiology. *J. Natl. Cancer Inst.* **1987**, *79*, 605–607.

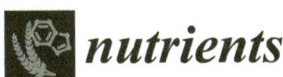

Systematic Review

The Prevalence of Sarcopenia in Chinese Older Adults: Meta-Analysis and Meta-Regression

Zi Chen, Wei-Ying Li, Mandy Ho and Pui-Hing Chau *

School of Nursing, The University of Hong Kong, Hong Kong, China; u1chenzi@connect.hku.hk (Z.C.); u3003886@connect.hku.hk (W.-Y.L.); mandyho1@hku.hk (M.H.)
* Correspondence: phchau@graduate.hku.hk; Tel.: +852-39-176-626

Abstract: Sarcopenia, with risk factors such as poor nutrition and physical inactivity, is becoming prevalent among the older population. The aims of this study were (i) to systematically review the existing data on sarcopenia prevalence in the older Chinese population, (ii) to generate pooled estimates of the sex-specific prevalence among different populations, and (iii) to identify the factors associated with the heterogeneity in the estimates across studies. A search was conducted in seven databases for studies that reported the prevalence of sarcopenia in Chinese older adults, aged 60 years and over, published through April 2020. We then performed a meta-analysis to estimate the pooled prevalence, and investigated the factors associated with the variation in the prevalence across the studies using meta-regression. A total of 58 studies were included in this review. Compared with community-dwelling Chinese older adults (men: 12.9%, 95% CI: 10.7–15.1%; women: 11.2%, 95% CI: 8.9–13.4%), the pooled prevalence of sarcopenia in older adults from hospitals (men: 29.7%, 95% CI:18.4–41.1%; women: 23.0%, 95% CI:17.1–28.8%) and nursing homes (men: 26.3%, 95% CI: 19.1 to 33.4%; women: 33.7%, 95% CI: 27.2 to 40.1%) was higher. The multivariable meta-regression quantified the difference of the prevalence estimates in different populations, muscle mass assessments, and areas. This study yielded pooled estimates of sarcopenia prevalence in Chinese older adults not only from communities, but also from clinical settings and nursing homes. This study added knowledge to the current epidemiology literature about sarcopenia in older Chinese populations, and could provide background information for future preventive strategies, such as nutrition and physical activity interventions, tailored to the growing older population.

Keywords: sarcopenia; prevalence; nutrition; physical activity; meta-analysis; meta-regression

Citation: Chen, Z.; Li, W.-Y.; Ho, M.; Chau, P.-H. The Prevalence of Sarcopenia in Chinese Older Adults: Meta-Analysis and Meta-Regression. *Nutrients* **2021**, *13*, 1441. https://doi.org/10.3390/nu13051441

Academic Editors: Cristiano Capurso and Maria Luz Fernandez

Received: 9 February 2021
Accepted: 21 April 2021
Published: 24 April 2021

Publisher's Note: MDPI stays neutral with regard to jurisdictional claims in published maps and institutional affiliations.

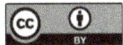

Copyright: © 2021 by the authors. Licensee MDPI, Basel, Switzerland. This article is an open access article distributed under the terms and conditions of the Creative Commons Attribution (CC BY) license (https:// creativecommons.org/licenses/by/ 4.0/).

1. Introduction

The speed of population ageing is accelerating globally. According to statistics from the World Health Organization (WHO), by 2050, the proportion of individuals over the age of 60 is expected almost to double (22%) compared with 12% in 2015 [1]. China is already witnessing this demographic trend; thus, the country's National Bureau of Statistics has predicted that the number of adults aged 65 years and above will increase from 166.58 million (11.9% of the total population) in 2018 to 366 million in 2050 [2].

Advancing age is marked by a series of physiological changes in body composition, including the decrease in skeletal muscle mass and increase in fat mass [3,4]. Sarcopenia is the age-related decline in skeletal muscle mass and function characterized by the loss of muscle strength and physical performance [5]. Accordingly, understanding more about its etiology and risk factors is of great interest. The onset and progression of sarcopenia can be attributed to numerous factors including physical inactivity and poor nutrition [6]. Therefore, most non-pharmacological interventions about sarcopenia mainly target these two modifiable factors. An umbrella review concluded that exercise training, especially resistance training, had a significant effect on the improvement of muscle mass, muscle strength, and physical performance [7]. Bloom et al. systematically reviewed observational evidence regarding the relationship of diet quality and sarcopenia, and concluded that a higher quality diet was associated with better physical performance among older adults [8]. Furthermore, a narrative review conducted by Tessier et al. examined the observational and interventional evidence regarding the association between some specific nutrients and sarcopenic components [9]. They found that some nutrients such as proteins, leucine, vitamin D, and n-3 polyunsaturated fatty acids (n-3 PUFAs) might have a protective impact on muscle health among older adults [9]. Previous research has associated sarcopenia with such adverse health outcomes as fractures, falls, functional decline, hospitalization, and even increased mortality [10,11]. Hence, early screening and identifying sarcopenia among older populations should be at the forefront of timely diet and/or exercise interventions for sarcopenia prevention and treatment.

Sarcopenia is diagnosed based on low muscle mass, low muscle strength, and diminished physical performance. However, no standard and unique diagnosis criteria for sarcopenia have yet been established. At present, several international groups, such as the European Working Group on Sarcopenia in Older People (EWGSOP), Asia Working Group for Sarcopenia (AWGS), International Working Group on Sarcopenia (IWGS), Foundation for the National Institutes of Health (FNIH) Sarcopenia Project, have provided their own diagnostic criteria for sarcopenia [12–14]. Estimates of sarcopenia prevalence are, in turn, dependent on the diagnostic criteria used to define it. For example, a longitudinal multi-center cohort research found the prevalence of sarcopenia among community-dwelling older adults ranged from 3.3% to 17.5% depending on the diagnostic criteria used (specifically, AWGS: 9.1%, EWGSOP: 17.5%, IWGS: 16.1%, and FNIH: 3.3%) [15]. Assessment of muscle mass is an essential part of sarcopenia diagnosis. Dual-energy X-ray absorptiometry (DXA) and bioelectrical impedance analysis (BIA) are both recommended to assess muscle mass in research and practice [12]. Therefore, estimates of the prevalence may also depend on different assessment approaches. For example, Beaudart et al. [16] compared the prevalence of sarcopenia (EWGSOP criterion) using different muscle mass assessments (DXA and BIA) among older adults over 65 years, and found the prevalence was lower when using the BIA technique (BIA vs. DXA: 12.8% vs. 21%). Likewise, there is evidence that the methods used to measure muscle strength and physical performance may yield inconsistent estimates of the prevalence of sarcopenia [17]. Furthermore, estimates of prevalence also varied across populations and areas [18–23]. Previous evidence revealed that hospitalized older adults and nursing-home residents had higher prevalence of sarcopenia compared with community-dwelling older residents [18]. Community-dwelling Chinese older adults residing outside mainland China (i.e., Hong Kong and Taiwan) showed a lower prevalence rate of sarcopenia than counterparts from the mainland [24].

At present, two systematic reviews have pooled the estimate of sarcopenia prevalence in community-dwelling Chinese older adults (17% and 11%, respectively) [24,25]. However, few systematic reviews have pooled the prevalence for Chinese older adults in other settings, such as clinical settings and nursing homes. Furthermore, no study has systematically investigated the factors contributing to the heterogeneity in the estimates of sarcopenia prevalence through meta-regression. Therefore, we conducted a meta-analysis and meta-regression to shed light on the prevalence of sarcopenia in Chinese older adults not only from communities, but also from clinical settings and nursing homes, and to explain the heterogeneity in sarcopenia prevalence across studies.

Information about the prevalence of sarcopenia is the first step to develop preventive routines or health services tailored to the growing older population. Meta-analysis and meta-regression of prevalence data are increasingly important for policy making and implementation of preventive measures in situations for which inconsistent prevalence estimates have been reported in the literature. This study could help policy makers and health practitioners make evidence-based decisions targeting the health issues of sarcopenia.

2. Methods

This review was conducted in accordance with the Preferred Reporting Items for Systematic Reviews and Meta Analyses (PRISMA) statement [26].

2.1. Search Methods

Two researchers (Z.C. and W.Y.L.) independently searched the following online electronic databases: PubMed, Cochrane Library, Embase (Ovid), CINAHL, Web of Science Core Collection, CNKI, and Wanfang (accessed on 15 April 2020); the latter two being Chinese. The search period was restricted from the earliest records to 15 April, 2020. Key search terms were "sarcopenia", "epidemiology", "prevalence", "aged", "elderly", "older", "China", and "Chinese". Logical operators (i.e., AND, OR) were used to shape the search strategy. Detailed search strategies for PubMed and Wanfang are presented in the Supplementary Materials as examples (S1: Search strategy). Relevant studies were identified through manual searches in the reference list of eligible studies.

Inclusion criteria were as followed: (1) the prevalence of sarcopenia was reported or could be calculated; (2) participants were of Chinese ethnicity; (3) the age was 60 years and over; (4) participants were recruited from the community, clinical settings, or nursing homes; (5) EWGOSP, AWGS, IWGS or FINH definitions of sarcopenia were adopted; (6) muscle mass was measured with DXA or BIA; (7) primary research irrespective of design. Exclusion criteria were (1) studies published as reviews, letters to editors, conference abstracts, expert opinions, case reports; (2) studies published in languages other than English and Chinese.

First, duplicate records were identified and removed. Then, titles and abstracts were screened to remove studies irrelevant to the research questions. Next, full-text articles were retrieved and reviewed for eligibility according to the selection criteria. When multiple papers came from the same dataset, we chose the one with the largest sample size which might be closer to the original cohort in order to avoid those using a particular subset of the whole dataset. The above process was performed independently by the two researchers (Z.C. and W.-Y.L.). Any discrepancies were adjudicated by a third researcher (P.-H.C.).

2.2. Data Extraction

The following details were extracted from each of the eligible studies: the year of publication, country or area in which the data were collected, research design, sample size, settings where participants were recruited, diagnostic criteria for sarcopenia, measurement of muscle mass, muscle strength, and physical performance and prevalence of sarcopenia. For cohort or intervention studies, only baseline data were extracted. For studies using more than one diagnostic criterion to define sarcopenia, all estimates of prevalence were extracted.

2.3. Critical Appraisal

Two researchers (Z.C. and W.Y.L.) independently assessed the quality of included studies using a validated tool developed by Hoy et al., which was tailored to assess the risk of bias for prevalence studies with different types of design [27]. The tool evaluates the risk of bias through 10 items. The first four items mainly focus on external validity, which involve the representativeness of the target population and the sampling frame, selection of the sample, and non-response bias. The remaining items address the issue of internal validity, which involves the use of proxy respondent or not, acceptable case definition, validated measurement, consistent mode of data collection, the length of the shortest prevalence period, and correct calculation of prevalence. Each item was rated as "low risk" or "high risk". When information in the article was not sufficient for judgement, that item was rated as "high risk". Following previous literature, the study was considered to have a low risk of bias when 9 or 10 items were rated "low risk"; a moderate risk of bias when 6 to 8 items were rated "low risk"; and a high risk of bias when 5 or less items were rated "low risk" [28,29].

2.4. Statistical Analysis

The prevalence of sarcopenia varied in different genders and populations recruited from different settings [18]. Accordingly, in this study, the pooled prevalence was obtained separately for each gender and for the population from each setting. For studies which recruited participants from mixed settings, only those which reported the prevalence for each setting were included in the meta-analysis. While more than one estimate was extracted from studies which used more than one diagnostic criterion to define sarcopenia, only the one that was more frequently used in other eligible studies was used for calculation of the pooled estimate.

Random-effect models take into account the possibility that the parameters for the population may vary among studies [30]. Therefore, because of the variations in populations, diagnosis criteria, muscle mass assessments, etc., among the eligible studies, we chose a random-effect model to calculate the pooled prevalence. The *metaprop* command in Stata 15.0 (Stata Corp, College Station, TX, USA) was used to obtain pooled estimates of prevalence [31,32].

We assessed the heterogeneity in the estimates across studies using Cochran's Q test, with a *p*-value < 0.10 indicating heterogeneity [33]. We quantified the heterogeneity using I-square, with I^2 statistics of 25%, 50%, and 75% set as the cut-offs for low, moderate, and high heterogeneity, respectively [33]. If heterogeneity existed, random-effect meta-regression was conducted to explore the potential source of variability in prevalence estimates across studies. Meta-regression can explore the effects of multiple study characteristics on the variance of pooled estimates simultaneously [30]. For this study, we performed multivariable meta-regression (using the *metareg* command) to model the adjusted association between multiple explanatory variables and prevalence estimates. Based on previous evidence, we considered the following study characteristics to be potential sources of heterogeneity: populations from different settings, diagnostic criteria for sarcopenia, assessment of muscle mass, muscle strength and physical performance, and the area of study. In order to have a sufficient power, meta-regression was only performed for covariates reported in at least ten studies [33].

Publication bias refers to the phenomenon that studies with significant results are more likely to get published than those with negative results, which can result in systematic differences between published and unpublished studies [34]. In the case of observational studies that report prevalence, however, there are no positive or negative results, and no well-established method is recommended to test for this bias in meta-analysis of prevalence studies. Therefore, in this study, we did not check for publication bias.

3. Results

3.1. Search Outcomes

We identified 459 records from databases and 6 records from the reference lists. After removing 139 duplicated records, we screened the titles and abstracts of the remaining 326 records, and removed another 168 irrelevant records, leaving 158 studies. Further reviewing the full texts of these studies for eligibility, we excluded another 100 for the reasons specified in Figure 1. We carried out the quantitative synthesis (i.e., meta-analysis and meta-regression) on the remaining 58 records.

The characteristics of the included studies are summarized in Table 1. Fifty-one (87.9%) studies were classified as having a moderate risk of bias and seven (12.1%) were classified as having a low risk of bias. None of the included studies recruited the nationwide representative sample. Twelve studies adopted random sampling [19,20,35–44]. One study was open to the non-response bias [35], Each study collected data of sarcopenia components directly from subjects and had a consistent mode of data collection. All included studies had acceptable case definition and correct calculation of prevalence. Details of the critical appraisal are presented in Supplementary Materials (Table S2).

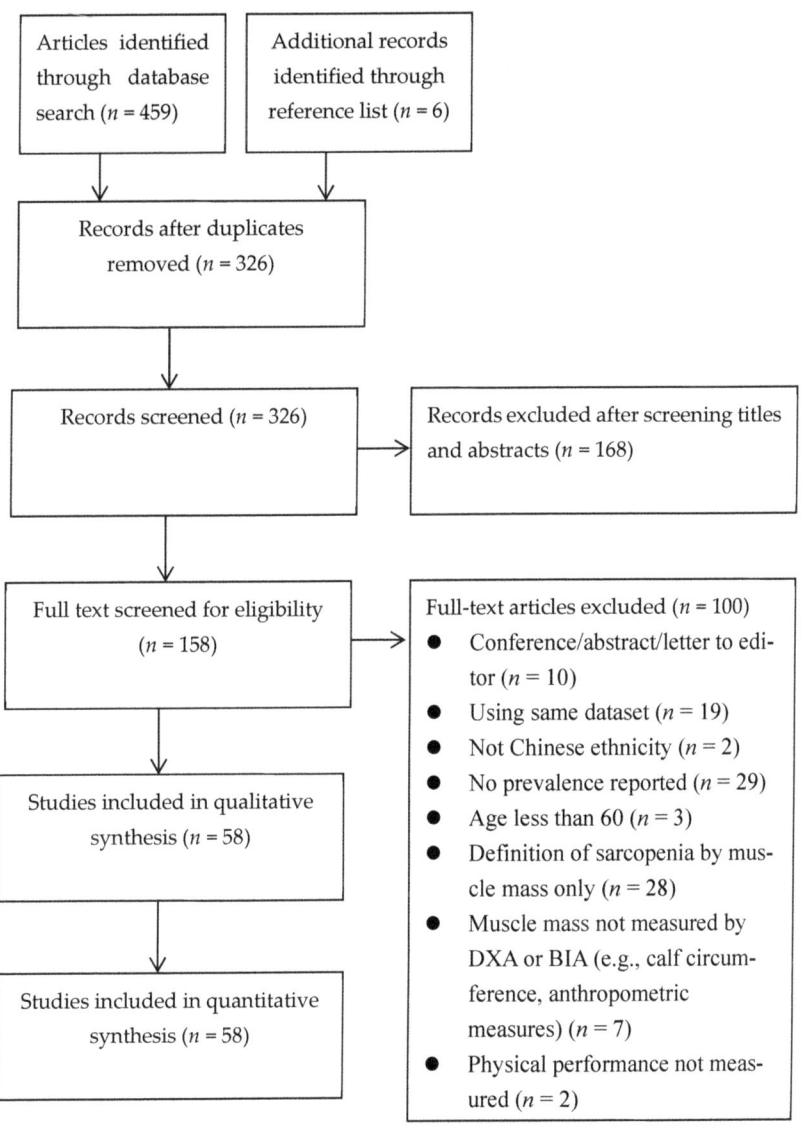

Figure 1. PRISMA flowchart.

Table 1. Characteristics of included studies (n = 58).

Study	Language	Region	Design	Sample Size			Assessment				Prevalence n (%)			Risk of Bias
				Total	Male	Female	Diagnostic Criteria	Muscle Mass	Muscle Strength	Physical Performance				
										Distance (m)	Gait Speed	Total	Male	Female	

Study	Language	Region	Design	Total	Male	Female	Diagnostic Criteria	Muscle Mass	Muscle Strength	Distance (m)	Gait Speed	Total	Male	Female	Risk of Bias
Community (n = 32)															
Meng et al., 2014 [45]	English	Mainland	Cross-sectional	101	101	—	EWGSOP	DXA	Dynamometer	6	Usual	46 (45.7)	46 (45.7)	—	Moderate
Wu et al., 2014 [46]	English	Taiwan	Cross-sectional	549	285	264	EWGSOP	BIA	Dynamometer	5	—	39 (7.1)	11 (3.9)	28 (10.6)	Moderate
Zhang et al., 2014 [47]	Chinese	Mainland	Cross-sectional	116	—	—	EWGSOP	DXA	Dynamometer	6	Usual	48 (41.4)	—	—	Moderate
Meng et al., 2015 [35]	English	Taiwan	Cross-sectional	771	412	359	EWGSOP	DXA	Dynamometer	5	Usual	44 (5.7)	35 (8.4)	9 (2.6)	Moderate
Wang et al., 2015 [48]	English	Mainland	Cross-sectional	316	164	152	AWGS	BIA	Dynamometer	4	Usual	94 (29.4)	43 (26.2)	51 (33.6)	Moderate
Wen et al., 2015 [36]	English	Mainland	Cross-sectional	286	136	150	IWGS / EWGSOP / AWGS	DXA	Dynamometer	6	Usual	17 (5.9) / 1 (0.3) / 9 (3.1)	10 (7.4) / 1 (0.8) / 8 (5.9)	7 (4.7) / — / 1 (0.7)	Moderate
Chan et al., 2016 [19]	English	HK	Cross-sectional	3957	1979	1878	AWGS	DXA	Dynamometer	6	Usual	290 (7.3)	185 (9.3)	105 (5.6)	Low
Han et al., 2016 [49]	English	Taiwan	Cross-sectional	878	402	476	EWGSOP	BIA	Dynamometer	7	Usual	29 (3.3)	27 (6.7)	2 (0.4)	Moderate
Han et al., 2016 [50]	English	Mainland	Cross-sectional	1069	467	602	AWGS	BIA	Dynamometer	4	Usual	99 (9.3)	30 (6.4)	69 (11.5)	Moderate
Huang et al., 2016 [20]	English	Taiwan	Cross-sectional	731	386	345	AWGS	DXA	Dynamometer	6	—	50 (6.8)	36 (9.3)	14 (4.1)	Low
Wang et al., 2016 [51]	English	Mainland	Cross-sectional	944	462	482	AWGS	BIA	Dynamometer	6	Usual	98 (10.4)	38 (8.2)	60 (12.5)	Moderate
Wang et al., 2016 [52]	English	Mainland	Cross-sectional	854	404	450	AWGS	BIA	Dynamometer	4	Usual	96 (11.2)	53 (13.1)	43 (9.6)	Low
Xia et al., 2016 [37]	Chinese	Mainland	Cross-sectional	683	239	444	AWGS	BIA	Dynamometer	4	—	137 (20.1)	41 (17.2)	96 (21.6)	Moderate
Fang et al., 2017 [53]	Chinese	Mainland	Cross-sectional	106	—	106	AWGS	DXA	Dynamometer	6	Usual	13 (12.2)	—	13 (12.2)	Moderate
Hai et al., 2017 [54]	English	Mainland	Cross-sectional	836	415	421	AWGS	BIA	Dynamometer	6	Usual	88 (10.5)	47 (11.3)	41 (9.7)	Moderate
Hua et al., 2017 [55]	Chinese	Mainland	Cross-sectional	300	168	132	AWGS	BIA	Dynamometer	6	Usual	54 (18.0)	38 (22.6)	16 (12.1)	Moderate
Meng et al., 2017 [56]	Chinese	Mainland	Cross-sectional	106	101	5	AWGS	BIA	Dynamometer	—	—	29 (27.4)	—	—	Moderate
Chu 2018 [57]	Chinese	Mainland	Cross-sectional	191	69	122	AWGS	BIA	Dynamometer	4	Maximal	28 (14.7)	8 (11.6)	20 (16.4)	Moderate
Wang et al., 2018 [23]	English	Mainland	Cross-sectional	865	427	438	AWGS	BIA	Dynamometer	6	Usual	71 (7.1)	28 (6.6)	33 (7.5)	Moderate
Yang et al., 2018 [58]	English	Mainland	Cross-sectional	384	160	224	EWGSOP	BIA	Dynamometer	4	Usual	45 (11.72)	17 (10.6)	28 (12.5)	Moderate
Zhang et al., 2018 [38]	Chinese	Mainland	Cross-sectional	1148	368	780	AWGS	BIA	Dynamometer	6	Usual	164 (14.3)	55 (14.9)	109 (14.0)	Low
Chen et al., 2019 [21]	English	Mainland	Prospective	691	304	387	AWGS	BIA	Dynamometer	4	—	55 (8.0)	—	—	Moderate

Table 1. Cont.

Study	Language	Region	Design	Sample Size			Diagnostic Criteria	Assessment				Prevalence n (%)			Risk of Bias
				Total	Male	Female		Muscle Mass	Muscle Strength	Physical Performance		Total	Male	Female	
										Distance (m)	Gait Speed				
Du et al., 2019 [22]	English	Mainland	Cross-sectional	631	213	418	AWGS	BIA	Dynamometer	6	Usual	77 (12.2)	41 (19.2)	36 (8.6)	Moderate
Liu et al., 2019 [39]	Chinese	Mainland	Cross-sectional	1723	915	808	AWGS	BIA	Dynamometer	6	Usual	121 (7.0)	96 (10.5)	25 (3.1)	Moderate
Liu 2019 [59]	Chinese	Mainland	Cross-sectional	769	416	353	AWGS	BIA	Dynamometer	6	Usual	32 (4.16)	12 (2.9)	20 (5.7)	Moderate
Wang et al., 2019 [60]	English	Mainland	Cross-sectional	945	465	480	AWGS	BIA	Dynamometer	6	Usual	276 (29.2)	123 (26.5)	153 (55.4)	Moderate
Xu et al., 2019 [40]	English	Mainland	Cross-sectional	2412	1012	1400	AWGS	BIA	Dynamometer	6	Usual	156 (6.5)	58 (5.7)	98 (7.0)	Moderate
Zhang et al., 2019 [61]	English	Mainland	Cross-sectional	1002	420	582	AWGS	BIA	Dynamometer	4	—	107 (10.7)	37 (8.8)	70 (12.0)	Moderate
Liu et al., 2020 [15]	English	Mainland	Cross-sectional	1712	—	—	AWGS	BIA	Dynamometer	4	Usual	556 (32.5)	—	—	Moderate
Rong et al., 2020 [62]	English	Mainland	Cross-sectional	450	266	184	AWGS	BIA	Dynamometer	6	Usual	89 (19.7)	50 (18.8)	39 (21.2)	Moderate
Xu et al., 2020 [63]	English	Mainland	Cross-sectional	582	246	336	AWGS	BIA	Dynamometer	6	Usual	15 (526.6)	82 (33.3)	73 (21.7)	Moderate
Yang et al., 2020 [64]	English	Mainland	Cross-sectional	483	184	299	FNIH IWGS AWGS EWGSOP1 EWGSOP2	BIA	Dynamometer	4	Usual	16 (3.3) 78 (16.1) 44 (9.1) 76 (15.7) 22 (4.6)	11 (6.0) 45 (24.5) 20 (10.9) 41 (22.3) 12 (6.5)	5 (1.7) 33 (11.0) 24 (8.0) 35 (11.7) 10 (3.3)	Moderate
Hospitals (n = 11)															
Wang et al., 2016 [52] [†]	English	Mainland	Cross-sectional	236	116	120	AWGS	BIA	Dynamometer	4	Usual	35 (14.8)	20 (17.2)	15 (12.5)	Low
Cui 2018 [65]	Chinese	Mainland	Cross-sectional	132	59	73	AWGS	DXA	Dynamometer	6	Usual	38 (28.8)	21 (35.6)	17 (23.3)	Moderate
Zhai et al., 2018 [66]	English	Mainland	Cross-sectional	494	216	278	AWGS	DXA	Dynamometer	6	—	158 (32.0)	87 (40.3)	71 (25.5)	Moderate
Chen et al., 2019 [67]	English	Mainland	Cross-sectional	118	92	26	AWGS	DXA	Dynamometer	6	Usual	71 (60.17)	65 (70.65)	6 (23.08)	Moderate
Wang 2019 [41]	Chinese	Mainland	Cross-sectional	119	64	55	AWGS	BIA	Dynamometer	—	—	26 (21.8)	17 (26.6)	9 (16.3)	Moderate
Yao 2019 [68]	Chinese	Mainland	Cross-sectional	378	153	225	AWGS	BIA	Dynamometer	6	Usual	47 (12.4)	15 (9.8)	32 (14.2)	Moderate
Yi et al., 2019 [69]	Chinese	Mainland	Cross-sectional	200	—	—	AWGS	BIA	Dynamometer	6	—	98 (49)	—	—	Moderate
Tan 2019 [70]	Chinese	Mainland	Cross-sectional	734	—	—	AWGS	BIA	Dynamometer	4	—	258 (35.1)	—	—	Moderate
Zhang et al., 2019 [71]	English	Mainland	Prospective	345	208	137	AWGS	BIA	Dynamometer	6	—	78 (22.6)	32 (15.4)	46 (33.6)	Moderate
Cui et al., 2020 [72]	English	Mainland	Cross-sectional	132	59	73	AWGS	DXA	Dynamometer	6	Usual	38 (28.8)	21 (55.3)	17 (44.7)	Moderate
Wang et al., 2020 [73]	Chinese	Mainland	Cross-sectional	236	144	92	AWGS	BIA	Dynamometer	6	—	63 (26.7)	28 (19.4)	35 (38.0)	Moderate

Table 1. Cont.

Study	Language	Region	Design	Sample Size			Diagnostic Criteria	Assessment				Prevalence n (%)			Risk of Bias
				Total	Male	Female		Muscle Mass	Muscle Strength	Physical Performance		Total	Male	Female	
										Distance (m)	Gait Speed				
Outpatient Services (n = 4)																
Li et al., 2014 [74]	Chinese	Mainland	Cross-sectional	169	169	—	IWGS	DXA	Dynamometer	6	Usual	106 (62.9)	106 (62.9)	—	Moderate
							EWGSOP				Usual	56 (33.3)	56 (33.3)		
Wang et al., 2016 [75]	Chinese	Mainland	Cross-sectional	410	—	—	EWGSOP	DXA	Dynamometer	6	Usual	80 (19.5)	—	—	Moderate
Fung et al., 2019 [42]	English	Singapore	Cross-sectional	266	—	—	AWGS	BIA	Dynamometer	6	Usual	70 (26.3)	—	—	low
Wang et al., 2019 [76]	Chinese	Mainland	Cross-sectional	430	191	239	EWGSOP	BIA	Dynamometer	6	Usual	95 (22.1)	32 (16.8)	63 (26.4)	Moderate
Nursing Home (n = 5)																
Hsu et al., 2014 [77]	English	Taiwan	Cross-sectional	353	353	—	EWGSOP	BIA	Dynamometer	6	Usual	109 (30.9)	109 (30.9)	—	Moderate
Wu et al., 2017 [43]	Chinese	Mainland	Cross-sectional	786	320	466	EWGSOP	BIA	Dynamometer	4	—	199 (25.3)	64 (20.0)	135 (29.0)	Moderate
Liao 2018 [78]	Chinese	Mainland	Cross-sectional	225	63	162	AWGS	BIA	Dynamometer	6	Usual	86 (38.2)	26 (41.3)	60 (37.0)	Moderate
Zeng et al., 2018 [79]	English	Mainland	Cross-sectional	277	83	194	FNIH	BIA	Dynamometer	4	Usual	87 (31.4)	19 (22.9)	68 (35.1)	Moderate
Yang et al., 2019 [80]	English	Mainland	Cross-sectional	316	112	204	AWGS	BIA	Dynamometer	4	—	91 (28.8)	34 (30.4)	57 (27.9)	Moderate
Mixed Settings: Communities and Nursing Homes (n = 2)																
Chen 2018 [81]	Chinese	Mainland	Cross-sectional	158	43	115	AWGS	BIA	Dynamometer	6	Usual	34 (21.5)	5 (11.4)	29 (25.4)	Moderate
Yang 2018 [44]	Chinese	Mainland	Cross-sectional	316	112	204	AWGS	BIA	Dynamometer	4	Usual	91 (28.8)	34 (30.4)	57 (27.9)	Low
Mixed Settings: Hospital and Outpatient Services (n = 5)																
Feng 2016 [82]	Chinese	Mainland	Cross-sectional	330	157	173	AWGS	BIA	Dynamometer	4	Maximal	35 (10.6)	21 (13.4)	14 (8.1)	Moderate
Ma 2017 [83]	Chinese	Mainland	Cross-sectional	764	550	214	AWGS	BIA	Dynamometer	4	Usual	138 (18.1)	82 (14.9)	56 (26.2)	Moderate
Zhou et al., 2018 [84]	Chinese	Mainland	Cross-sectional	163	100	63	IWGS	DXA	Dynamometer	3	Maximal	26 (16.0)	—	—	Moderate
Zhang et al., 2019 [85]	Chinese	Mainland	Cross-sectional	223	—	—	AWGS	BIA	Dynamometer	6	Usual	49 (22.0)	—	—	Moderate
Yang 2019 [86]	Chinese	Mainland	Cross-sectional	102	51	51	AWGS	BIA	Dynamometer	4	Maximal	17 (16.0)	—	—	Moderate

†: This study provided sarcopenia prevalence for older adults from communities and clinical settings separately.

3.2. Prevalence in Older Men

In the 46 studies that reported the prevalence of sarcopenia in older men, the overall prevalence was 18% (95% CI: 15.7 to 20.4%, $I^2 = 95.2\%$). For participants from different settings, the pooled prevalence rates were 12.9% (95% CI: 10.7 to 15.1%, $I^2 = 93.7\%$) in community-dwelling older men ($n = 27$), 29.7% (95% CI: 18.4 to 41.1%, $I^2 = 95.5\%$) for hospitalized older men ($n = 9$), and 26.3% (95% CI: 19.1 to 33.4%, $I^2 = 83.7\%$) in nursing-home residents ($n = 5$). We did not pool the prevalence for outpatients due to an insufficient number of studies ($n = 2$). Substantial heterogeneity in prevalence estimates was found across the studies, with all of the I-square values being greater than 80%.

3.3. Prevalence in Older Women

In the 44 studies that reported the prevalence of sarcopenia in older women, the overall prevalence was 16.4% (95% CI: 14.1 to 18.8%, $I^2 = 97.3\%$). For participants from different settings, the prevalence was 11.2% (95% CI: 8.9 to 13.4%, $I^2 = 97.1\%$) in community-dwelling older women, ($n = 27$), 23.0% (95% CI: 17.1 to 28.8%, $I^2 = 80.9\%$) for hospitalized older women ($n = 9$), and 33.7% (95% CI: 27.2 to 40.1%, $I^2 = 78.4\%$) for those from nursing homes ($n = 4$). Because only one study reported the prevalence for female outpatients, we did not perform meta-analysis for outpatients. Similarly, considerable heterogeneity was found across studies.

3.4. Meta-Regression Analysis

We performed a multivariable meta-regression to explore the potential sources of the considerable heterogeneity in the estimates of sarcopenia prevalence across studies. The results of the regression indicated that, irrespective of gender, the hospitalized patients and nursing-home residents had a higher prevalence of sarcopenia than community-dwelling older adults. For older men, the prevalence rate was lower when muscle mass was assessed using the BIA method rather than the DXA method. Furthermore, those from mainland China appeared to have a higher prevalence of sarcopenia compared with those from Hong Kong or Taiwan. For older women, only the participants from different settings showed a significant association with the prevalence of sarcopenia (Table 2).

Table 2. Multivariable meta-regression.

Covariates	Males ($n = 43$)			Females ($n = 41$)		
	Exp (β)	95% CI	p-Value	Exp (β)	95% CI	p-Value
Populations						
Community-dwelling (ref)	1.00			1.00		
Outpatients	1.29	(0.52, 3.17)	0.570	2.28	(0.67, 7.73)	0.180
Hospitalized people	1.69	(1.01, 2.86)	0.047	2.10	(1.17, 3.78)	0.015
Nursing-home residents	2.50	(1.35, 4.66)	0.005	2.73	(1.38, 5.38)	0.005
Diagnosis criteria						
AWGS (ref)	1.00			1.00		
EWGSOP	1.23	(0.67, 2.27)	0.490	0.92	(0.39, 2.15)	0.840
Assessment of muscle mass						
DXA (ref)	1.00			1.00		
BIA	0.58	(0.35, 0.98)	0.044	1.17	(0.60, 2.29)	0.640
Area						
Mainland (ref)	1.00			1.00		
Out of mainland	0.47	(0.22, 0.98)	0.045	0.51	(0.18, 1.43)	0.190
Walk distance						
6 m (ref)	1.00			1.00		
4 m	0.84	(0.53, 1.32)	0.440	1.12	(0.68, 1.83)	0.650
Others	0.81	(0.34, 1.93)	0.630	0.73	(0.24, 2.25)	0.580

4. Discussion

This meta-analysis provided a comprehensive picture of the prevalence of sarcopenia in Chinese older adults. It filled the knowledge gap by extending the existing reviews of sarcopenia prevalence in Chinese older adults from communities to other settings (clinical settings and nursing homes) as well. We also systematically investigated factors that contributed to the significant heterogeneity in pooled prevalence estimates using multivariable meta-regression. Our findings contribute to the epidemiological literature on sarcopenia in Chinese older adults, and can provide a starting point for future research and efforts in sarcopenia prevention among Chinese populations.

For community-dwelling Chinese older adults, we obtained similar estimates of prevalence (12.9% in men vs. 11.2% in women) compared with previous reports (11% in men vs. 10% in women; 14% in men vs. 9% in women) [24,25]. When compared with the prevalence in Europeans (13% in men vs. 14% in women), our estimates were comparable with them [18]. However, Papadopoulou et al. [18] found non-Asian groups seemed more prone to sarcopenia than Asian groups. The difference in ethnic characteristics, body size, and dietary regimes etc., between Asians and non-Asians might be possible reasons for the potential disparity in the sarcopenia prevalence. As for gender difference, our result was similar to the previous evidence that higher prevalence of sarcopenia was shown in Chinese community-dwelling older males than females [15,22,25]. However, in western countries, the evidence of gender difference was controversial depending on the EWGSOP cut-off values applied [13,87]. For hospitalized older adults, we found the prevalence to be 29.7% in men and 23.0% in women. To our knowledge, this is the first systematic review to pool the prevalence of sarcopenia for Chinese older adults who are hospitalized. Our findings revealed a relatively higher prevalence in this group compared with that from communities. Compared with the pooled estimates of hospitalized older adults mainly from Europe (23% in men and 24% in women), our findings were higher in hospitalized men and comparable in hospitalized women [18]. For outpatients, considering that Cochran's Q is not very informative and tends to be biased when the number of studies is small, we did not perform meta-analysis for this group [88]. For those residing in nursing homes, similarly, no meta-analysis synthesized the prevalence of sarcopenia in this Chinese group before. Shen et al. [28] conducted a systematic review pooling the prevalence of sarcopenia in nursing-home populations from 16 studies. However, they only included one original study that targeted the Chinese population [28]. Compared with Shen et al.'s results (43% in men vs. 46% in women), we obtained lower pooled estimates (26.3% in men vs. 33.7% in women) [28]. Nevertheless, the above evidence suggested the high risk of prevalent sarcopenia in nursing-home residents. Institutionalized populations may be more prone to malnutrition [89,90]. A recent cross-sectional study found that malnutrition and physical frailty were highly prevalent among institutionalized older residents and malnutrition was associated with an increased risk of physical frailty among institutionalized Chinese older adults [89]. Hence, nutrition and exercise intervention should be promoted to the institutionalized population to prevent or reverse muscle function for this population.

Multivariable meta-regression indicated that the populations being from different settings was a significant factor contributing to the variation in the pooled prevalence estimates for both genders. Compared with community-dwelling older residents, those who were hospitalized were at 1.69 to 2.10 times the risk of prevalent sarcopenia, and nursing-home residents had 2.50 to 2.73 times the risk. The much higher prevalence rate of sarcopenia in older adults from hospitals and nursing homes was also reported by Papadopoulou and colleagues [18]. However, while Papadopoulou and colleagues reported variation in the pooled prevalence estimates for older adults from different settings, they did not perform meta-regression to quantify it. Our study provided the evidence regarding how much the risk of prevalence increased for older adults who were hospitalized or residing in a nursing home compared with their community-dwelling counterparts. Our findings suggest that hospitalized older adults and those living in nursing homes are particularly vulnerable to this muscle disorder. Therefore, these populations should be prioritized in sarcopenia-screening and early-prevention efforts. Furthermore, intervention studies of sarcopenia targeting hospitalized older adults and those in nursing homes are warranted to inform evidence-based prevention and management efforts such as exercise and/or nutrition interventions for these susceptible groups. Meta-regression did not show significant difference in the prevalence estimate between the community-dwelling and outpatient groups for both genders. However, there were a small number of studies targeting outpatients, which might reduce the statistical power. Future research could further examine the risk of prevalent sarcopenia in this group of older adults.

We found the prevalence estimate in older men varied depending on the method used to assess muscle mass. Specifically, compared with the DXA method, the risk of prevalence was lower (OR: 0.58, 95% CI: 0.35 to 0.98) when using the BIA method. However, no such difference was detected in older women. There is some evidence that the BIA method tends to yield higher estimates of muscle mass, and therefore lower estimates of the prevalence of sarcopenia than the DXA method [91]. Wu and Li [24] synthesized the prevalence estimates from 16 original studies targeting community-dwelling Chinese older adults and obtained similar prevalence estimates irrespective of muscle mass assessments (DXA: 13%, BIA: 12%). However, they did not perform a meta-regression to further examine whether different muscle mass assessments could result in significantly different prevalence estimates after adjusting other covariates. In fact, the measurement of muscle mass remains a challenge in primary care settings; and, while DXA is the standard and more accurate method, BIA is preferred in primary care settings and research because it is more available, easier to use, and less expensive [92]. There are different types of equipment and frequencies of BIA. Based on previous study, BIA with a multifrequency device showed better agreement with the DXA method than that with other devices when assessing appendicular skeletal muscle mass [51]. The updated AWGS consensus in 2019 also recommended the use of multifrequency BIA [93]. However, the "model" of BIA measurement was not always stated explicitly in previous studies. Therefore, in future research, if the BIA method is used to assess muscle mass, the multifrequency type should be used and clearly documented.

Our study also found the risk of prevalent sarcopenia in older Chinese men living outside the mainland, specifically, in Hong Kong and Taiwan, to be nearly half that of their counterparts living on the mainland (OR: 0.47, 95% CI: 0.23 to 0.98). However, this difference was not significant in the case of older Chinese women. Regional variation in the prevalence of sarcopenia among community-dwelling Chinese older adults was also reported in a previous systematic review, with 17% in mainland and 6% in Hong Kong and Taiwan [24]. However, that review did not conduct meta-regression to quantify the regional variation in the prevalence of sarcopenia. Possible explanations for the variation between mainland Chinese and those living outside the mainland might be attributed to the different levels of economic development, different healthcare and dietary regimes, etc. [94]. Future studies could further explore the reasons why the prevalence of sarcopenia among older adults living outside the mainland is lower than for those in mainland China. Furthermore, as mainland China has a huge area with diverse geographic and climate variations, the prevalence of sarcopenia might also vary across different geographic locations. Until now, no study has investigated the epidemiological characteristics of sarcopenia among different geographic areas within China. Therefore, we further divided the area into 4 regions (south and east of mainland, west of mainland, north of mainland, and outside of mainland) and ran the univariable mate-regression. Findings showed that significant difference in the prevalence of sarcopenia was only presented between mainland areas and outside of the mainland; there was no difference among different geographic locations within mainland China in both genders (Supplementary Materials, Table S3). Therefore, we only divided the area into two regions (mainland and outside of the mainland) in the main analysis.

Previous observational studies found that older age was significantly associated with sarcopenia and severe sarcopenia in Chinese older adults [46,50]. However, less than half of included studies reported the gender-specific age (Supplementary Materials, Table S4). Therefore, our main results did not consider the age in the multivariable meta-regression.

Instead, we conducted a supplementary analysis to fit the univariable meta-regression for age (details are presented in Supplementary Materials, Table S5). Findings indicated that the age group of 80 years and over showed a higher prevalence of sarcopenia compared with that of 60 to 70 years, which is consistent with current knowledge that the advanced age is an important risk factor of sarcopenia [50]. Body mass index (BMI) was also reported to be associated with the prevalence of sarcopenia in some literature, with a higher BMI relating to the lower prevalence of sarcopenia [46,50]. In this systematic review, BMI values reported in articles were all above 23 kg/m^2 for both genders (Supplementary Materials, Table S4). We did not include BMI in the meta-regression, considering that the comparison between overweight and obesity might be less meaningful. For other possible factors which might influence the variance of prevalence reported, such as rural-urban regions, comorbidities, and others (e.g., type of dynamometer, protocol of gait speed test), due to limited information reported in the articles, we could not analyze them through meta-regression.

The present study was subject to several limitations. Firstly, a few of the included studies reported the prevalence by different age groups, so we could not pool the prevalence rate by age subgroup. However, age is a well-established factor of sarcopenia. The lower bound of age for participants in the studies included in this review ranged considerably, from 60 to 80 years. Therefore, age may be a significant source of the substantial heterogeneity that we found across studies. Future epidemiological research of sarcopenia is encouraged to report age-specific prevalence. Secondly, due to the small number of studies which reported the prevalence of sarcopenia for outpatients, we were unable to obtain a pooled prevalence rate for this group. Thirdly, we did not include all of the possible covariates in our meta-regression analysis to investigate the source of considerable variations in sarcopenia prevalence. For example, all of the included studies used dynamometers to assess muscle strength, but we had insufficient information to investigate the potential influence of the type of dynamometer used on the prevalence rate. We were likewise unable to analyze the influence of different measurement protocols used for the gait speed tests due to insufficient information. Finally, our results should be interpreted with caution because most of the included studies had a moderate risk of bias and significant heterogeneity.

5. Conclusions

This meta-analysis and meta-regression provides a comprehensive synthesis of sarcopenia prevalence in current literature targeting Chinese older populations not only from communities, but also from clinical settings and nursing homes. This is, to our knowledge, the first study to report pooled prevalence in Chinese older populations from clinical settings and nursing homes, and to examine the impact of populations from different settings, diagnostic criteria, muscle mass assessments, areas and walk distance of gait speed test on the prevalence estimate of sarcopenia via meta-regression analysis. Despite the variations in prevalence estimate across studies, this study revealed a certain proportion of Chinese older adults suffering from sarcopenia, especially for those who were hospitalized and residing in nursing homes. Considering the accelerating pace of aging, efforts should be made to implement early screening and lifestyle interventions such as nutrition and physical activity promotion to prevent this increasingly widespread age-related geriatric syndrome, especially for vulnerable groups.

Supplementary Materials: The following are available online at https://www.mdpi.com/article/10.3390/nu13051441/s1, S1: Search strategy; Table S2 Critical Appraisal of Study Quality; Table S3 Univariable meta-regression for regions; Table S4 Age and BMI reported in studies; Table S5 Univariable meta-regression for age.

Author Contributions: Conceptualization, P.-H.C., Z.C., and M.H.; acquisition of data, Z.C. and W.-Y.L.; formal analysis, Z.C. and P.-H.C.; writing—original draft preparation, Z.C.; writing—review and editing, P.-H.C., M.H., Z.C., and W.-Y.L.; supervision, P.-H.C. All authors have read and agreed to the published version of the manuscript.

Funding: This research received no external funding.

Institutional Review Board Statement: Not applicable.

Informed Consent Statement: Not applicable.

Data Availability Statement: Data sharing not applicable.

Conflicts of Interest: The authors declare no conflict of interest.

References

1. WHO. Ageing and Health. Available online: https://www.who.int/news-room/fact-sheets/detail/ageing-and-health (accessed on 13 May 2020).
2. National Bureau of Statistics. 2019 China Statistical Yearbook. Available online: http://www.stats.gov.cn/tjsj/ndsj/2019/indexeh.htm (accessed on 17 August 2020).
3. Larsson, L.; Degens, H.; Li, M.; Salviati, L.; Lee, Y.I.; Thompson, W.; Kirkland, J.L.; Sandri, M. Sarcopenia: Aging-related loss of muscle mass and function. *Physiol. Rev.* **2019**, *99*, 427–511. [CrossRef] [PubMed]
4. Sakuma, K.; Yamaguchi, A. Sarcopenic obesity and endocrine adaptation with age. *Int. J. Endocrinol.* **2013**, *2013*, 204164. [CrossRef] [PubMed]
5. Santilli, V.; Bernetti, A.; Mangone, M.; Paoloni, M. Clinical definition of sarcopenia. *Clin. Cases Miner. Bone Metab.* **2014**, *11*, 177–180. [CrossRef] [PubMed]
6. Anton, S.D.; Hida, A.; Mankowski, R.; Layne, A.; Solberg, L.M.; Mainous, A.G.; Buford, T. Nutrition and Exercise in Sarcopenia. *Curr. Protein Pept. Sci.* **2018**, *19*, 649–667. [CrossRef]
7. Beckwée, D.; Delaere, A.; Aelbrecht, S.; Baert, V.; Beaudart, C.; Bruyere, O.; de Saint-Hubert, M.; Bautmans, I. Exercise Interventions for the Prevention and Treatment of Sarcopenia. A Systematic Umbrella Review. *J. Nutr. Health Aging* **2019**, *23*, 494–502. [CrossRef]
8. Bloom, I.; Shand, C.; Cooper, C.; Robinson, S.; Baird, J. Diet Quality and Sarcopenia in Older Adults: A Systematic Review. *Nutrients* **2018**, *10*, 308. [CrossRef]
9. Tessier, A.J.; Chevalier, S. An Update on Protein, Leucine, Omega-3 Fatty Acids, and Vitamin D in the Prevention and Treatment of Sarcopenia and Functional Decline. *Nutrients* **2018**, *10*, 1099. [CrossRef]
10. Beaudart, C.; Zaaria, M.; Pasleau, F.; Reginster, J.-Y.; Bruyère, O. Health outcomes of sarcopenia: A systematic review and meta-analysis. *PLoS ONE* **2017**, *12*, e0169548. [CrossRef]
11. Pamoukdjian, F.; Bouillet, T.; Lévy, V.; Soussan, M.; Zelek, L.; Paillaud, E. Prevalence and predictive value of pre-therapeutic sarcopenia in cancer patients: A systematic review. *Clin. Nutr.* **2018**, *37*, 1101–1113. [CrossRef]
12. Chen, L.K.; Liu, L.K.; Woo, J.; Assantachai, P.; Auyeung, T.W.; Bahyah, K.S.; Chou, M.Y.; Chen, L.Y.; Hsu, P.S.; Krairit, O.; et al. Sarcopenia in Asia: Consensus report of the Asian Working Group for Sarcopenia. *J. Am. Med. Dir. Assoc.* **2014**, *15*, 95–101. [CrossRef]
13. Fielding, R.A.; Vellas, B.; Evans, W.J.; Bhasin, S.; Morley, J.E.; Newman, A.B.; Abellan van Kan, G.; Andrieu, S.; Bauer, J.; Breuille, D.; et al. Sarcopenia: An undiagnosed condition in older adults. Current consensus definition: Prevalence, etiology, and consequences. International working group on sarcopenia. *J. Am. Med. Dir. Assoc.* **2011**, *12*, 249–256. [CrossRef]
14. Studenski, S.A.; Peters, K.W.; Alley, D.E.; Cawthon, P.M.; McLean, R.R.; Harris, T.B.; Ferrucci, L.; Guralnik, J.M.; Fragala, M.S.; Kenny, A.M.; et al. The FNIH sarcopenia project: Rationale, study description, conference recommendations, and final estimates. *J. Gerontol. A Biol. Sci. Med. Sci.* **2014**, *69*, 547–558. [CrossRef] [PubMed]
15. Liu, X.; Hou, L.; Xia, X.; Liu, Y.; Zuo, Z.; Zhang, Y.; Zhao, W.; Hao, Q.; Yue, J.; Dong, B. Prevalence of sarcopenia in multi ethnics adults and the association with cognitive impairment: Findings from West-China health and aging trend study. *BMC Geriatr.* **2020**, *20*, 63. [CrossRef]
16. Beaudart, C.; Reginster, J.Y.; Slomian, J.; Buckinx, F.; Dardenne, N.; Quabron, A.; Slangen, C.; Gillain, S.; Petermans, J.; Bruyère, O. Estimation of sarcopenia prevalence using various assessment tools. *Exp. Gerontol.* **2015**, *61*, 31–37. [CrossRef]
17. Bruyère, O.; Beaudart, C.; Reginster, J.Y.; Buckinx, F.; Schoene, D.; Hirani, V.; Cooper, C.; Kanis, J.A.; Rizzoli, R.; McCloskey, E.; et al. Assessment of muscle mass, muscle strength and physical performance in clinical practice: An international survey. *Eur. Geriatr. Med.* **2016**, *7*, 243–246. [CrossRef]
18. Papadopoulou, S.K.; Tsintavis, P.; Potsaki, P.; Papandreou, D. Differences in the Prevalence of Sarcopenia in Community-Dwelling, Nursing Home and Hospitalized Individuals. A Systematic Review and Meta-Analysis. *J. Nutr. Health Aging* **2020**, *24*, 83–90. [CrossRef] [PubMed]
19. Chan, R.; Leung, J.; Woo, J. A prospective cohort study to examine the association between dietary patterns and sarcopenia in Chinese community-dwelling older people in Hong Kong. *J. Am. Med. Dir. Assoc.* **2016**, *17*, 336–342. [CrossRef]
20. Huang, C.Y.; Hwang, A.C.; Liu, L.K.; Lee, W.J.; Chen, L.Y.; Peng, L.N.; Lin, M.H.; Chen, L.K. Association of dynapenia, sarcopenia, and cognitive impairment among community-dwelling older Taiwanese. *Rejuvenation Res.* **2016**, *19*, 71–78. [CrossRef]
21. Chen, X.; Guo, J.; Han, P.; Fu, L.; Jia, L.; Yu, H.; Yu, X.; Hou, L.; Wang, L.; Zhang, W.; et al. Twelve-month incidence of depressive symptoms in suburb-dwelling Chinese older adults: Role of sarcopenia. *J. Am. Med. Dir. Assoc.* **2019**, *20*, 64–69. [CrossRef]

22. Du, Y.; Wang, X.; Xie, H.; Zheng, S.; Wu, X.; Zhu, X.; Zhang, X.; Xue, S.; Li, H.; Hong, W.; et al. Sex differences in the prevalence and adverse outcomes of sarcopenia and sarcopenic obesity in community dwelling elderly in East China using the AWGS criteria. *BMC Endocr. Disord.* **2019**, *19*, 109. [CrossRef] [PubMed]
23. Wang, H.; Hai, S.; Liu, Y.; Cao, L.; Liu, Y.; Liu, P.; Zhou, J.; Yang, Y.; Dong, B. Association between depressive symptoms and sarcopenia in older Chinese community-dwelling individuals. *Clin. Interv. Aging* **2018**, *13*, 1605–1611. [CrossRef]
24. Wu, L.J.; Li, J.X. Prevalence of sarcopenia in the community-dwelling elder people in China: A systematic review and meta-analysis. *Modern Prev. Med.* **2019**, *46*, 18. (In Chinese)
25. Tian, S.; Xu, Y.; Han, F. Prevalence of sarcopenia in the community-dwelling, elderly Chinese population: A systematic review and meta-analysis. *Lancet* **2017**, *390*, S35. [CrossRef]
26. Moher, D.; Liberati, A.; Tetzlaff, J.; Altman, D.G. Preferred reporting items for systematic reviews and meta-analyses: The PRISMA statement. *PLoS Med.* **2009**, *6*, e1000097. [CrossRef]
27. Hoy, D.; Brooks, P.; Woolf, A.; Blyth, F.; March, L.; Bain, C.; Baker, P.; Smith, E.; Buchbinder, R. Assessing risk of bias in prevalence studies: Modification of an existing tool and evidence of interrater agreement. *J. Clin. Epidemiol.* **2012**, *65*, 934–939. [CrossRef] [PubMed]
28. Shen, Y.; Chen, J.; Chen, X.; Hou, L.; Lin, X.; Yang, M. Prevalence and Associated Factors of Sarcopenia in Nursing Home Residents: A Systematic Review and Meta-analysis. *J. Am. Med. Dir. Assoc.* **2019**, *20*, 5–13. [CrossRef] [PubMed]
29. Mogire, R.M.; Mutua, A.; Kimita, W.; Kamau, A.; Bejon, P.; Pettifor, J.M.; Adeyemo, A.; Williams, T.N.; Atkinson, S.H. Prevalence of vitamin D deficiency in Africa: A systematic review and meta-analysis. *Lancet Glob. Health* **2020**, *8*, e134–e142. [CrossRef]
30. Higgins, J.; Thomas, J.; Chandler, J.; Cumpston, M.; Li, T.; Page, M.; Welch, V. *Cochrane Handbook for Systematic Reviews of Interventions*, 2nd ed.; John Wiley & Sons: Chichester, UK, 2019.
31. StataCorp. *Stata Statistical Software: Release 15*; StataCorp LP: College Station, TX, USA, 2017.
32. Nyaga, V.N.; Arbyn, M.; Aerts, M. Metaprop: A Stata command to perform meta-analysis of binomial data. *Arch. Public Health* **2014**, *72*, 39. [CrossRef]
33. Higgins, J.P.; Thompson, S.G.; Deeks, J.J.; Altman, D.G. Measuring inconsistency in meta-analyses. *BMJ* **2003**, *327*, 557–560. [CrossRef]
34. Easterbrook, P.J.; Berlin, J.A.; Gopalan, R.; Matthews, D.R. Publication bias in clinical research. *Lancet* **1991**, *337*, 867–872. [CrossRef]
35. Meng, N.H.; Li, C.I.; Liu, C.S.; Lin, C.H.; Lin, W.Y.; Chang, C.K.; Li, T.C.; Lin, C.C. Comparison of height- and weight-adjusted sarcopenia in a Taiwanese metropolitan older population. *Geriatr. Gerontol. Int.* **2015**, *15*, 45–53. [CrossRef]
36. Wen, X.; An, P.; Chen, W.C.; Lv, Y.; Fu, Q. Comparisions of sarcopenia prevalence based on different diagnostic criteria in Chinese older adults. *J. Nutr. Health Aging* **2015**, *19*, 342–347. [CrossRef]
37. Xia, Z.W.; Meng, L.C.; Man, Q.Q.; Li, L.X.; Song, P.K.; Li, Y.Q.; Gao, Y.X.; Jia, S.S.; Zhang, J. Analysis of the dietary factors on sarcopenia in elderly in Beijing. *J. Hyg. Res.* **2016**, *45*, 388–393. (In Chinese) [CrossRef]
38. Zhang, Y.; Tan, Y.T.; Huang, X.X.; Zhang, Z.H.; Bai, J.J.; Zhang, M.; Huang, Y.Q.; Chen, J.; Wang, J.F.; Bao, Z.J. Prevalence of Sarcopenia and the Associated Risk Factors in Community Elderly in Shanghai. *Geriatr. Health Care* **2018**, *24*, 608–613. (In Chinese)
39. Liu, J.L.; Cai, Y.Y. Investigation of prevalence among community-dwelling older adults in Shanghai. *China Health Vis.* **2016**, 248–249. (In Chinese) [CrossRef]
40. Xu, H.Q.; Shi, J.P.; Shen, C.; Liu, Y.; Liu, J.M.; Zheng, X.Y. Sarcopenia-related features and factors associated with low muscle mass, weak muscle strength, and reduced function in Chinese rural residents: A cross-sectional study. *Arch. Osteoporos.* **2018**, *14*, 2. [CrossRef]
41. Wang, Z.T. Correlation Analysis of Coronary Heart Disease and Sarcopenia in Elderly Inpatients. Master's Thesis, Southern Medical University, Guangzhou, China, 2019.
42. Fung, F.Y.; Koh, Y.L.E.; Malhotra, R.; Ostbye, T.; Lee, P.Y.; Shariff Ghazali, S.; Tan, N.C. Prevalence of and factors associated with sarcopenia among multi-ethnic ambulatory older Asians with type 2 diabetes mellitus in a primary care setting. *BMC Geriatr.* **2019**, *19*, 1–10. [CrossRef]
43. Wu, Z.L.; Wang, Y.B.; Su, F.Q.; Song, B.; Li, G.; Zhu, H.M. Epidemiological investigation of sarcopenia in the nursing homes in Fengxian District and analysis of their risk factors. *Shanghai Med. Pharm. J.* **2017**, *38*, 37–40. (In Chinese)
44. Yang, L.J. Research on Sarcopenia and Its Relative factors in Elderly Population in Suzhou. Master's Thesis, Nanjing Medical University, Suzhou, China, 2018.
45. Meng, P.; Hu, Y.X.; Fan, L.; Zhang, Y.; Zhang, M.X.; Sun, J.; Liu, Y.; Li, M.; Yang, Y.; Wang, L.H.; et al. Sarcopenia and sarcopenic obesity among men aged 80 years and older in Beijing: Prevalence and its association with functional performance. *Geriatr. Gerontol. Int.* **2014**, *14* (Suppl. 1), 29–35. [CrossRef]
46. Wu, C.H.; Chen, K.T.; Hou, M.T.; Chang, Y.F.; Chang, C.S.; Liu, P.Y.; Wu, S.J.; Chiu, C.J.; Jou, I.M.; Chen, C.Y. Prevalence and associated factors of sarcopenia and severe sarcopenia in older Taiwanese living in rural community: The Tianliao Old People study 04. *Geriatr. Gerontol. Int.* **2014**, *14* (Suppl. 1), 69–75. [CrossRef]
47. Zhang, Y.; Hu, Y.X.; Fan, L.; Zhang, M.X.; Sun, J.; Han, X.Q.; Ma, X.N.; Dong, H.Y.; Li, M. Relationship between site-specific loss of bodr skeletal muscle mass and gait performance in very old men in Beijing. *Chin. J. Health Care Med.* **2014**, *16*, 421–425. (In Chinese) [CrossRef]

48. Wang, Y.J.; Wang, Y.; Zhan, J.K.; Tang, Z.Y.; He, J.Y.; Tan, P.; Deng, H.Q.; Huang, W.; Liu, Y.S. Sarco-Osteoporosis: Prevalence and Association with Frailty in Chinese Community-Dwelling Older Adults. *Int. J. Endocrinol.* **2015**, *2015*, 482940. [CrossRef]
49. Han, D.S.; Chang, K.V.; Li, C.M.; Lin, Y.H.; Kao, T.W.; Tsai, K.S.; Wang, T.G.; Yang, W.S. Skeletal muscle mass adjusted by height correlated better with muscular functions than that adjusted by body weight in defining sarcopenia. *Sci. Rep.* **2016**, *6*, 19457. [CrossRef]
50. Han, P.; Kang, L.; Guo, Q.; Wang, J.; Zhang, W.; Shen, S.; Wang, X.; Dong, R.; Ma, Y.; Shi, Y.; et al. Prevalence and Factors Associated With Sarcopenia in Suburb-dwelling Older Chinese Using the Asian Working Group for Sarcopenia Definition. *J. Gerontol. Ser. A Biol. Sci. Med. Sci.* **2016**, *71*, 529–535. [CrossRef] [PubMed]
51. Wang, H.; Hai, S.; Cao, L.; Zhou, J.; Liu, P.; Dong, B.R. Estimation of prevalence of sarcopenia by using a new bioelectrical impedance analysis in Chinese community-dwelling elderly people. *BMC Geriatr.* **2016**, *16*, 216. [CrossRef]
52. Wang, T.; Feng, X.; Zhou, J.; Gong, H.; Xia, S.; Wei, Q.; Hu, X.; Tao, R.; Li, L.; Qian, F.; et al. Type 2 diabetes mellitus is associated with increased risks of sarcopenia and pre-sarcopenia in Chinese elderly. *Sci. Rep.* **2016**, *6*, 38937. [CrossRef]
53. Fang, Y.; Pan, L.; Chen, L.; Chen, J.Y.; Peng, Y.D.; Gu, W.S.; You, L. Sarcopenia screening for older women with low body-weight and low handgrip strength is more urgently. *Chin. J. Endocrinol. Metab.* **2017**, *33*, 1043–1046. (In Chinese)
54. Hai, S.; Cao, L.; Wang, H.; Zhou, J.; Liu, P.; Yang, Y.; Hao, Q.; Dong, B. Association between sarcopenia and nutritional status and physical activity among community-dwelling Chinese adults aged 60 years and older. *Geriatr. Gerontol. Int.* **2017**, *17*, 1959–1966. [CrossRef]
55. Hua, C.; Chen, G.L.; Wen, X.L.; Liu, C.; Zhang, J. HMB intervention of muscle loss in community-dwelling elders with malnutrition. *Electron. J. Metab. Nutr. Cancer* **2017**, *4*, 72–77. (In Chinese) [CrossRef]
56. Meng, L.; Shi, J.; Zou, C.S.; Tan, X.; Zhou, B.Y.; Duan, C.B.; Shi, H.; Xi, H. Correlation of frailty severity with muscle mass and physical function in Chinese older adults:preliminary findings. *Chin. J. Geriatr.* **2017**, *36*, 1313–1317. (In Chinese) [CrossRef]
57. Chu, X.J. Osteopenia and Sarcopenia in Chinese Elderly. Master's Thesis, Jiangsu University, Suzhou, China, 2018.
58. Yang, M.; Hu, X.; Xie, L.; Zhang, L.; Zhou, J.; Lin, J.; Wang, Y.; Li, Y.; Han, Z.; Zhang, D.; et al. Validation of the Chinese version of the Mini Sarcopenia Risk Assessment questionnaire in community-dwelling older adults. *Medicine* **2018**, *97*, e12426. [CrossRef]
59. Liu, L.L. Prevalence and Risk Factors of Sarcopenia in Meddle-Aged and Elderly Population in Urban Area of Chongqing, China. Master's Thesis, Chongqing Medical University, Chongqing, China, 2019.
60. Wang, H.; Hai, S.; Liu, Y.X.; Cao, L.; Liu, Y.; Liu, P.; Yang, Y.; Dong, B.R. Associations between Sarcopenic Obesity and Cognitive Impairment in Elderly Chinese Community-Dwelling Individuals. *J. Nutr. Health Aging* **2019**, *23*, 14–20. [CrossRef]
61. Zhang, L.; Guo, Q.; Feng, B.L.; Wang, C.Y.; Han, P.P.; Hu, J.; Sun, X.D.; Zeng, W.F.; Zheng, Z.X.; Li, H.S.; et al. A Cross-Sectional Study of the Association between Arterial Stiffness and Sarcopenia in Chinese Community-Dwelling Elderly Using the Asian Working Group for Sarcopenia Criteria. *J. Nutr. Health Aging* **2019**, *23*, 195–201. [CrossRef]
62. Rong, Y.D.; Bian, A.L.; Hu, H.Y.; Ma, Y.; Zhou, X.Z. A cross-sectional study of the relationships between different components of sarcopenia and brachial ankle pulse wave velocity in community-dwelling elderly. *BMC Geriatr.* **2020**, *20*, 115. [CrossRef] [PubMed]
63. Xu, W.; Chen, T.; Cai, Y.; Hu, Y.; Fan, L.; Wu, C. Sarcopenia in Community-Dwelling Oldest Old Is Associated with Disability and Poor Physical Function. *J. Nutr. Health Aging* **2020**, *24*, 339–345. [CrossRef]
64. Yang, L.; Yao, X.; Shen, J.; Sun, G.; Sun, Q.; Tian, X.; Li, X.; Li, X.; Ye, L.; Zhang, Z.; et al. Comparison of revised EWGSOP criteria and four other diagnostic criteria of sarcopenia in Chinese community-dwelling elderly residents. *Exp. Gerontol.* **2020**, *130*, 110798. [CrossRef] [PubMed]
65. Cui, M.Z. Clinical Characteristics of Sarcopenia among Patients with Type2 Diabetes. Master's Thesis, Jilin University, Changchun, China, 2018.
66. Zhai, Y.; Xiao, Q.; Miao, J. The Relationship between NAFLD and Sarcopenia in Elderly Patients. *Can. J. Gastroenterol. Hepatol.* **2018**, *2018*, 5016091. [CrossRef]
67. Chen, Q.; Hao, Q.; Ding, Y.; Dong, B. The Association between Sarcopenia and Prealbumin Levels among Elderly Chinese Inpatients. *J. Nutr. Health Aging* **2019**, *23*, 122–127. [CrossRef]
68. Yao, S.H. Prevalence of Sarcopenia and Osteoporosis and Analysis of Their Risk Factors and Correlation in Elderly Hospitalized Patients. Master's Thesis, Jishou University, Jishou, China, 2019.
69. Yi, H.W.; Li, W.L.; Yu, Y.L.; Ma, D.B. The relative factors analysis of malnutrition status and sarcopenia in elderly patients. *Electron. J. Metab. Nutr. Cancer* **2019**, *6*. (In Chinese) [CrossRef]
70. Tan, Z.Q. Study on the Influencing Factors of Sarcopenia in Elderly Patients with HFpEF, HFmrEF, and HFrEF. Master's Thesis, Chengdu Medical College, Chengdu, China, 2019.
71. Zhang, N.; Zhu, W.L.; Liu, X.H.; Chen, W.; Zhu, M.L.; Kang, L.; Tian, R. Prevalence and prognostic implications of sarcopenia in older patients with coronary heart disease. *J. Geriatr. Cardiol.* **2019**, *16*, 756–763. [CrossRef] [PubMed]
72. Cui, M.; Gang, X.; Wang, G.; Xiao, X.; Li, Z.; Jiang, Z.; Wang, G. A cross-sectional study: Associations between sarcopenia and clinical characteristics of patients with type 2 diabetes. *Medicine* **2020**, *99*, e18708. [CrossRef]
73. Wang, L.; Wei, Y.L.; Liu, J.; Wang, J.T. Related factors for sarcopenia in elderly hospitalized patients with chronic diseases. *Chin. General. Practic.* **2020**, *23*, 611–616. (In Chinese) [CrossRef]

74. Li, M.; Hu, Y.X.; Dong, H.Y.; Zhang, Y.; Fan, L.; Zhang, M.X.; Sun, J.; Han, X.Q.; Liu, Y.X.; Ma, X.N. Compare different measurement for prevalence of sarcopenia in a cohort of healthy community-dwelling older men in Beijing area. *Chin. J. Health Care Med.* **2014**, *16*, 426–429. (In Chinese) [CrossRef]
75. Wang, R.; Hu, Y.X.; Fan, L.; Cui, H.; Gao, L.G.; Zhang, Y.; Gao, D.W.; Cao, J.; Gong, W.Q. Effect of sarcopenia on the rate of rehospitalization in elderly male patients. *Chin. J. Health Care Med.* **2016**, *18*, 106–109. (In Chinese) [CrossRef]
76. Wang, Y.N.; Song, H.L.; Gu, Y.H.; Xu, J.L. Influencing factors of sarcopenia among older adults with type2 diabetes. *Prev. Med.* **2019**, *31*, 582–585. (In Chinese) [CrossRef]
77. Hsu, Y.H.; Liang, C.K.; Chou, M.Y.; Liao, M.C.; Lin, Y.T.; Chen, L.K.; Lo, Y.K. Association of cognitive impairment, depressive symptoms and sarcopenia among healthy older men in the veterans retirement community in southern Taiwan: A cross-sectional study. *Geriatr. Gerontol. Int.* **2014**, *14* (Suppl. 1), 102–108. [CrossRef]
78. Liao, S.W. Prevalence and Risk Factors of Sarcopenia among Older Adults Living in Nursing Homes in Chongqing. Master's Thesis, Chongqing Medical University, Chongqing, China, 2018.
79. Zeng, Y.; Hu, X.; Xie, L.; Han, Z.; Zuo, Y.; Yang, M. The Prevalence of Sarcopenia in Chinese Elderly Nursing Home Residents: A Comparison of 4 Diagnostic Criteria. *J. Am. Med. Dir. Assoc.* **2018**, *19*, 690–695. [CrossRef] [PubMed]
80. Yang, L.J.; Wu, G.H.; Yang, Y.L.; Wu, Y.H.; Zhang, L.; Wang, M.H.; Mo, L.Y.; Xue, G.; Wang, C.Z.; Weng, X.F. Nutrition, Physical Exercise, and the Prevalence of Sarcopenia in Elderly Residents in Nursing Homes in China. *Med. Sci. Monit.* **2019**, *25*, 4390–4399. [CrossRef]
81. Chen, J.M. The Associated Factors of Traditional Chinese Medicine Syndromes in Older Adults with Sarcopenia. Master's Thesis, Beijing University of Chinese Medicine, Beijing, China, 2018.
82. Feng, X. The Occurrence of Sarcopenia and Related Factors Analysis in Elderly Patients with Type 2 Diabetes Mellitus. Master's Thesis, Jiangsu Univeristy, Suzhou, China, 2016.
83. Ma, Y. The Occurence and Associated Factors of Sarcopenic Obesity in Older Adults. Master's Thesis, Tianjin University of Traditional Chinese Medicine, Tianjin, China, 2017.
84. Zhou, X.L.; Wang, S.; Xu, T.Y. Correlation between chronic atrophic gastritis and sarcopenia in elderly population. *Med. J. Natl. Defending Forces Southwest China* **2018**, *28*, 329–331. [CrossRef]
85. Zhang, T.; Gu, Y.H. Effect of abdominal obesity on sarcopenia and osteoporosis in elderly people with normal body mass index. *Chin. J. Clin. Med.* **2019**, *26*, 754–758. [CrossRef]
86. Yang, P.P. Investigation on the Current Status of Sarcopenia in Middle-Aged and Elderly Patients with T2DM. Master's Thesis, Nanchang University, Nanchang, China, 2019.
87. Beaudart, C.; Reginster, J.Y.; Slomian, J.; Buckinx, F.; Locquet, M.; Bruyère, O. Prevalence of sarcopenia: The impact of different diagnostic cut-off limits. *J. Musculoskelet. Neuronal. Interact.* **2014**, *14*, 425–431. [CrossRef]
88. Von Hippel, P.T. The heterogeneity statistic I(2) can be biased in small meta-analyses. *BMC Med. Res. Methodol.* **2015**, *15*, 35. [CrossRef]
89. Liu, W.; Chen, S.; Jiang, F.; Zhou, C.; Tang, S. Malnutrition and Physical Frailty among Nursing Home Residents: A Cross-Sectional Study in China. *J. Nutr. Health Aging* **2020**, *24*, 500–506. [CrossRef]
90. Pigłowska, M.; Guligowska, A.; Kostka, T. Nutritional Status Plays More Important Role in Determining Functional State in Older People Living in the Community than in Nursing Home Residents. *Nutrients* **2020**, *12*, 2042. [CrossRef]
91. Janssen, I.; Heymsfield, S.B.; Baumgartner, R.N.; Ross, R. Estimation of skeletal muscle mass by bioelectrical impedance analysis. *J. Appl. Physiol.* **2000**, *89*, 465–471. [CrossRef]
92. Yilmaz, O.; Bahat, G. Suggestions for assessment of muscle mass in primary care setting. *Aging Male* **2017**, *20*, 168–169. [CrossRef]
93. Chen, L.K.; Woo, J.; Assantachai, P.; Auyeung, T.W.; Chou, M.Y.; Iijima, K.; Jang, H.C.; Kang, L.; Kim, M.; Kim, S.; et al. Asian Working Group for Sarcopenia: 2019 Consensus Update on Sarcopenia Diagnosis and Treatment. *J. Am. Med. Dir. Assoc.* **2020**, *21*, 300–307.e2. [CrossRef]
94. Tyrovolas, S.; Koyanagi, A.; Olaya, B.; Ayuso-Mateos, J.L.; Miret, M.; Chatterji, S.; Tobiasz-Adamczyk, B.; Koskinen, S.; Leonardi, M.; Haro, J.M. Factors associated with skeletal muscle mass, sarcopenia, and sarcopenic obesity in older adults: A multi-continent study. *J. Cachexia Sarcopenia Muscle* **2016**, *7*, 312–321. [CrossRef]

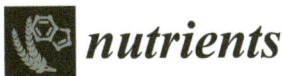

Article

Dairy Product Intake and Long-Term Risk for Frailty among French Elderly Community Dwellers

Berna Rahi [1,†], Hermine Pellay [2,3,†], Virginie Chuy [2,4], Catherine Helmer [2], Cecilia Samieri [2] and Catherine Féart [2,*]

1. Department of Natural Sciences, School of Arts and Sciences, Lebanese American University, Byblos 36, Lebanon; berna.rahi@gmail.com
2. Institut National de la Santé et de la Recherche Médicale (INSERM), University Bordeaux, INSERM, BPH, U1219, F-33000 Bordeaux, France; hermine.pellay@u-bordeaux.fr (H.P.); virginie.chuy@u-bordeaux.fr (V.C.); catherine.helmer@u-bordeaux.fr (C.H.); cecilia.samieri@u-bordeaux.fr (C.S.)
3. CNIEL, Service Recherche Nutrition-Santé, F-75009 Paris, France
4. Department of Dentistry and Oral Health, CHU Bordeaux, University Bordeaux, F-33000 Bordeaux, France
* Correspondence: catherine.feart-couret@u-bordeaux.fr
† These authors have equally contributed to this work.

Abstract: Dairy products (DP) are part of a food group that may contribute to the prevention of physical frailty. We aimed to investigate DP exposure, including total DP, milk, fresh DP and cheese, and their cross-sectional and prospective associations with physical frailty in community-dwelling older adults. The cross-sectional analysis was carried out on 1490 participants from the Three-City Bordeaux cohort. The 10-year frailty risk was examined in 823 initially non-frail participants. A food frequency questionnaire was used to assess DP exposure. Physical frailty was defined as the presence of at least 3 out of 5 criteria of the frailty phenotype: weight loss, exhaustion, slowness, weakness, and low physical activity. Among others, diet quality and protein intake were considered as confounders. The baseline mean age of participants was 74.1 y and 61% were females. Frailty prevalence and incidence were 4.2% and 18.2%, respectively. No significant associations were observed between consumption of total DP or DP sub-types and frailty prevalence or incidence (OR = 1.40, 95%CI 0.65–3.01 and OR = 1.75, 95%CI 0.42–1.32, for a total DP consumption >4 times/d, respectively). Despite the absence of beneficial associations of higher DP consumption on frailty, older adults are encouraged to follow the national recommendations regarding DP.

Keywords: dairy products; frailty; older adults; cohort study

Citation: Rahi, B.; Pellay, H.; Chuy, V.; Helmer, C.; Samieri, C.; Féart, C. Dairy Product Intake and Long-Term Risk for Frailty among French Elderly Community Dwellers. *Nutrients* **2021**, *13*, 2151. https://doi.org/10.3390/nu13072151

Academic Editor: Emmanuel Biver

Received: 5 May 2021
Accepted: 21 June 2021
Published: 23 June 2021

Publisher's Note: MDPI stays neutral with regard to jurisdictional claims in published maps and institutional affiliations.

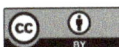

Copyright: © 2021 by the authors. Licensee MDPI, Basel, Switzerland. This article is an open access article distributed under the terms and conditions of the Creative Commons Attribution (CC BY) license (https://creativecommons.org/licenses/by/4.0/).

1. Introduction

In recent years, the world has been experiencing a steady increase in the aging population. It is expected that by 2050, one in six people will be over the age of 65, including one in four in Europe and northern America [1]. This increased life expectancy is associated with a higher risk of morbidities. In fact, nearly a quarter (23%) of the overall global burden of death and illness is in people aged over 60, and much of this burden is attributable to long-term illnesses [2]. Advancing age is indeed accompanied by common geriatric syndromes, such as frailty [3]. Frailty is characterized by a depletion in the functional reserves of physiological systems, which limits the possibility to adapt to changes in the environment over time, leading to falls, hospitalization, disability, and death [4]. Nevertheless, frailty can be prevented, and diet appears to be a major determinant of its development [5,6]. Several studies have reported that particular macronutrients [7,8], food groups [9–11] and dietary patterns are associated with frailty [12–17]. Particularly, our group has previously reported the relevance of protein intake (>1 g/d being associated with a lower prevalence of frailty) [18], of fruit and vegetable intake (>5 servings/d being associated with a lower risk of frailty) [9], and of the Mediterranean diet (a higher adherence being associated with a lower frailty risk) [17]. In line with our findings, several other longitudinal studies have showed that a higher protein intake is protective against frailty [19–21].

Dietary sources of protein include dairy products (DP), which are also important sources of calcium and vitamin D. Interestingly, recent studies have showed that higher DP consumption was associated with better age-related health outcomes, and particularly lower risks of type 2 diabetes [22,23], cardiovascular diseases and mortality [24,25]. The type of DP (i.e., milk, fresh DP and cheese) appears to be key component of such associations. In fact, a meta-analysis on 938,415 participants and 93,518 mortality cases reported an absence of association between total dairy (high- or low-fat) and milk with the risk of death, while total fermented dairy (including sour milk products, yogurt or cheese; +20 g/day) were associated with a significant 2% reduced risk of all-cause mortality and cardiovascular diseases [26]. While two systematic reviews also observed that higher DP intakes were associated with higher appendicular muscle mass, improved balance-test scores, and an attenuation of the loss of muscle strength [27,28], the direct potential benefit of DP on frailty as a whole has scarcely been studied. To the best of our knowledge, a single prospective study implemented in the Spanish Seniors-ENRICA cohort [29] reported that consuming seven or more servings per week of low-fat milk was associated with a significantly lower risk of frailty compared with consuming less than one serving per week. The external validity of such results remains uncertain. Indeed, the SHARE database demonstrated significant heterogeneity in DP consumption across Europe, with higher levels in central and northern countries and in Spain, and the lowest prevalence of dairy intake in eastern European countries [30]. Of note, high cheese consumption is a hallmark of French dietary habits, and France is also characterized by low milk consumption. Finally, several socio-demographic, nutritional characteristics and lifestyle factors have been associated with the French DP consumption, with specificities according to each DP sub-type [31]. Altogether, it is conceivable that the featured consumption of DP sub-types among French older adults could be differentially associated with frailty.

Therefore, our objective was to assess the cross-sectional and prospective associations between total DP and DP sub-types (milk, fresh DP and cheese) consumption and the 10-year frailty risk among older adults of the Three-City (3C) Bordeaux cohort.

2. Methods

2.1. Study Overview

The 3C-study is a French population-based prospective study initiated in 1999–2000 to study the vascular risk factors of dementia [32]. Its protocol was approved by the Consultative Committee for the Protection of Persons participating in Biomedical Research at Kremlin-Bicêtre and all participants gave written informed consent. Participants were randomly sampled from electoral rolls from three French cities (Bordeaux, Dijon, and Montpellier). Eligible participants had to be 65 years and older at the time of recruitment and not institutionalized. Among the 9294 participants included at baseline, 2104 were from the Bordeaux center, which completed the initial data collection in 2001–2002 (wave 1). A comprehensive dietary survey of 1597 participants was also performed. This dietary survey served as the baseline for the present study, where DP frequency of consumption and frailty were assessed.

2.2. Assessment of Dairy Products

Dietary data were obtained from a semi-quantitative Food Frequency Questionnaire (FFQ) administered during face-to-face interviews by dietitians. This allowed the assessment of the daily frequency of consumption of 148 foods and beverages (with frequencies assessed in 11 classes, from "never or less than once a month" to "7 times per week") during each of the six meals/snacks of the day, as previously detailed [33]. Data from the FFQ was validated against a 24-h dietary recall in an independent subsample of the 3C-study [34]. DP consumption was considered using the frequency of consumption of milk, fresh DP, and cheese. The milk consumption variable included the consumption of "milk", "coffee with milk", "tea with milk", "chocolate", "chicory", and "natural milk or with cereal". Consumption of "yogurt and cottage cheese" was classified as fresh DP while frequency of consumption of "cheese" was considered as the cheese category. As already described by Pellay et al. (2020), we considered the DPs' frequency of consumption as four main exposures, including total DP, milk, fresh DP, and cheese [31]. For each DP component, three categories were created based on the quartile distribution of consumption (low frequency: first quartile; intermediate frequency: quartiles 2 and 3; high frequency: fourth quartile). This classification ensured the differentiation between the most infrequent and frequent consumers, as previously described [31].

2.3. Assessment of Frailty

At baseline and at the 10-year follow-up, frailty was defined following the Cardiovascular Health Study frailty index [4], the tool recommended by the International Conference of Frailty and Sarcopenia Research [35]. Nevertheless, minor modifications were made to adapt this tool to the available data in our cohort study, as already published [17,18]. Briefly, (1) weight loss was defined as self-reported unintentional loss of 3 kg or more or, if missing, as a body mass index (BMI) <21 kg/m^2; (2) exhaustion was evaluated using the following statements from the Center for Epidemiologic Studies-Depression scale (CES-D): "I felt that everything I did was an effort" and "I could not get going". Participants were considered frail for this criterion when they answered "a moderate amount of the time" or "most of the time" to either of these statements [36]; (3) walking speed was determined based on a 6-m walking test, adjusting for height and gender. Participants in the highest quintile were considered slow. When this information was missing, participants were considered frail for this criterion when they reported being unable to walk between 500 m and 1 km or to walk up and down a flight of stairs based on the Rosow–Breslau scale [37]. This proxy has been shown to be strongly associated with walking [38]; (4) weakness was identified in different ways at baseline and at the 10-year follow-up, depending on availability of data. At the 10-year follow-up, weakness was identified using the handgrip strength quartiles stratified by sex and BMI, as recommended [4]. At baseline, weakness was identified using the chair standing method, shown to be a good proxy for handgrip strength [39]; (5) physical activity was assessed in a face-to-face interview via an open-ended questionnaire. Low physical activity was defined as less than 1 h of sports activities or less than 3.5 h of leisure activities per week, as previously described [17,18].

Older adults with three or more criteria out of five were considered as frail, otherwise they were considered as non-frail. Prevalent frail participants at baseline were excluded for the prospective analyses.

The FRAIL scale was also used to define frailty in sensitivity analyses [40]. The FRAIL scale includes five self-reported components: Fatigue, Resistance, Ambulation, Illnesses and Loss of weight. Fatigue and weight loss were evaluated similarly to those of the frailty index. Resistance and Ambulation were evaluated using the Rosow–Breslau scale, as recommended. Resistance was assessed by asking participants if they could walk up and down a flight of stairs and Ambulation by asking if they could walk between 500 m and 1 km; "no" responses were each scored as 1 point. Lastly, Illnesses was scored 1 for respondents who reported 5 or more chronic conditions out of 13 including hypertension, diabetes, hypercholesterolemia, cardio- and cerebro-vascular diseases (myocardial infarction or cardiac and vascular surgery, or arteritis or stroke), Parkinson's disease, cognitive decline and dyspnea. Cancer was considered when reports were available, i.e., at the 10-year follow-up. The FRAIL score ranged from 0–5, with those scoring three or more considered as frail and those scoring two or less as non-frail.

2.4. Assessment of Disability

Dependency in basic Activities of Daily Living (ADLs) was assessed using the five following items of the Katz scale: bathing, dressing, toileting, transferring from bed to chair, and eating [41]. An individual was considered dependent if they could not perform at least one activity without a given level of assistance, as defined in the original instrument. All identified dependent participants at baseline and at 10-year follow-up were excluded from the analyses because frailty is considered as risk factor for dependency [35].

2.5. Covariates

The covariates included age, sex, marital status, education, smoking status, polypharmacy (dichotomous variable with 6 medications/d as a cut-off), multimorbidity (dichotomous variable with 2 chronic diseases or more as a cut-off point), and global cognitive performances using the Mini-Mental State Examination (MMSE) [42] (0–30 points; higher scores indicate better cognitive status). A diet quality score was also computed. This score included seven components: pulses, raw fruits, raw vegetables, cooked fruits and vegetables, fish, alcohol and olive oil. Each component was dichotomized into meeting the current dietary recommendations versus not. The total score of 7 was also dichotomized into having a good diet quality (score > 3) versus not (score $\leq$ 3). Finally, total protein intake was evaluated from a single 24-h dietary recall that was administered at home in addition to the FFQ [43].

2.6. Statistical Analysis

Baseline demographic, clinical and dietary characteristics were compared between prevalent frail and non-frail (i.e., sample used in the cross-sectional analysis) and incident frail and non-frail (i.e., sample used in the longitudinal analysis) older adults using the student's *t*-test or chi-square test, depending on the type of the variables.

Logistic regression models were used to estimate odds ratio (OR) and 95% confidence intervals (95% CI) for the association between consumption of total DP or DP sub-type (milk, fresh DP, or cheese) and frailty, both cross-sectionally and prospectively. For each DP exposure, intermediate frequency consumption (quartiles 2 and 3) and high frequency consumption (quartile 4) were compared to the reference category of low frequency consumption (quartile 1).

Model 1 was adjusted for age, sex, education and marital status. Model 2 was additionally adjusted for smoking status, multimorbidity, polypharmacy, diet quality score, total protein intake and global cognitive performances. Finally, two sets of sensitivity analyses were performed. First, we assessed frailty using the FRAIL scale and the same multivariate models were applied, except excluding multimorbidity as a covariate from model 2 as this variable is a component of the FRAIL scale. Second, we retained all ADL dependent individuals as we assumed that those who are ADL dependent might already be frail, both in the cross-sectional analysis and the prospective one. All statistical analyses were performed with the SAS Statistical package (Version 9.4 SAS Institute) and statistical significance was set at $p < 0.05$.

3. Results

3.1. Sample Characteristics

Among 1597 participants who answered the dietary survey at baseline, 107 were excluded from all analyses for the following reasons: 20 were ADL dependent at baseline, 67 could not be classified for frailty, 9 had missing information about DP consumption and 11 participants had missing information for covariates. Therefore, the final sample for the cross-sectional analysis comprised 1490 participants (including 1427 non-frail). Among those participants, 979 (69%) were followed up at 10 years (during the follow-up, 355 participants died). An additional 156 participants were excluded from longitudinal analyses ($n = 79$ participants were identified as dependent and $n = 77$ with missing frailty status at 10 years). Thus, 823 participants were prospectively analyzed (Figure 1).

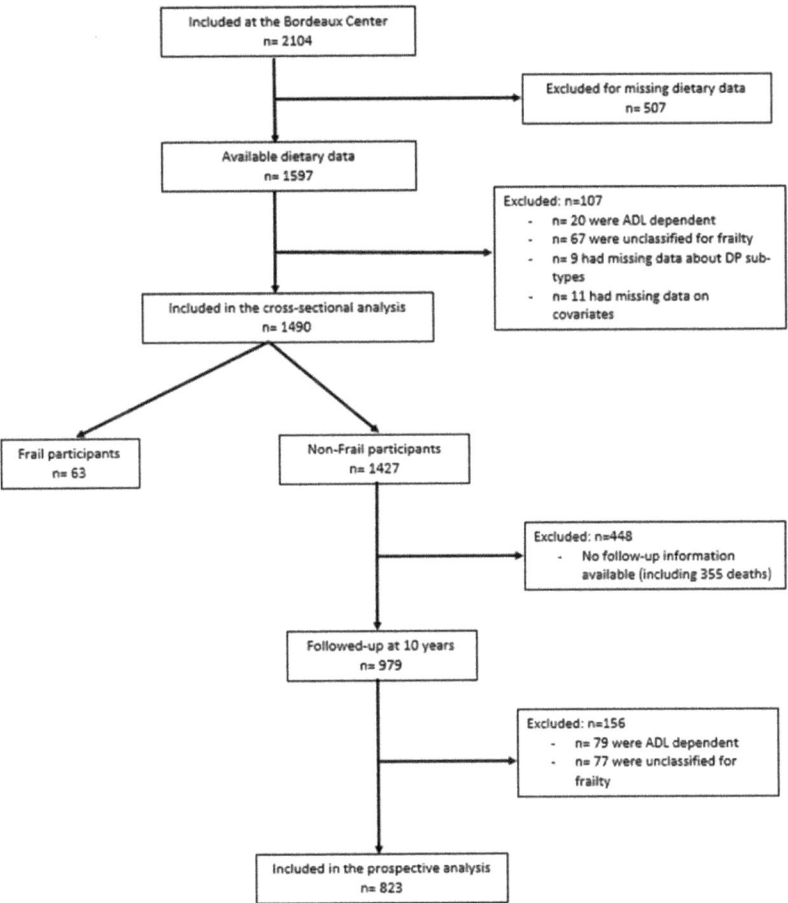

Figure 1. Flow chart of the cross-sectional and the prospective studied samples. Three-City Bordeaux Study, 2000–2010.

In cross-sectional analyses, the studied sample (n = 1490) constituted mainly of females (n = 906, 60.8%) and had an average age of 74.1 ± 4.9 (standard deviation) years (Table 1). Half the sample was married (57%) and reported multimorbidity (48%), and a third (32%) was taking 6 medications/d or more. Prevalence of frailty was 4.2% (n = 63). The most prevalent frailty criterion was low physical activity (n = 234, 20.1%) followed by slow walking speed (n = 281, 19%) while the least prevalent frailty criterion was muscle weakness (n = 77, 5.3%) followed by weight loss (n = 82, 5.5%). Those included in prospective analyses (n = 823) were non-frail participants at baseline, mainly females (65.0%) and were on average 72.8 ± 4.4 years old. A total of 150 participants (18.2%) exhibited frailty at the 10-year follow-up and the most incident frailty criterion was low physical activity (n = 473, 58.2%) followed by muscle weakness (n = 199, 26.6%). The least incident frailty criterion was weight loss (n = 69, 8.4%) followed by exhaustion (n = 138, 17.6%).

Table 1. Socio-demographic, clinical, dietary, and lifestyle characteristics according to the frailty prevalence (cross-sectional sample, n = 1490 in 2000) and incidence (prospective sample, n = 823 between 2000–2010) of older adults from the Three-City study, Bordeaux (France).

	Cross-Sectional Analyses				Prospective Analyses			
	Overall (n = 1490)	Frail at Baseline (n = 63)	Non-Frail at Baseline (n = 1427)	p^a	Overall (n = 823)	Non-Frail at Follow-Up (n = 673)	Incident Frail (n = 150)	p^a
Demographic characteristics (n, %) *								
Sex (females)	906 (60.81)	43 (68.25)	863 (60.48)	0.22	535 (65.01)	433 (64.34)	102 (68.00)	0.40
Age (y), mean (SD)	74.10 (4.90)	77.69 (5.24)	73.95 (4.82)	<0.0001	72.80 (4.35)	72.20 (4.08)	75.49 (4.50)	<0.0001
Education				0.27				0.11
No/Primary	478 (32.10)	26 (41.27)	452 (31.67)		232 (28.19)	180 (26.75)	52 (34.67)	
Secondary or high	731 (49.10)	26 (41.27)	705 (49.40)		424 (51.52)	357 (53.05)	67 (44.67)	
University	281 (18.90)	11 (17.46)	270 (18.92)		167 (20.29)	136 (20.21)	31 (20.67)	
Marital Status				0.053				0.001
Married	849 (57.00)	26 (41.27)	823 (57.67)		471 (57.23)	402 (59.73)	69 (46.00)	
Divorced/separated	118 (7.90)	5 (7.94)	113 (7.92)		64 (7.78)	56 (8.32)	8 (5.33)	
Widowed	429 (28.80)	27 (42.86)	402 (28.17)		228 (27.70)	168 (24.96)	60 (40.00)	
Single	94 (6.30)	5 (7.94)	89 (6.24)		60 (7.29)	47 (6.98)	13 (8.67)	
Clinical characteristics (n, %) *								
Smoking status				0.45				0.54
Never smoker	937 (62.90)	44 (69.84)	893 (62.58)		540 (65.61)	442 (65.68)	98 (65.33)	
Ex-smoker	472 (31.70)	17 (26.98)	455 (31.89)		242 (29.40)	195 (28.97)	47 (31.33)	
Current	81 (5.40)	2 (3.17)	79 (5.54)		41 (4.98)	36 (5.35)	5 (3.33)	
MMSE score [b], mean (SD)	27.52 (1.98)	26.43 (2.34)	27.57 (1.96)	<0.0001	27.84 (1.79)	27.89 (1.76)	27.61 (1.90)	0.08
Medications/d ≥ 6	480 (32.20)	38 (60.31)	442 (30.97)	<0.0001	220 (26.73)	155 (23.03)	65 (43.33)	<0.0001
Multimorbidity	727 (48.8)	41 (65.08)	686 (48.07)	0.008	395 (48.00)	299 (44.43)	96 (64.00)	<0.0001
Nutritional and dietary characteristics								
BMI (kg/m²) (m = 18)	26.33 (4.16)	27.51 (6.10)	26.28 (4.06)	0.03	26.25 (3.95)	26.15 (3.83)	26.68 (4.43)	0.15
BMI categories				0.16				0.63
<23	307 (20.86)	12 (21.05)	295 (20.85)		172 (21.00)	142 (21.19)	30 (20.13)	
23–27	577 (39.20)	16 (28.07)	561 (39.65)		329 (40.17)	273 (40.75)	56 (37.58)	
>27	588 (39.95)	29 (50.88)	559 (39.51)		318 (38.83)	255 (38.06)	63 (42.28)	
Total protein (g/d)	75.75 (26.80)	72.14 (27.05)	75.91 (26.79)	0.27	75.36 (26.22)	76.05 (25.98)	72.23 (27.12)	0.11
Diet index (n, % high quality)	761 (51.1)	32 (50.79)	729 (51.09)	0.96	423 (51.40)	357 (53.05)	66 (44.00)	0.05
Items of the phenotype of frailty								
Weight loss	82 (5.51) (m = 1)	27 (43.55)	55 (3.85)	<0.0001	69 (8.42) m = 4	35 (5.22)	34 (22.97)	<0.0001
Exhaustion	223 (15.12) (m = 15)	53 (84.13)	170 (12.04)	<0.0001	138 (17.56) m = 37	54 (8.32)	84 (61.31)	<0.0001
Muscle weakness	77 (5.25) (m = 24)	35 (58.33)	42 (2.99)	<0.0001	199 (26.57) m = 74	107 (17.31)	92 (70.23)	<0.0001
Walking speed	281 (18.90) (m = 3)	53 (84.12)	228 (16.01)	<0.0001	209 (25.49) m = 3	81 (12.09)	128 (85.33)	<0.0001
Physical activity	234 (20.05) (m = 323)	36 (78.26)	198 (17.66)	<0.0001	473 (58.18) m = 10	329 (49.47)	144 (97.30)	<0.0001

* All data are presented as n (%) except for age, MMSE, BMI, and protein intake where the mean (SD) is presented; [a] Baseline differences between prevalent frail and non-frail (n = 1490) and incident frail and non-frail (n = 823) participants tested by t-tests or chi square tests depending on the type of the variable; [b] Mini-Mental State Examination; m = missing.

Prevalent and incident frail older adults were significantly older, were more likely to be depressed, to take 6 medications/day or more, and to have comorbidities at baseline compared with prevalent non-frail participants, and with participants free from frailty over time, respectively (Table 1). Moreover, prevalent frail participants exhibited a significantly higher BMI on average than non-frail participants, and the daily consumption of proteins was not significantly different between the frail and non-frail participants at baseline (i.e., cross-sectional sample). Regarding the sample enrolled in prospective analyses, incident frail participants had a similar BMI compared to those who remained free from frailty, while a higher percentage of incident frail participants had a lower diet quality score compared with participants who remained free from frailty (53% vs. 44%, $p = 0.045$).

Frequencies of consumption of DP (total DP, milk, fresh DP, and cheese) are presented in Table 2 for both cross-sectional and prospective samples. No significant differences were observed between prevalent frail and non-frail or incident frail and non-frail participants regarding the frequency of total DP and DP-subtypes consumption at baseline.

Table 2. Frequency of consumption of dairy products (total and sub-types) according to the frailty prevalence (cross-sectional sample, n = 1490 in 2000) and incidence (prospective sample, n = 823 between 2000–2010) of older adults from the Three-City study, Bordeaux (France).

	Cross-Sectional Analyses				Prospective Analyses			
	Overall (n = 1490)	Frail at Baseline (n = 63)	Non-Frail at Baseline (n = 1427)	p [a]	Overall (n = 823)	Non-Frail at Follow-Up (n = 673)	Incident Frail (n = 150)	p [a]
Total Dairy Products				0.37				0.58
Low: ≤2 times/d	375 (25.17)	13 (20.63)	362 (25.37)		198 (24.06)	157 (23.33)	41 (27.33)	
Intermediate: 2–4 times/d	769 (51.61)	31 (49.21)	738 (51.72)		439 (53.34)	362 (53.79)	77 (51.33)	
High: ≥4 times/d	346 (23.22)	19 (30.16)	327 (22.92)		186 (22.60)	154 (22.88)	32 (21.33)	
Milk				0.37				0.54
Low: 0 times/d	433 (29.06)	17 (26.98)	416 (29.15)		229 (27.83)	182 (27.04)	47 (31.33)	
Intermediate: 0–1 times/d	716 (48.05)	27 (42.86)	689 (48.28)		383 (46.54)	318 (47.25)	65 (43.33)	
High: >1 times/d	341 (22.89)	19 (30.16)	322 (22.56)		211 (25.64)	173 (25.71)	38 (25.33)	
Fresh dairy products				0.52				0.46
Low: <0.5 times/d	408 (27.38)	16 (25.40)	392 (27.47)		207 (25.15)	167 (24.81)	40 (26.67)	
Intermediate: 0.5–1.5 times/d	723 (48.52)	28 (44.44)	695 (48.70)		419 (50.91)	339 (50.37)	80 (53.33)	
High: >1.5 times/d	359 (24.09)	19 (30.16)	340 (23.83)		197 (23.94)	167 (24.81)	30 (20.00)	
Cheese				0.39				0.31
Low: ≤0.5 times/d	297 (19.93)	16 (19.69)	281 (19.69)		174 (21.14)	143 (21.25)	31 (20.67)	
Intermediate: 0.5–1.5 times/d	779 (52.28)	28 (52.63)	751 (52.63)		477 (54.31)	372 (55.27)	75 (50.00)	
High: >1.5 times/d	414 (27.79)	19 (30.16)	395 (27.68)		202 (24.54)	158 (23.48)	44 (29.33)	

All data are presented as n (%); [a] Baseline differences between prevalent frail and non-frail (n = 1490) and incident frail and non-frail (n = 823) participants tested by t-tests or chi square tests depending on the type of the variable; m = missing.

3.2. Associations between Spectrum of DP Exposure and Prevalence of Frailty

In models adjusted for age, sex, marital status and education, we did not observe any significant association between total DP and DP sub-types and frailty prevalence, when comparing the highest frequency to the lowest frequency consumption of DP (Table 3). In models additionally adjusted for smoking status, multimorbidity, polypharmacy, protein intake, diet quality and global cognitive score, all associations with the prevalence of frailty remained not significant for all DP exposures: total DP (OR = 1.08, 95% CI = 0.54–2.17 and 1.40, 95% CI = 0.65–3.01 for intermediate and high consumption vs. low, respectively), milk (OR = 1.13, 95% CI = 0.56–2.31), fresh DP (OR = 1.13, 95% CI= 0.54–2.33), and cheese (OR = 0.89; 95% CI = 0.43–1.88) for high vs. low frequency of consumption.

3.3. Associations between Spectrum of DP Exposure and Incidence of Frailty

When focusing on the 10-year risk for frailty, we observed that baseline frequencies of consumption of total DP and DP sub-types were not significantly associated with the frailty risk when we compared the lowest frequency to the highest frequency of consumption of total DP (OR = 0.74, 95% CI = 0.42–1.30), milk (OR = 0.80, 95% CI = 0.48–1.35), fresh DP (OR = 0.68, 95% CI = 0.38–1.20) and cheese consumption (OR = 1.19, 05% CI = 0.68–2.10) in fully adjusted models (Table 4).

3.4. Sensitivity Analyses

The FRAIL scale was also implemented to alternatively identify prevalent and incident frail participants. Sixty out of 1552 participants (3.9%) were considered as frail at baseline according to this scale. In fully adjusted models (i.e., model 2), all associations with the prevalence of frailty were not significant for all DP exposures: total DP (OR = 1.42, 95% CI = 0.64–3.13), milk (OR= 1.11, 95% CI = 0.54–2.32), fresh DP (OR = 0.96, 95% CI= 0.46–1.98), and cheese (OR = 0.86; 95% CI = 0.39–1.88) for high vs. low frequency of consumption. Among 1492 non-frail non-dependent, 1006 were followed at the 10-year follow-up (lost to follow-up n = 486). Among those, an additional 87 were excluded from the analysis because they were ADL dependent and another 23 were excluded because they were unclassified for the FRAIL scale, leading to a final sample size of 896, with 45 (5.0%) classified as frail on the FRAIL scale. Regarding the spectrum of DP exposures, we only observed that the highest, compared with the lowest, frequency of consumption of fresh DP was associated with lower frailty risk in the fully adjusted model (OR = 0.35, 95% CI = 0.13–0.97, p = 0.04, p global = 0.13) while all other associations were non-significant, for instance, total DP (OR = 1.66, 95% CI = 0.26–1.67), milk (OR= 1.21, 95% CI = 0.49–2.98), and cheese (OR = 1.25; 95% CI = 0.49–3.21) for high vs. low frequency of consumption.

Second, when all ADL dependent individuals were maintained in analytic samples, 1501 and 885 participants were included for the cross-sectional and prospective analyses, respectively. Among those 1501 participants, 68 (4.5%) were identified as frail. None of the total DP or DP sub-types exposures were associated with frailty prevalence in the fully adjusted models: total DP (OR = 1.44, 95% CI = 0.68–3.04), milk (OR= 1.04, 95% CI = 0.52–2.1), fresh DP (OR = 1.21, 95% CI= 0.59–2.48), and cheese (OR = 0.85; 95% CI = 0.42–1.74) for high vs. low frequency of consumption. Among those 1433 non-frail at baseline, 449 were lost at the 10-year follow-up and 99 were unclassified for frailty incidence, leading to a final sample size of 885 for the prospective analyses. At the 10-year follow-up, 195 participants (22%) were identified as frail. Regarding the spectrum of DP exposures, none of the frequency of consumption of total DP or DP sub-types were significantly associated with frailty risk in the fully adjusted models: total DP (OR = 0.65, 95% CI = 0.39–1.09), milk (OR = 0.61, 95% CI = 0.38–1.00), fresh DP (OR = 0.64, 95% CI = 0.39–1.08), and cheese (OR = 1.4; 95% CI = 0.83–2.41) for high vs. low frequency of consumption.

Table 3. Multivariate association between baseline frequencies of consumption of total DP, milk, fresh DP, and cheese and frailty prevalence among older adults in the Three-City Study, Bordeaux (n = 1490, 2000).

	Total Dairy Products Frequency of Consumption					
	n frail/Total	Model 1 OR (95% CI)	p		Model 2 OR (95% CI)	p
Low: ≤2 times/d	13/375	Ref			Ref	
Intermediate: 2–4 times/d	31/769	1.07 (0.54–2.09)	0.84		1.08 (0.54–2.17)	0.82
High: ≥4 times/d	19/346	1.50 (0.72–3.13)	0.28		1.40 (0.65–3.01)	0.39
Global p			0.45			0.62
	Milk Frequency of Consumption					
	n frail/Total	Model 1 OR (95% CI)	p		Model 2 OR (95% CI)	p
Low: 0 times/d	17/433	Ref			Ref	
Intermediate: 0–1 times/d	27/716	0.91 (0.49–1.71)	0.77		0.83 (0.44–1.58)	0.57
High: >1 times/d	19/341	1.21 (0.61–2.41)	0.58		1.13 (0.56–2.31)	0.73
Global p			0.66			0.62
	Fresh Dairy Products Frequency of Consumption					
	n frail/Total	Model 1 OR (95% CI)	p		Model 2 OR (95% CI)	p
Low: <0.5 times/d	16/408	Ref			Ref	
Intermediate: 0.5–1.5 times/d	28/723	0.90 (0.47–1.72)	0.76		0.83 (0.43–1.62)	0.57
High: >1.5 times/d	19/359	1.22 (0.60–2.48)	0.58		1.13 (0.54–2.33)	0.74
Global p			0.62			0.62
	Cheese Frequency of Consumption					
	n frail/Total	Model 1 OR (95% CI)	p		Model 2 OR (95% CI)	p
Low: ≤0.5 times/d	16/297	Ref			Ref	
Intermediate: 0.5–1.5 times/d	28/779	0.66 (0.35–1.27)	0.22		0.68 (0.38–1.32)	0.25
High: >1.5 times/d	19/414	0.92 (0.45–1.86)	0.81		0.89 (0.43–1.88)	0.77
Global p			0.38			0.45

OR: Odds ratio, CI: Confidence Intervals; Model 1: Model adjusted for age, sex, marital status and education; Model 2: Model 1 + additional adjustment for smoking status, multimorbidity, polypharmacy, total protein, diet quality score, and Mini-Mental State Examination.

Table 4. Multivariate association between baseline frequencies of consumption of total DP, milk, fresh DP, and cheese and the 10-year frailty risk among older adults in the Three-City Study, Bordeaux (n = 823, 2000–2010).

		Total Dairy Products Frequency of Consumption				
	n frail/Total	Model 1 OR (95% CI)	p	Model 2 OR (95% CI)	p	
Low: ≤2 times/d	41/198	Ref		Ref		
Intermediate: 2–4 times/d	77/439	0.70 (0.44–1.09)	0.11	0.73 (0.46–1.16)	0.19	
High: ≥ 4 times/d	32/186	0.76 (0.44–1.30)	0.19	0.75 (0.42–1.32)	0.32	
Global p			0.28		0.40	
		Milk Frequency of Consumption				
	n frail/Total	Model 1 OR (95% CI)	p	Model 2 OR (95% CI)	p	
Low: 0 times/d	47/229	Ref		Ref		
Intermediate: 0–1 times/d	65/383	0.47 (0.50–1.21)	0.26	0.79 (0.50–1.22)	0.28	
High: >1 times/d	38/211	0.75 (0.45–1.24)	0.26	0.78 (0.46–1.31)	0.34	
Global p			0.43		0.50	
		Fresh Dairy Products Frequency of Consumption				
	n frail/Total	Model 1 OR (95% CI)	p	Model 2 OR (95% CI)	p	
Low: <0.5 times/d	40/207	Ref		Ref		
Intermediate: 0.5–1.5 times/d	80/419	0.92 (0.58–1.44)	0.71	0.91 (0.57–1.45)	0.68	
High: >1.5 times/d	30/197	0.66 (0.38–1.16)	0.15	0.65 (0.57–1.16)	0.15	
Global p			0.31		0.31	
		Cheese Frequency of Consumption				
	n frail/Total	Model 1 OR (95% CI)	p	Model 2 OR (95% CI)	p	
Low: ≤0.5 times/d	31/174	Ref		Ref		
Intermediate: 0.5–1.5 times/d	75/447	0.86 (0.53–1.40)	0.54	0.86 (0.52–1.41)	0.54	
High: >1.5 times/d	44/202	1.31 (0.76–2.27)	0.33	1.25 (0.71–2.21)	0.44	
Global p			0.17		0.27	

OR: Odds ratio, CI: Confidence Intervals; Model 1: Model adjusted for age, sex, marital status and education; Model 2: Model 1 + additional adjustment for smoking status, multimorbidity, polypharmacy, total protein, diet quality score, and Mini-Mental State Examination.

4. Discussion

In the present analysis of French community-dwelling older adults enrolled in the 3C-Bordeaux study, the frequency of DP consumption was not significantly associated with frailty, assessed using proxies of the frailty phenotype, in either cross-sectional or prospective analyses. In particular, total DP, milk, fresh DP and cheese were not associated with frailty prevalence at baseline. Similarly, these food groups were not associated with frailty risk at 10 years. Similar results were observed when frailty was assessed using the FRAIL scale, strengthening our conclusions.

Several studies have evaluated the association between DP and age-related chronic diseases and mortality [22,23,44]. Nevertheless, to our knowledge, very few studies have evaluated the relationship between DP and frailty and their results were mixed. A cross-sectional study evaluated the association between dairy intake and physical function among 1456 older women aged 70 to 85 years [45]. The authors observed that compared to those in the lowest tertile of dairy consumption, those in the highest tertile of consumption had significantly higher handgrip strength and lower odds for a poor Timed Up and Go while no differences were observed in the prevalence of falls. In a sample of 1871 Spanish older adults enrolled in the Seniors-ENRICA cohort [29], greater consumption of low-fat dairy products and low-fat milk in particular was associated with lower frailty risk over 3.5 years of follow-up, while no significant results were observed for whole milk, yogurt, cheese and low-fat yogurt. Contrary to the presented studies, our findings did not show any association with frailty prevalence or risk at the 10-year follow-up. Interestingly, our results are similar to a recent analysis of the InCHIANTI study where the main objective was to evaluate the associations between adherence to a Mediterranean-type diet (MeDi) and frailty index at baseline and at the 10-year follow-up [46]. In a sub-analysis, the authors investigated the effect of individual components of the MeDi and frailty, and they observed that DP intake was not significantly associated with frailty in both the cross-sectional and prospective analyses.

Several possible explanations could justify the absence of associations between DP and frailty in our sample. First, the FFQ used to collect dietary data assessed the frequency of consumption only, while information about the quantities, which could have been interesting, were only assessed by a single 24-h dietary recall (which questions its relevance). Therefore, despite the higher consumption frequency, this intake might have been below what is recommended and therefore affected our results. In fact, in a recent analysis of the 3C-study participants describing their DP intake at baseline, it was observed that participants with the highest frequency of total DP per day consumed lower than the recommended intakes [31]. These results were in line with a previous national report where it was observed that 64% of participants aged 55 to 79 years old reported consumption below recommendations [47]. Second, in the 3C-study, total DP consumption and its sub-types have been previously shown to be associated with different eating patterns [31]. Although we have adjusted for diet quality in our analyses, we cannot exclude the possibility of some residual confounding that has led to an absence of significance. This is noteworthy as it was observed that higher total DP consumption was associated with a higher consumption of biscuits, sweets and cooked vegetables, and higher frequency of milk consumption was significantly associated with higher intakes of biscuit and sweets, a dietary pattern described as "biscuits and snacking" in the 3C-study. Moreover, it was observed that the highest frequency consumers of fresh DP had a low total energy intake. Finally, the highest frequency of cheese consumption was associated with a high consumption of cereals and grains, sweets, charcuterie, meat, poultry, and alcohol [31]. These results showed that the higher consumption of total DP or sub-types was associated with less-than-optimal diets, rich in sugar and saturated fatty acids, part of a western-type diet [48] and potential risk factors for frailty [14,49,50]. For instance, in a cross-sectional NHANES study including 4062 participants ≥ 50 y of age, a higher percentage of saturated fatty acid intake was associated with higher frailtyprevalence [50]. Therefore, we speculated that the null association between highest DP consumption and frailty observed here might be the result of possible positive effects of some favorable nutrients on frailty (i.e., higher protein and energy intake), but attenuated by the possible negative effects of saturated fatty acid intake and the overall diet quality, although we have controlled for components of the diet in the analyses. Third, no information was available about the quality of DP, whether they were natural or sweetened, or fermented or not. In fact, flavored milk, whole yogurt and fermented milk, dairy desserts and sweetened cheeses are all sources of added sugars, which were shown to be associated with an increased risk of frailty in an analysis of the Seniors ENRICA cohort [49]. The highest tertile of added sugars consumption was associated with a higher frailty risk (i.e., multiplied by 2.3) compared to those in the lowest tertile. Finally, unlike the analyses from the Seniors-ENRICA cohort study [29], we were not able to differentiate between types of DP consumed based on their fat content. Nevertheless, the 24-h dietary recall administered at baseline of the 3C-Bordeaux study showed that only 7% of the participants had whole-fat milk and among those, only 10% reported regular consumption of whole-fat milk while up to 25% of the sample consumed whole fresh DP and 19% consumed flavored fresh DP or yogurt with fruits (unpublished data). This might imply that factors other than the fat content of DP might play a role in the association between DP and frailty. Altogether, we speculated that the observed null association between highest DP consumption (whatever the subtypes) and frailty might be the results of interactions between the different concentrations of beneficial and harmful ingredients leading to an unbalanced quality of DP and of related dietary patterns.

The present study has some methodological limitations. First, as previously stated, we had no detailed information about the portion sizes and this would have affected our results as national recommendations emphasize the quantity consumed rather than frequency. Moreover, a high frequency consumption does not necessarily mean reaching the recommended levels, as older adults might have frequent but smaller intakes. Therefore, the inability to evaluate the portion sizes might have hindered any potential association of DP with frailty status. We also did not assess DP intake from mixed dishes, and this might have led to underestimation of the DP consumption frequency. This is an important issue to consider in future studies as milk is a recurrent constituent of several French recipes. Another limitation is that we did not adjust for important micronutrients related to DP and associated with frailty, namely, vitamin D [51,52]. Furthermore, recall bias cannot be excluded as it can lead to under or overestimation of DP intakes despite meticulous data collection. Regarding the assessment of frailty, we complemented slowness and handgrip strength with the Rosow–Breslau scale and the chair stand test, respectively, to minimize the loss of participants due to missing data. Indeed, the Rosow–Breslau scale has been shown to be strongly associated with walking [38] and the chair stand test was shown to be a good proxy for handgrip strength [39,53]. Furthermore, we were not able to check frailty incidence over 10-years at different waves of follow-up because the frailty phenotype could not be calculated at each time interval. Nevertheless, this limit was toned down when using the FRAIL scale, which identified a lower number of frail participants, but provided similar results on the DP-frailty associations in both the cross-sectional and prospective analyses. Despite these similarities, we speculate that the imbalance between frail and non-frail groups might have led to underpowered comparisons, hindering the observation of real differences if any. In addition, a selection bias cannot be dismissed, since not included participants (cross-sectional sample) were older, had lower educational levels and cognitive performance, had more frequent depressive symptoms, multi-morbidities, polypharmacy, and worse diet scores than included participants (data not shown). Finally, although we adjusted for several major covariates, some residual confounding factors cannot be dismissed. In fact, we acknowledge that the collected dietary data dates back to 2000, which is old, and this might affect the relevance of our results. Nevertheless, the French RDA applied to the year of data collection (2000–2001) is still applied till now and it has been previously reported that intakes of major food groups appeared to be relatively stable during follow-up in 3C Bordeaux [54].

Despite these limitations, the current study has several strengths. First, we focused our analyses on a large sample of French elderly consumers, known to exhibit distinctive DP consumption, notably cheese [31], within a population-based setting while adjusting for major confounders (note, less than 0.1% of 3C-Bordeaux participants were consumers of food supplements at baseline, which precluded using this data as a confounder). Second, survival analyses were performed to check if there is any competitive risk with death (data not shown). We observed that DP exposures were not significantly associated with mortality, eliminating the selection bias leading to survival effect often faced in prospective studies involving older adults. Moreover, we confirmed our main results using a different scale to assess frailty and when keeping participants who exhibited dependency in both cross-sectional and prospective studied samples, which allowed us to further decrease the selection bias (i.e., frailty being considered as a pre-dependency stage and risk factor for disability [35,55]).

In conclusion, we did not observe any association between DP consumption, whatever the sub-types, and frailty prevalence or incidence among this sample of French older adults. Studies on this topic are scarce and future studies are still needed while taking into consideration the identified limitations, such as the potential benefits/risks ratio of DP nutrient contents. In the meantime, and beyond frailty, older adults are encouraged to follow French nutritional recommendations for DP consumption (2 to 3 times/d) as their benefits on the general well-being of older adults to prevent osteoporosis and malnutrition are well established, and recent large-scale settings have also suggested their protective ability to prevent chronic diseases and mortality.

Author Contributions: Conceptualization, C.F.; Formal analysis, H.P.; Methodology, B.R., H.P. and C.F.; Project administration, C.H. and C.F.; Resources, C.S. and C.F.; Supervision, C.F.; Validation, C.F.; Writing—original draft, B.R. and H.P.; Writing—review & editing, V.C., C.H., C.S. and C.F. All authors have read and agreed to the published version of the manuscript.

Funding: This research received no external funding.

Institutional Review Board Statement: The 3C study was approved by the Consultative Committee for the Protection of Persons participating in Biomedical Research at Kremlin-Bicêtre.

Informed Consent Statement: Informed consent was obtained from all subjects involved in the study.

Data Availability Statement: Data described in the manuscript, code book and analytic code will be made available upon request: http://www.three-city-study.com/ancillary-studies.php (accessed on 5 April 2021).

Acknowledgments: The Three-City Study is conducted under a partnership agreement between the Institut National de la Santé et de la Recherche Médicale (INSERM), Victor Segalen—Bordeaux2 University and the Sanofi-Synthélabo company. The Fondation pour la Recherche Médicale funded the preparation and beginning of the study. The 3C-Study is also sponsored by the Caisse Nationale Maladie des Travailleurs Salariés, Direction Générale de la Santé, Conseils Régionaux of Aquitaine and Bourgogne, Fondation de France, Ministry of Research-INSERM Program Cohortes et collections de données biologiques, the Fondation Plan Alzheimer (FCS 2009–2012), the Caisse Nationale pour la Solidarité et l'Autonomie (CNSA) and the "Programme Longévité et vieillissement", COGICARE 07-LVIE 003 01, the FRAILOMIC Initiative (FP7-HEALTH-2012-Proposal No. 305483-2).

Conflicts of Interest: The authors declare no conflict of interest regarding the current work.

References

1. Department of Economic and Social Affairs, U.N. World Population Prospects 2019: Highlights. Available online: https://population.un.org/wpp/Publications/Files/WPP2019_10KeyFindings.pdf (accessed on 5 April 2021).
2. World Health Organization. "Ageing Well" Must Be a Global Priority. Available online: https://http://www.who.int/news/item/06-11-2014--ageing-well-must-be-a-global-priority (accessed on 5 April 2021).
3. Tabue-Teguo, M.; Grasset, L.; Avila-Funes, J.A.; Genuer, R.; Proust-Lima, C.; Péres, K.; Féart, C.; Amieva, H.; Harmand, M.G.; Helmer, C.; et al. Prevalence and Co-Occurrence of Geriatric Syndromes in People Aged 75 Years and Older in France: Results From the Bordeaux Three-city Study. *J. Gerontol. Ser. A Biol. Sci. Med Sci.* **2017**, *73*, 109–116. [CrossRef]
4. Fried, L.P.; Tangen, C.M.; Walston, J.; Newman, A.B.; Hirsch, C.; Gottdiener, J.; Seeman, T.; Tracy, R.; Kop, W.J.; Burke, G.; et al. Frailty in older adults: Evidence for a phenotype. *J. Gerontol. Ser. A Biol. Sci. Med Sci.* **2001**, *56*, M146–M156. [CrossRef] [PubMed]
5. Mareschal, J.; Genton, L.; Collet, T.H.; Graf, C. Nutritional Intervention to Prevent the Functional Decline in Community-Dwelling Older Adults: A Systematic Review. *Nutrients* **2020**, *12*, 2820. [CrossRef]
6. Feart, C. Nutrition and frailty: Current knowledge. *Prog. Neuro Psychopharmacol. Biol. Psychiatry* **2019**, *95*, 109703. [CrossRef]
7. Sandoval-Insausti, H.; Pérez-Tasigchana, R.F.; López-García, E.; García-Esquinas, E.; Rodríguez-Artalejo, F.; Guallar-Castillón, P. Macronutrients Intake and Incident Frailty in Older Adults: A Prospective Cohort Study. *J. Gerontol. Ser. A Biol. Sci. Med Sci.* **2016**, *71*, 1329–1334. [CrossRef]
8. Shikany, J.M.; Barrett-Connor, E.; Ensrud, K.E.; Cawthon, P.M.; Lewis, C.E.; Dam, T.T.; Shannon, J.; Redden, D.T. Macronutrients, diet quality, and frailty in older men. *J. Gerontol. Ser. A Biol. Sci. Med Sci.* **2014**, *69*, 695–701. [CrossRef]
9. García-Esquinas, E.; Rahi, B.; Peres, K.; Colpo, M.; Dartigues, J.F.; Bandinelli, S.; Feart, C.; Rodríguez-Artalejo, F. Consumption of fruit and vegetables and risk of frailty: A dose-response analysis of 3 prospective cohorts of community-dwelling older adults. *Am. J. Clin. Nutr.* **2016**, *104*, 132–142. [CrossRef]
10. Fung, T.T.; Struijk, E.A.; Rodriguez-Artalejo, F.; Willett, W.C.; Lopez-Garcia, E. Fruit and vegetable intake and risk of frailty in women 60 years old or older. *Am. J. Clin. Nutr.* **2020**, *112*, 1540–1546. [CrossRef] [PubMed]
11. Del Brutto, O.H.; Mera, R.M.; Ha, J.E.; Gillman, J.; Zambrano, M.; Sedler, M.J. Dietary Oily Fish Intake and Frailty. A Population-Based Study in Frequent Fish Consumers Living in Rural Coastal Ecuador (the Atahualpa Project). *J. Nutr. Gerontol. Geriatr.* **2020**, *39*, 88–97. [CrossRef]
12. Rashidi Pour Fard, N.; Amirabdollahian, F.; Haghighatdoost, F. Dietary patterns and frailty: A systematic review and meta-analysis. *Nutr. Rev.* **2019**, *77*, 498–513. [CrossRef]
13. Feng, Z.; Lugtenberg, M.; Franse, C.; Fang, X.; Hu, S.; Jin, C.; Raat, H. Risk factors and protective factors associated with incident or increase of frailty among community-dwelling older adults: A systematic review of longitudinal studies. *PLoS ONE* **2017**, *12*, e0178383. [CrossRef]

14. Leon-Munoz, L.M.; Garcia-Esquinas, E.; Lopez-Garcia, E.; Banegas, J.R.; Rodriguez-Artalejo, F. Major dietary patterns and risk of frailty in older adults: A prospective cohort study. *BMC Med.* **2015**, *13*, 11. [CrossRef]
15. Struijk, E.A.; Hagan, K.A.; Fung, T.T.; Hu, F.B.; Rodríguez-Artalejo, F.; Lopez-Garcia, E. Diet quality and risk of frailty among older women in the Nurses' Health Study. *Am. J. Clin. Nutr.* **2020**, *111*, 877–883. [CrossRef] [PubMed]
16. Lorenzo-López, L.; Maseda, A.; de Labra, C.; Regueiro-Folgueira, L.; Rodríguez-Villamil, J.L.; Millán-Calenti, J.C. Nutritional determinants of frailty in older adults: A systematic review. *BMC Geriatr.* **2017**, *17*, 108. [CrossRef]
17. Rahi, B.; Ajana, S.; Tabue-Teguo, M.; Dartigues, J.F.; Peres, K.; Feart, C. High adherence to a Mediterranean diet and lower risk of frailty among French older adults community-dwellers: Results from the Three-City-Bordeaux Study. *Clin. Nutr.* **2018**, *37*, 1293–1298. [CrossRef]
18. Rahi, B.; Colombet, Z.; Gonzalez-Colaco Harmand, M.; Dartigues, J.F.; Boirie, Y.; Letenneur, L.; Feart, C. Higher Protein but Not Energy Intake Is Associated With a Lower Prevalence of Frailty Among Community-Dwelling Older Adults in the French Three-City Cohort. *J. Am. Med Dir. Assoc.* **2016**, *17*, 672.e7–672.e11. [CrossRef]
19. Coelho-Júnior, H.J.; Rodrigues, B.; Uchida, M.; Marzetti, E. Low Protein Intake Is Associated with Frailty in Older Adults: A Systematic Review and Meta-Analysis of Observational Studies. *Nutrients* **2018**, *10*, 1334. [CrossRef] [PubMed]
20. Mendonça, N.; Kingston, A.; Granic, A.; Jagger, C. Protein intake and transitions between frailty states and to death in very old adults: The Newcastle 85+ study. *Age Ageing* **2019**, *49*, 32–38. [CrossRef] [PubMed]
21. Isanejad, M.; Sirola, J.; Rikkonen, T.; Mursu, J.; Kröger, H.; Qazi, S.L.; Tuppurainen, M.; Erkkilä, A.T. Higher protein intake is associated with a lower likelihood of frailty among older women, Kuopio OSTPRE-Fracture Prevention Study. *Eur. J. Nutr.* **2020**, *59*, 1181–1189. [CrossRef] [PubMed]
22. Drouin-Chartier, J.P.; Li, Y.; Ardisson Korat, A.V.; Ding, M.; Lamarche, B.; Manson, J.E.; Rimm, E.B.; Willett, W.C.; Hu, F.B. Changes in dairy product consumption and risk of type 2 diabetes: Results from 3 large prospective cohorts of US men and women. *Am. J. Clin. Nutr.* **2019**, *110*, 1201–1212. [CrossRef]
23. Mitri, J.; Mohd Yusof, B.N.; Maryniuk, M.; Schrager, C.; Hamdy, O.; Salsberg, V. Dairy intake and type 2 diabetes risk factors: A narrative review. *Diabetes Metab. Syndr.* **2019**, *13*, 2879–2887. [CrossRef] [PubMed]
24. Dehghan, M.; Mente, A.; Rangarajan, S.; Sheridan, P.; Mohan, V.; Iqbal, R.; Gupta, R.; Lear, S.; Wentzel-Viljoen, E.; Avezum, A.; et al. Association of dairy intake with cardiovascular disease and mortality in 21 countries from five continents (PURE): A prospective cohort study. *Lancet* **2018**, *392*, 2288–2297. [CrossRef]
25. Ding, M.; Li, J.; Qi, L.; Ellervik, C.; Zhang, X.; Manson, J.E.; Stampfer, M.; Chavarro, J.E.; Rexrode, K.M.; Kraft, P.; et al. Associations of dairy intake with risk of mortality in women and men: Three prospective cohort studies. *BMJ Clin. Res. Ed.* **2019**, *367*, l6204. [CrossRef]
26. Guo, J.; Astrup, A.; Lovegrove, J.A.; Gijsbers, L.; Givens, D.I.; Soedamah-Muthu, S.S. Milk and dairy consumption and risk of cardiovascular diseases and all-cause mortality: Dose-response meta-analysis of prospective cohort studies. *Eur. J. Epidemiol.* **2017**, *32*, 269–287. [CrossRef] [PubMed]
27. Cuesta-Triana, F.; Verdejo-Bravo, C.; Fernández-Pérez, C.; Martín-Sánchez, F.J. Effect of Milk and Other Dairy Products on the Risk of Frailty, Sarcopenia, and Cognitive Performance Decline in the Elderly: A Systematic Review. *Adv. Nutr.* **2019**, *10*, S105–S119. [CrossRef] [PubMed]
28. Hanach, N.I.; McCullough, F.; Avery, A. The Impact of Dairy Protein Intake on Muscle Mass, Muscle Strength, and Physical Performance in Middle-Aged to Older Adults with or without Existing Sarcopenia: A Systematic Review and Meta-Analysis. *Adv. Nutr.* **2019**, *10*, 59–69. [CrossRef]
29. Lana, A.; Rodriguez-Artalejo, F.; Lopez-Garcia, E. Dairy Consumption and Risk of Frailty in Older Adults: A Prospective Cohort Study. *J. Am. Geriatr. Soc.* **2015**, *63*, 1852–1860. [CrossRef]
30. Ribeiro, I.; Gomes, M.; Figueiredo, D.; Lourenço, J.; Paúl, C.; Costa, E. Dairy Product Intake in Older Adults across Europe Based On the SHARE Database. *J. Nutr. Gerontol. Geriatr.* **2019**, *38*, 297–306. [CrossRef]
31. Pellay, H.; Marmonier, C.; Samieri, C.; Feart, C. Socio-Demographic Characteristics, Dietary, and Nutritional Intakes of French Elderly Community Dwellers According to Their Dairy Product Consumption: Data from the Three-City Cohort. *Nutrients* **2020**, *12*, 3418. [CrossRef]
32. 3C Study Group. Vascular factors and risk of dementia: Design of the Three-City Study and baseline characteristics of the study population. *Neuroepidemiology* **2003**, *22*, 316–325. [CrossRef]
33. Samieri, C.; Jutand, M.A.; Féart, C.; Capuron, L.; Letenneur, L.; Barberger-Gateau, P. Dietary patterns derived by hybrid clustering method in older people: Association with cognition, mood, and self-rated health. *J. Am. Diet. Assoc.* **2008**, *108*, 1461–1471. [CrossRef]
34. Simermann, J.; Barberger-Gateau, P.; Berr, C. Validation of a Food Frequency Questionnaire in older population. In Proceedings of the 25th annual congress of SFNEP: Clinical Nutrition and Metabolism, Montpellier, France, 28–30 November 2007.
35. Dent, E.; Morley, J.E.; Cruz-Jentoft, A.J.; Woodhouse, L.; Rodríguez-Mañas, L.; Fried, L.P.; Woo, J.; Aprahamian, I.; Sanford, A.; Lundy, J.; et al. Physical Frailty: ICFSR International Clinical Practice Guidelines for Identification and Management. *J. Nutr. Health Aging* **2019**, *23*, 771–787. [CrossRef]
36. Radloff, L.S. The CES-D scale a self-report depression scale for research in the general population. *Appl. Psychol. Meas.* **1977**, *1*, 385–401. [CrossRef]
37. Rosow, I.; Breslau, N. A Guttman health scale for the aged. *J. Gerontol.* **1966**, *21*, 556–559. [CrossRef]

38. Alexander, N.B.; Guire, K.E.; Thelen, D.G.; Ashton-Miller, J.A.; Schultz, A.B.; Grunawalt, J.C.; Giordani, B. Self-reported walking ability predicts functional mobility performance in frail older adults. *J. Am. Geriatr. Soc.* **2000**, *48*, 1408–1413. [CrossRef] [PubMed]
39. Avila-Funes, J.A.; Helmer, C.; Amieva, H.; Barberger-Gateau, P.; Le Goff, M.; Ritchie, K.; Portet, F.; Carriere, I.; Tavernier, B.; Gutierrez-Robledo, L.M.; et al. Frailty among community-dwelling elderly people in France: The three-city study. *J. Gerontol. Ser. A Biol. Sci. Med Sci.* **2008**, *63*, 1089–1096. [CrossRef] [PubMed]
40. Morley, J.E.; Malmstrom, T.K.; Miller, D.K. A simple frailty questionnaire (FRAIL) predicts outcomes in middle aged African Americans. *J. Nutr. Health Aging* **2012**, *16*, 601–608. [CrossRef]
41. Katz, S.; Ford, A.B.; Moskowitz, R.W.; Jackson, B.A.; Jaffe, M.W. Studies of Illness in the Aged. The Index of ADL: A Standardized Measure of Biological and Psychosocial Function. *JAMA J. Am. Med Assoc.* **1963**, *185*, 914–919. [CrossRef] [PubMed]
42. Folstein, M.F.; Folstein, S.E.; McHugh, P.R. "Mini-mental state". A practical method for grading the cognitive state of patients for the clinician. *J. Psychiatr. Res.* **1975**, *12*, 189–198. [CrossRef]
43. Feart, C.; Jutand, M.A.; Larrieu, S.; Letenneur, L.; Delcourt, C.; Combe, N.; Barberger-Gateau, P. Energy, macronutrient and fatty acid intake of French elderly community dwellers and association with socio-demographic characteristics: Data from the Bordeaux sample of the Three-City Study. *Br. J. Nutr.* **2007**, *98*, 1046–1057. [CrossRef]
44. Gil, Á.; Ortega, R.M. Introduction and Executive Summary of the Supplement, Role of Milk and Dairy Products in Health and Prevention of Noncommunicable Chronic Diseases: A Series of Systematic Reviews. *Adv. Nutr.* **2019**, *10*, S67–S73. [CrossRef] [PubMed]
45. Radavelli-Bagatini, S.; Zhu, K.; Lewis, J.R.; Dhaliwal, S.S.; Prince, R.L. Association of dairy intake with body composition and physical function in older community-dwelling women. *J. Acad. Nutr. Diet.* **2013**, *113*, 1669–1674. [CrossRef] [PubMed]
46. Tanaka, T.; Talegawkar, S.A.; Jin, Y.; Bandinelli, S.; Ferrucci, L. Association of Adherence to the Mediterranean-Style Diet with Lower Frailty Index in Older Adults. *Nutrients* **2021**, *13*, 1129. [CrossRef] [PubMed]
47. Agence Nationale de Sécurité Sanitaire de L'alimentation, d.l.e.e.d.t.A. INCA 3 : Evolution des Habitudes et Modes de Consommation, de Nouveaux Enjeux en Matière de Sécurité Sanitaire et de Nutrition. Available online: https://http://www.anses.fr/fr/content/inca-3-evolution-des-habitudes-et-modes-de-consommation-de-nouveaux-enjeux-en-mati%C3%A8re-de (accessed on 5 April 2021).
48. Hu, F. Dietary pattern analysis: A new direction in nutritional epidemiology. *Curr. Opin. Lipidol.* **2002**, *13*, 3–9. [CrossRef]
49. Laclaustra, M.; Rodriguez-Artalejo, F.; Guallar-Castillon, P.; Banegas, J.R.; Graciani, A.; Garcia-Esquinas, E.; Ordovas, J.; Lopez-Garcia, E. Prospective association between added sugars and frailty in older adults. *Am. J. Clin. Nutr.* **2018**, *107*, 772–779. [CrossRef] [PubMed]
50. Jayanama, K.; Theou, O.; Godin, J.; Cahill, L.; Rockwood, K. Association of fatty acid consumption with frailty and mortality among middle-aged and older adults. *Nutrition* **2020**, *70*, 110610. [CrossRef] [PubMed]
51. Artaza-Artabe, I.; Sáez-López, P.; Sánchez-Hernández, N.; Fernández-Gutierrez, N.; Malafarina, V. The relationship between nutrition and frailty: Effects of protein intake, nutritional supplementation, vitamin D and exercise on muscle metabolism in the elderly. A systematic review. *Maturitas* **2016**, *93*, 89–99. [CrossRef]
52. Bruyère, O.; Cavalier, E.; Buckinx, F.; Reginster, J.Y. Relevance of vitamin D in the pathogenesis and therapy of frailty. *Curr. Opin. Clin. Nutr. Metab. Care* **2017**, *20*, 26–29. [CrossRef]
53. Rantanen, T.; Era, P.; Kauppinen, M.; Heikkinen, E. Maximal isometric muscle strength and socioeconomic status, health, and physical activity in 75-year-old persons. *J. Aging Phys. Act.* **1994**, *2*, 206–220. [CrossRef]
54. Pelletier, A.; Barul, C.; Feart, C.; Helmer, C.; Bernard, C.; Periot, O.; Dilharreguy, B.; Dartigues, J.F.; Allard, M.; Barberger-Gateau, P.; et al. Mediterranean diet and preserved brain structural connectivity in older subjects. *Alzheimer Dement. J. Alzheimer Assoc.* **2015**, *11*, 1023–1031. [CrossRef]
55. Liu, H.X.; Ding, G.; Yu, W.J.; Liu, T.F.; Yan, A.Y.; Chen, H.Y.; Zhang, A.H. Association between frailty and incident risk of disability in community-dwelling elder people: Evidence from a meta-analysis. *Public Health* **2019**, *175*, 90–100. [CrossRef] [PubMed]

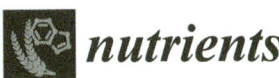

Article

Dietary Patterns and Risk Factors of Frailty in Lebanese Older Adults

Nathalie Yaghi [1], Cesar Yaghi [2,3], Marianne Abifadel [4], Christa Boulos [1] and Catherine Feart [5,*]

[1] Department of Nutrition & Dietetics, Faculty of Pharmacy, Saint Joseph University of Beirut, P.O. Box 17-5208 Mar Mikhael, Beirut 1104 2020, Lebanon; nathalie.yaghi@usj.edu.lb (N.Y.); christa.boulos@usj.edu.lb (C.B.)
[2] Department of Gastroenterology, Faculty of Medicine, Saint Joseph University of Beirut, P.O. Box 17-5208 Mar Mikhael, Beirut 1104 2020, Lebanon; cesar.yaghi@usj.edu.lb
[3] Hotel-Dieu de France of Beirut University Hospital, P.O. Box 166830, Alfred Naccache Blvd, Beirut, Lebanon
[4] Laboratory of Biochemistry and Molecular Therapeutics, Faculty of Pharmacy, Pôle Technologie-Santé, Saint Joseph University of Beirut, P.O. Box 17-5208 Mar Mikhael, Beirut 1104 2020, Lebanon; marianne.abifadel@usj.edu.lb
[5] LEHA team, INSERM U1219, Université de Bordeaux, F-33000 Bordeaux, France
* Correspondence: catherine.feart-couret@u-bordeaux.fr; Tel.: +33-(0)5-47-304-204

Abstract: Factors associated with frailty, particularly dietary patterns, are not fully understood in Mediterranean countries. This study aimed to investigate the association of data-driven dietary patterns with frailty prevalence in older Lebanese adults. We conducted a cross-sectional national study that included 352 participants above 60 years of age. Sociodemographic and health-related data were collected. Food frequency questionnaires were used to elaborate dietary patterns via the K-mean cluster analysis method. Frailty that accounted for 15% of the sample was twice as much in women (20%) than men (10%). Identified dietary patterns included a Westernized-type dietary pattern (WDP), a high intake/Mediterranean-type dietary pattern (HI-MEDDP), and a moderate intake/Mediterranean-type dietary pattern (MOD-MEDDP). In the multivariate analysis, age, waist to height ratio, polypharmacy, age-related conditions, and WDP were independently associated with frailty. In comparison to MOD-MEDDP, and after adjusting for covariates, adopting a WDP was strongly associated with a higher frailty prevalence in men (OR = 6.63, 95% (CI) (1.82–24.21) and in women (OR = 11.54, 95% (CI) (2.02–65.85). In conclusion, MOD-MEDDP was associated with the least prevalence of frailty, and WDP had the strongest association with frailty in this sample. In the Mediterranean sample, a diet far from the traditional one appears as the key deleterious determinant of frailty.

Keywords: frailty; dietary pattern; malnutrition; food groups; Mediterranean dietary pattern; Westernized dietary pattern; older adults; cross-sectional study

1. Introduction

The frailty phenotype is a multifactorial syndrome associated with aging, characterized by unintentional weight loss, self-reported exhaustion, muscular weakness, slow walking speed, and low physical activity [1]. Physical frailty is also recognized as a risk factor for mortality, increased morbidity [2], malnutrition [2], and falls [3,4]. If not managed, frailty can lead to disability and dependency [5,6], and become a burden to the individual, caregivers, and public health authorities. This process, which moves from robustness to frailty, disability, then dependency, is preventable, and could even improve in some aspects, if addressed in the early stages (i.e., in the prefrail state) [7–10].

Frailty, being a multifactorial condition, is related to several sociodemographic-, lifestyle-, and health-related factors. Associations were found between frailty risk and marital status [11], education [12], depression [13], polypharmacy [14], and nutritional status [2,15].

Gender discrepancies have also been reported regarding the risk of frailty. Although women tend to live longer, their health status is poorer than men and biological and socio-behavioral factors may contribute to a higher frailty predisposition [16,17]. In many studies, the prevalence and incidence of frailty in women was found to be greater than in men [18].

Among other risk factors for frailty, anthropometric, nutritional, and dietary risk factors are often mentioned [17]. Frailty is also closely related to body composition and nutritional status. It is well established that malnutrition and the risk of malnutrition, characterized by low mini-nutritional assessment (MNA) scores, increase the risk of frailty in older adults [19,20]. BMI was also associated with frailty in a U shape trend, with both low and high BMI being associated with higher incidence of frailty [21–25]. Furthermore, central obesity characterized by a high waist circumference (WC), has also been linked to frailty risk, and recent studies even reported that the association between BMI and frailty was in part mediated by waist to height ratio (WHTR) [26–28].

According to several authors, current recommended dietary allowances (RDA) for protein intake at 0.8 g/kg (BW) appears to be insufficient to prevent muscle loss with aging [29]. The protein intake that showed a better muscle preservation and was linked to lower frailty risk was proposed at protein intakes between 1 and 1.5 g/kg BW [29–32].

Apart from the nutritional status, dietary patterns were also linked with risk of frailty in older adults. Rashidi et al. showed that people adopting a healthy dietary pattern, characterized by a high consumption of fruits, vegetables, and whole grains, had 31% less chance of becoming frail [33]. Pooled results showed that a greater adherence to a Mediterranean diet, evaluated by the Mediterranean Diet Score (MDS), was associated with a significantly lower risk of frailty compared to poorer adherence [34,35]. Similar findings from the Hellenic Longitudinal Investigation on Aging and Diet (HELIAD) showed that each additional unit in the MDS was associated with a 5–7% decrease in the odds of frailty, depending on the tools used in the evaluation of frailty [36]. In Spain, a higher prevalence of frailty was observed in older adults adopting an unhealthy dietary pattern (DP) compared to individuals adopting a healthy dietary pattern [37]. In England, a longitudinal study showed that a dietary pattern characterized by a high fat intake and low fiber intake was associated with a higher risk of frailty in men. Following a prudent diet and having a higher adherence to a Mediterranean dietary pattern was also found to decrease the likelihood of frailty [38]. The Rotterdam cohort study showed that a higher adherence to national dietary guidelines was associated with lower risk of frailty over time, and a traditional dietary pattern characterized by a high consumption of legumes, eggs, and savory snacks was the only one protecting against frailty; health-conscious dietary patterns and high meat patterns failed to be associated with frailty [39]. Results from the 12-year follow-up, three-city study, showed that men following the dietary pattern characterized by a "pasta" pattern, and women adopting the "biscuits and snacking" pattern had a significantly higher risk of frailty compared with those following the "healthy" pattern (characterized by higher fish intake in men and higher fruits and vegetables intake in women) [40]. In the multicentric, 1 year NU-AGE interventional study, the administration of a Mediterranean diet for a 1year period, by modulating the microbiome ecosystem was linked with lower frailty incidence in older adults [41].

Several studies showed that prevalence of frailty and pre-frailty in low- to middle-income countries (LMIC) was higher than in high income countries (HIC) [18,42]. In Lebanon, one of the countries bordering the Mediterranean basin with an aging population, few studies have yet been interested in the frailty status among its elderly population. In 2016, the prevalence of frailty (including pre-frailty) was estimated to 66.8% in rural living older individuals, aged 65 years and more, with a higher prevalence of frailty among individuals considered undernourished or at risk of malnutrition according to MNA [19,43]. However, no data is available on the association between nutritional status, dietary patterns, and frailty in this population.

The aims of the present study were (i) to determine the prevalence of frailty and its covariates among older Lebanese adults, and (ii) to explore the association between dietary patterns and frailty among these individuals.

2. Materials and Methods

2.1. Study Design and Participants

We conducted a national, cross-sectional study in seven of the eight governorates of Lebanon. Recruitment of participants and data collection were carried out in collaboration with the Ministry of Social Affairs (MOSA) through 77 medico-social centers serving low to middle class income families, from October 2017 to October 2019. The sample was weighed according to the proportion of older adults over 60 years in each governorate and was randomly selected based on the sample previously drawn for the validation of the Arabic version of Mini-Mental State Examination (MMSE) [44,45].

As shown in Figure 1, a sample of 600 individuals was initially targeted. Individuals were included in the present study if they were aged 60 years and above, community dwelling, and attending the MOSA socio-medical centers for medical care and social assistance. Non-inclusion criteria included artificial feeding, total dependency, major hearing and visual impairment, active cancer disease, end stage kidney disease with hemodialysis, and advanced liver disease, as diagnosed by the center medical team. Once contact was initiated, 159 individuals were either unable to be reached, refused to participate, or were deceased after randomization, and six were excluded because of newly discovered cancer or major disability. Data were finally retained for 401 participants, of whom, 352 (88%) had a valid Food Frequency Questionnaire (FFQ).

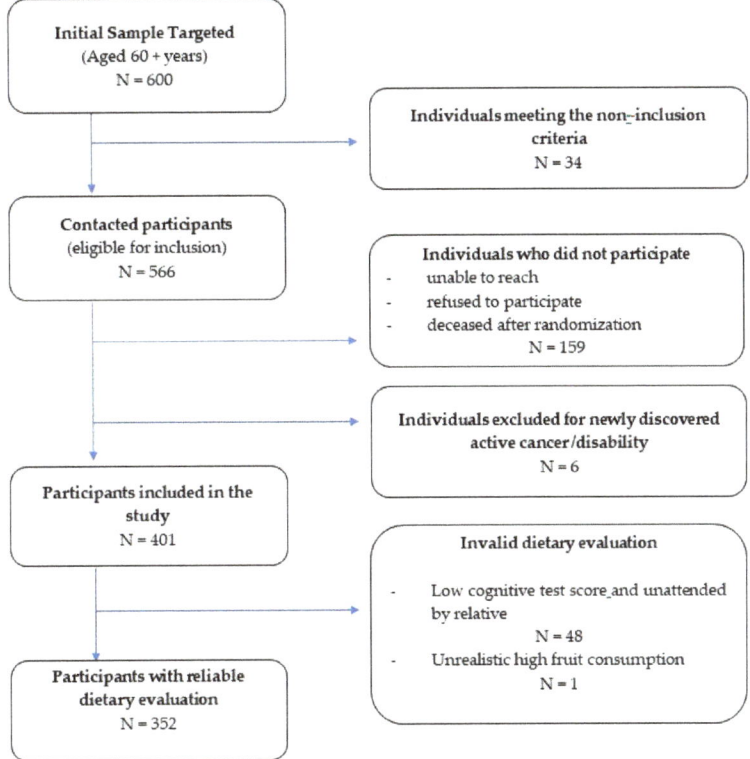

Figure 1. Study Flow chart.

Participants were contacted (via phone) by social workers or nurses working in the MOSA centers and were invited to attend the MOSA center. Information was collected by 10 dietitians living in the area surrounding the MOSA centers and who were familiar with the dietary habits of the local inhabitants. All investigators underwent several training sessions before starting the survey. To decrease investigator bias, all filled questionnaires were reviewed by the principal and field investigators before data entry. Each person was interviewed at the center near his/her home, and for participants unable to attend, the interview was performed by the research team at home. The interview with each participant or caretaker lasted around 30–45 min. Depending on literacy, the cognitive functions of each participant were assessed either through the Mini-Mental State Examination (MMSE) [44] or "Test des Neufs Images" (TNI) [46]. In case of significant cognitive decline, then the accompanying person was asked to fill the questionnaire on behalf of the participant.

The study was conducted in accordance with the Declaration of Helsinki, and the protocol of the study was approved by the Ethics Committee of Saint Joseph University of Beirut (USJ 2016-99). Written informed consent was signed by each participant, prior to completion of the interview.

2.2. Data Collected

2.2.1. Frailty and FRAIL Scale

Frail status of the participants was assessed based on the five criteria of FRAIL scale including fatigue, resistance, ambulation, illness, and loss of weight [47]. Fatigue was measured by asking respondents how much time during the past 4 weeks they felt tired, with responses of "all of the time" or "most of the time" scoring 1 point. Resistance was assessed by asking participants if they had any difficulty walking up 10 steps alone without resting and without aids, and ambulation, by asking if they had any difficulty walking several hundred yards alone and without aids; "yes" responses were each scored as 1 point. Illness was scored 1 for respondents who reported 5 or more illnesses out of the 11 following illnesses: heart attack, congestive heart failure, angina, asthma, arthritis, stroke, kidney disease, hypertension, diabetes, cancer, and chronic lung disease. Weight loss was scored 1 for respondents with a self-reported weight decline of 5% or greater within the past 12 months. Frail scale scores range from 0–5 and represent frail (score = 3–5), pre-frail (score = 1–2), and robust (score = 0) health status [47]. For data analysis, the studied sample was further categorized to frail versus non-frail (robust or prefrail).

2.2.2. Sociodemographic and Health-Related Data

Information regarding age and gender, living conditions, marital status, and economic situation were collected. Participants were asked to state whether they live alone or with any relative, spouse, family members, or friends. Educational level and literacy were evaluated and classified into two categories: >7 years and ≤7 years of education.

Number and type of diseases and health conditions were reported by each participant or its caregiver: cardiovascular diseases, diabetes, hypertension, heart failure and arrhythmia, renal disease, thyroid disorder, gastrointestinal diseases, anemia, osteoarthritis and arthritis, and osteoporosis. The presence of these diseases was ascertained based on: (a) self-reports linked to previous diagnoses, and/or (b) available medical records kept in the MOSA center, and/or (c) available medical prescriptions. The number of diseases was summed and categorized to multimorbidity defined as the simultaneous presence of two or more diseases in the same individual. Hearing or visual impairment, poor oral health, and sleep disorders were grouped as age-related conditions. Results were then dichotomized based on the presence of two or more of these age-related conditions. Current medications were recorded by caregiver, and polypharmacy was defined as the regular use of six or more prescription medications daily.

Since cognitive decline might influence reporting in the elderly population, cognitive impairment was evaluated depending on literacy, using population specific cut-offs based on age, educational level and sex, of MMSE for literate participants, and a score of TNI, Total Recall ≤ 9, for illiterate participants [44,46,48].

2.2.3. Anthropometric and Functional Measurements

Data included height, weight, body mass index (BMI), waist circumference (WC), and waist to height ratio (WHR). BMI was categorized according to the Lipchitz classification (<22, 22–27, and >27 kg/m^2) [49], Hand grip strength (HGS) was measured using the handgrip electronic dynamometer (Camry EH101). Handgrip strength was performed 3 times and the average of the three measurements was the reported result. We then used the BMI and gender specific cut-off values of HGS as classified by Fried phenotype, to classify as low or good HGS measurements [50].

Physical activity was evaluated using the Rapid Assessment of Physical Activity (RAPA) 2 scale. The nine-item questionnaire covered all ranges of activity, from sedentary to regular and vigorous physical activity in addition to strength training and flexibility adapted to the elderly [51]. Respondent's score was initially categorized into five levels of physical activity. For data analysis, these levels were then classified into three categories: sedentary, regular active and optimal active. Responses to the strength training and flexibility items were scored separately [51].

2.2.4. Nutritional and Dietary Data

Nutritional status was estimated using the Mini-Nutritional Assessment Short Form (MNA-SF) [52], classifying individuals into three levels: normal nutritional status (score above 12), at risk of malnutrition (scores 8–11), and malnutrition (scores below 8). Participants were then classified into two categories: the first category named "poor nutritional status" included participants that were considered malnourished and at risk of malnutrition by the MNA-SF, and the second category named "normal nutritional status" included participants who had a normal nutritional status according to MNA-SF.

Dietary assessment and food consumption was measured using a population based FFQ, reporting the consumption of a list of 90 food items (validation in progress of publication) and representing all food groups, consumed the previous year: bread and cereals, milk and dairy, vegetables and fruits, meat, poultry and fish, fats and oils, sweets and desserts, and non-alcoholic beverages. Consumption of these items was reported as daily, weekly, or monthly, as usual portion size. A manual illustrating the usual servings and portions of foods listed in the FFQ was developed for the study to help investigators and participants better estimate quantities consumed. The portions consumed were then translated into daily consumption in grams. Daily consumption was later analyzed by Nutrilog software (Nutrilog, version 3.20, France) to extract daily nutrient intake. To extract dietary patterns, the 90 foods listed in the FFQ were then grouped into 20 predefined categories based on similarities in nutrient composition and consumption characteristics (Supplemental Material: Table S1). These categories were then entered in the K-mean cluster analysis to determine the dietary patterns of our population.

For all the categories of food, except for sweets, reported portions used to estimate consumption were based on standard portions adopted in the dietary guidelines 2015–2020 [53]. Sweetened soft drinks were added to sugars and jams after sugar content estimation was made. As for sweets and desserts, usual serving size was adopted for cluster analysis.

2.3. Statistical Analysis

Statistical analysis was performed using the SPSS program version 21.0. Difference between genders and frailty status for sociodemographic, nutritional, dietary, health-related, and anthropometric data, were compared using the non-parametric tests, Mann–Whitney and Kruskal–Wallis for numeric variables that are not normally distributed, and chi-square test for categorical variables. K-means clustering was used to regroup participants with similar dietary patterns. Differences in food intake between dietary patterns was calculated by Kruskal–Wallis test. Cut-offs for age, polypharmacy, multimorbidity, age-related conditions, and waist to height ratio (WHTR) were determined through classification tree and used for subsequent multivariate analysis. In the multivariate analyses, we proceeded to several models of binary logistic regression using dichotomized frailty variable as the dependent variable. Odds-ratios with 95% confidence intervals were calculated. The main explanatory variables reaching significance level identified in each model were added to the following model. Age category, marital status, education level, and living conditions were entered first (model 1). From this model, we retained covariates significantly associated with frailty and then added anthropometric variables including MNA-SF, BMI, and waist to height ratio categories (model 2). From model 2, we retained all covariates significantly associated with frailty and then added health-related covariates (multimorbidity, polypharmacy, and age-related conditions (model 3). From model 3, we retained all covariates significantly associated with frailty and finally added food dietary patterns (model 4). Each Model was rerun with the food patterns groups in order to adjust for the variables identified respectively in each model. The multivariate analysis was rerun for each gender. The level of significance was fixed at a $p = 0.05$ for all analyses.

3. Results

3.1. Sample Characteristics

The present analysis included 352 participants, with 50% being women. Details of the sample characteristics are shown in Table 1.

Table 1. Sociodemographic and clinical characteristics of the total sample, and stratified by gender ($N = 352$).

		Total ($N = 352$)	Men ($N = 176$)	Women ($N = 176$)	p Value
		Sociodemographic Status			
Age (years)		73 (67–79)	73 (67.3–80)	73 (67–78)	0.288
Marital status	Married	232 (65.9)	143 (81.3)	89 (50.6)	<0.001
	Divorced	10 (2.8)	4 (2.3)	6 (3.4)	
	Single	18 (5.1)	6 (3.4)	12 (6.8)	
	Widowed	92 (26.1)	23 (13.1)	69 (39.2)	
Living conditions	Living Alone	53 (15.1)	16 (9.1)	37 (21)	<0.001
	Living with partner	202 (57.4)	131 (74.4)	71 (30.3)	
	Living with others	97 (27.6)	29 (16.5)	68 (38.6)	
Education	Low level	149 (42.3)	65 (36.9)	84 (47.7)	0.04
Economic status	Insufficient income	198 (56.3)	98 (55.7)	100 (56.8)	0.159
		Health and Functional Status			
Frailty status	Frail	53 (15.1)	18 (10.2)	35 (19.9)	0.01
	Not frail	299 (84.9)	158 (89.8)	141 (80.1)	
Cognitive Status	Low cognitive test	116 (33)	57 (32.4)	59 (33.5)	0.821
Polypharmacy	≥6 drugs	254 (73.8)	133 (77.8)	121 (69.9)	0.098
Multi-morbidity	≥2 chronic illnesses	270 (76.9)	127 (72.6)	143 (81.3)	0.054
Age-related conditions	≥2 conditions	189 (53.7)	84 (47.7)	105 (59.7)	0.025
Physical Activity	Sedentary	275 (78.1)	146 (83)	129 (73.3)	0.301
	Regular Active	74 (21)	30 (17)	44 (25)	
	Optimal active	3 (0.9)	0 (0)	3 (1.7)	
Strength	HGS (kg)	23.1 (17.8–31.2)	31 (24.5–35.7)	18.3 (13.6–22.3)	<0.001
		Nutritional Status and Nutrient Intake			
BMI	BMI(kg/m^2)	28.2 (25–32.8)	27.5 (24.3–31.2)	29.7 (25.9–35.1)	<0.001
	BMI < 22	109 (31)	64 (36.4)	45 (25.6)	0.042
	BMI (22–27)	30 (8.5)	17 (9.7)	13 (7.4)	
	BMI > 27	213 (60.5)	95 (54)	118 (67)	

Table 1. Cont.

		Total (N = 352)	Men (N = 176)	Women (N = 176)	p Value
WTHR		0.64 (0.59–0.70)	0.62 (0.57–0.67)	0.67 (0.61–0.75)	<0.001
Nutritional status (MNA-SF score)	Normal	225 (63.9)	114 (64.8)	111 (63.1)	0.74
	Poor	127 (36.1)	62 (35.2)	65 (36.9)	
Energy and macronutrients intake	Energy (Kcal/d)	1824 (1509–2299)	2031 (1638–2447)	1726 (1408–2094)	<0.001
	Calories (Kcal/kg BW)	25.3 (20.1–31.8)	26.1 (20.1–31.8)	24.5 (19.5–31.9)	0.214
	Carbohydrates (g/d)	201 (161.3–258)	226 (178.5–293)	185.5 (145.3–218.5)	<0.001
	Proteins (g/d)	66.7 (50.1–84.1)	72.3 (58.9–92.3)	59.6 (46.1–73.2)	<0.001
	Proteins (g/kg BW)	0.91 (0.68–1.15)	0.94 (0.73–1.17)	0.85 (0.65–1.13)	0.022
	Fats (g/d)	89.2 (72.5–111)	90.4 (74.1–112.8)	86.3 (70.6–109.8)	0.076

Abbreviations: BMI: body mass index; WC: waist circumference; WHTR: waist to height ratio; HSG: handgrip strength; Kcal/d: Calories per day; Calories/kg BW: Calories per kg body weight; Protein/kg BW: Proteins per kg body weight. Numeric variables are represented as median (interquartile range). Categorical variables are represented as N (percentage).

The sample accounted for 15.1% frail individuals, with more women being classified as frail compared to men: 35 (19.9%) and 18 (10.2%), respectively. In addition, women had more age-related conditions compared to men and more women than men had a low educational level.

Median BMI for the total sample was 28.2 kg/m^2, with 60.5% of the sample having a BMI > 27 kg/m^2. Women had a significantly higher median BMI 29.7 (25.9–35.1) kg/m^2 compared to men 27.5 (24.3–31.2) kg/m^2. Median WHTR was also significantly higher among women. With 63.9% of the sample having a normal nutritional status as evaluated by MNA-SF, no difference was found between nutritional statuses among gender.

Median energy intake of the participants was 1824 Kcal/d. Energy, carbohydrates, and protein intakes were lower in women compared to men. Median protein intake per kg body weight (g/kg BW) was also lower in women (0.85 g/kg BW) compared to men (0.94 g/kg BW). Caloric intake per kg body weight (Kcal/kg BW) was nonetheless not different between the two sexes.

3.2. Dietary Patterns

As shown in Table 2, three dietary patterns were identified in the total sample. The first, named Westernized-type dietary pattern (WDP), followed by 11.9% of the participants (29 men and 13 women), was characterized by the highest caloric intake, consumption of refined flour products, sugar and sweets, dairy products, as well as processed and saturated fats and the lowest olive, seeds, and oleaginous fruits and whole cereal products intake. The second pattern, named high intake/Mediterranean-type dietary pattern (HI-MEDDP), adopted by 23% of participants (21 men and 60 women), was characterized by a relatively high caloric intake, a higher consumption of vegetables, fruits, legumes than the other 2 DPs, and the highest consumption of foods rich in monounsaturated fats. Median consumption of olive, seeds, and oleaginous fruits in the HI-MEDDP group was above nine teaspoons of oil equivalent per day. This pattern also had the lowest consumption of refined flour products, and the highest consumption of whole cereal products. Finally, the third pattern, named moderate intake/Mediterranean-type dietary pattern (MOD-MEDDP), represented the highest proportion of our sample (65.1% of the sample, with 126 men and 106 women), and was characterized by a diversified and balanced DP. Consumption of most foods in this pattern was either intermediate or lower compared to the other two patterns, with the lowest consumption of sweets and sugar among the three patterns.

Table 2. Consumption of predefined food categories according to dietary patterns for the overall sample. N = 352.

	WDP	HI-MEDDP	MOD-MEDDP	p Value
	N = 42 (11.9%)	N = 81 (23%)	N = 229 (65.1%)	
Kilocalories/day	2261 (1953–2845)	2028 (1652–2473)	1743 (1453–2123)	<0.001
Refined flour products	5.09 (3.38–7.84)	2.25 (0.7–5.09)	3.32 (1.15–5.11)	<0.001
Whole breads and cereals (including burghul)	0.35 (0.11–1.46)	1.49 (0.36–2.82)	0.76 (0.18–2.33)	0.008
Potato	0.4 (0.14–0.78)	0.27 (0.1–0.51)	0.25 (0.1–0.43)	0.024
Vegetables	2.9 (2.1–3.84)	3.74 (2.59–5.23)	2.93 (2.09–4.52)	0.002
Fruits	2.1 (1.09–2.78)	2.45 (1.52–3.4)	1.89 (1.25–2.86)	0.033
Legumes	0.3 (0.18–0.57)	0.57 (0.24–0.86)	0.29 (0.13–0.57)	0.006
Meat and poultry	2.26 (1.49–3.6)	2.02 (1.5–2.94)	1.93 (1.2–3.03)	0.137
Eggs	0.57 (0.25–0.86)	0.29 (0.18–0.57)	0.29 (0.1–0.57)	0.002
Fish and shellfish	0.42 (0.08–0.78)	0.43 (0.17–0.83)	0.4 (0.13–0.73)	0.568
Milk and dairy products	1.89 (1.05–2.61)	1.71 (0.99–2.43)	1.39 (0.85–2.05)	0.002
Vegetable oils	3 (0.94–4)	3 (1–3.62)	3 (2–3.08)	0.704
Olive, seeds and oleaginous fruits	4.03 (3–6.04)	9.87 (8.02–12.67)	4.16 (3.07–6.18)	<0.001
Processed and saturated fats	0.02 (0–1)	0 (0–0.17)	0 (0–0.18)	0.024
Low fat sweets	0.49 (0.07–2.11)	0.43 (0.08–1.33)	0.14 (0–0.36)	<0.001
High fat sweets	0.19 (0.07–0.49)	0.14 (0–0.43)	0.07 (0–0.26)	<0.001
Sugars and jams	8.5 (6.05–12.36)	3 (0.96–5.37)	1 (0.15–2.13)	<0.001

Abbreviations: WDP: Westernized dietary pattern; HI-MEDDP: high-intake Mediterranean dietary pattern; MOD-Med: moderate-intake Mediterranean dietary pattern. Caloric intake and intake of food groups per day are represented as Median (interquartile range). Values represent the cluster centers of each food group in the three identified food patterns, expressed in portions/day.

Gender-specific food consumption characteristics of the 3 DP, showed that women following the WDP consumed more sugar portions (median consumption of 13 teaspoons of sugars and jams) than men (equivalent to almost seven teaspoons of added sugar) in this same pattern, although median energy intake was on average lower in women compared to men. Men and women adopting the HI-MEDDP had the highest median consumption of olive, seeds, and oleaginous fruits (12 and 9 teaspoons equivalent of fat, respectively) (data in Supplementary Table S2).

3.3. Frailty

3.3.1. Frailty Association with Sociodemographic and Health-Related Factors

Sociodemographic, health, and nutritional characteristics of the study sample according to the frailty status are represented in Table 3. Factors associated with frailty included higher age, female gender, and lower educational level (<7 years at school); the latter was not associated to frailty in men.

Table 3. Sociodemographic and health-related factors associated with frailty in total sample and stratified by gender.

		Total			Men			Women		
		N = 352			176 (50)			176 (50)		
		Non-Frail	Frail	p Value	Non-Frail	Frail	p Value	Non-Frail	Frail	p Value
N (%)		299 (84.9)	53 (15.1)		158 (89.8)	18 (10.2)		141 (80.1)	35 (19.9)	
		Sociodemographic Parameters								
Age (years)		72 (60–93)	78 (60–91)	<0.001	72 (60–93)	82 (60–88)	0.003	72 (60–90)	76 (65–91)	0.001
Education	Elementary and lower	116 (38.8)	33 (62.3)	0.001	57 (36.1)	8 (44.4)	0.486	59 (41.8)	25 (71.4)	0.002

Table 3. Cont.

	Total			Men			Women		
				Health-Related Parameters					
Polypharmacy	61 (21)	29 (54.7)	<0.001	32 (20.9)	6 (33.3)	0.231	29 (21)	23 (65.7)	<0.001
Multi-morbidity	218 (73.2)	52 (98.1)	<0.001	110 (70.1)	17 (94.4)	0.028	108 (76.6)	35 (100)	<0.001
Age-related conditions	148 (49.5)	41 (77.4)	<0.01	74 (46.8)	10 (55.6)	0.483	74 (52.5)	31 (88.6)	<0.001
				Anthropometric Parameters					
BMI (kg/m^2)	28.1 (16.5–49.4)	29.8 (18.5–46.2)	0.096	27.5 (16.5–40)	26.1 (18.5–34)	0.173	28.9 (18.2–49.4)	32.4 (19.6–46.1)	0.018
WHTR	0.64 (0.42–0.99)	0.69 (0.49–1)	<0.001	0.62 (0.42–0.41)	0.6 (0.52–0.69)	0.705	0.65 (0.5–0.99)	0.75 (0.49–1)	<0.001
				Nutritional Status, Strength, and Activity					
Low HGS		127 (45)	44 (86.3)	<0.001	64 (43)	13 (81.2)	0.004	63 (47.4)	31 (88.6)	<0.001
Physical activity	Sedentary	224 (74.9)	51 (96.2)		128 (81)	18 (100)		96 (68.1)	33 (94.3)	
	Regular	72 (24.1)	2 (3.8)	<0.001	30 (19)	0 (0)	0.042	42 (29.8)	2 (5.7)	<0.001
	Optimal	3 (1)	0 (0.0)		0 (0)	0 (0)		3 (2.1)	0 (0)	
Poor nutritional status		96 (32.1)	31 (58.5)	<0.001	51 (32.3)	10 (55.6)	<0.001	44 (31.2)	21 (60)	<0.001

Abbreviations: BMI: body mass index; WC: waist circumference; WHTR: waist to height ratio; HSG: handgrip strength; MNA-SF: Mini-Nutritional Assessment-Short Form. Numeric variables are represented as median (interquartile range). Categorical variables are represented as N (%).

Taking more than five medications, having more than one disease, more than one age-related condition, and having a higher WHTR was associated with frailty in the total sample and in women. In men, only multimorbidity was found to be associated with frailty, whereas no association with health and anthropometric parameters was observed.

Regarding nutritional status evaluated by MNA-SF, we identified a significant association with frailty, with a higher prevalence of poor nutritional status (malnutrition and risk of malnutrition) among frail individuals in both genders.

3.3.2. Frailty and Dietary Patterns

Table 4 displays the dietary patterns and food intake associated with frailty.

Table 4. Dietary patterns, food, and nutrient intake associated with frailty in the total sample and stratified by gender.

	Total (N = 352)			Men (N = 176)			Women (N = 176)		
	Non-Frail 299 (85)	Frail 53 (15)	p	Non-Frail 158 (90)	Frail 18 (10)	p	Non-Frail 141 (80)	Frail 35 (20)	p
				Food Patterns					
WDP	33 (11)	9 (17)	0.125	26 (16.5)	3 (16.7)	0.673	7 (5)	6 (17.1)	0.01
HI-MEDDP	65 (21.7)	16 (30.2)		20 (12.7)	1 (5.6)		45 (31.9)	15 (42.9)	
MOD-MEDDP	201 (67.2)	28 (52.8)		112 (70.9)	14 (77.8)		89 (63.1)	14 (40)	
				Food Intake					
Sugars and jams	1.8 (0.29–4)	2 (0.36–5.5)	0.21	1.64 (0.32–4)	2.14 (0.25–4)	0.794	1.93 (0.3–3.75)	1.85 (0.43–6.7)	0.204
Low fat sweets	0.17 (0.01–0.59)	0.3 (0.08–1.08)	0.037	0.13 (0–0.47)	0.15 (0.04–0.5)	0.53	0.24 (0.04–0.8)	0.37 (0.14–1.3)	0.097
Fruits and Vegetables	5.6 (4.1–7.4)	4.8 (3.1–6.6)	0.022	5.8 (4.08–7.35)	4.7 (3.8–6.9)	0.196	5.6 (4.2–7.5)	5.2 (3.1–6.4)	0.07
Vegetable oils	3 (1.5–3.1)	3 (2.5–4)	0.027	3 (1.5–3.16)	3 (1–3)	0.96	3 (1.5–3.08)	3 (3–4)	0.009

Table 4. Cont.

	Total (N = 352)			Men (N = 176)			Women (N = 176)		
Olive, seeds and oleaginous fruits	5.04 (3.3–7.7)	6 (3.6–8.3)	0.513	5.2 (3.3–7.5)	5.1 (3.96–6.7)	0.786	4.8 (3.4–7.82)	6.4 (3.4–9.1)	0.305
Energy and Macronutrients									
Caloric intake (Cal/d)	1851 (1543–2349)	1763 (1398–2075)	0.039	2077.5 (1667–2487)	1734 (1422–1900)	0.025	1709 (1416–2082)	1763 (1388–2120)	0.859
Kilocalories/kg BW	25.63 (20.1–32.1)	23.1 (19.4–30.3)	0.095	26.5 (21.03–32.1)	22.4 (18.2–29.9)	0.107	24.93 (19.84–31.9)	23.7 (19.4–31.7)	0.457
Carbohydrates (g)	204 (166–263)	184 (143–217)	0.009	237.5 (181–295)	198.5 (152–233)	0.038	188 (149–219)	167 (129–217)	0.356
Proteins (g)	67.8 (51.3–84.8)	57.4 (44.9–70.5)	0.006	74.05 (60.4–94.1)	62 (51.8–84.6)	0.033	61.1 (46.3–77.4)	54.4 (44.1–70.5)	0.295
Protein/kg BW	0.93 (0.69–1.17)	0.81 (0.66–0.97)	0.016	0.96 (0.74–1.18)	0.81 (0.73–1.07)	0.133	0.87 (0.65–1.16)	0.81 (0.63–1)	0.161
FAT (g)	89.5 (74.1–111)	84.9 (66.2–113)	0.328	91.65 (75.8–115)	81.25 (63.8–107)	0.058	85.8 (70.7–107)	90.9 (70–119)	0.638

Abbreviations: WDP: Westernized dietary pattern. HI-MEDDP: high-intake Mediterranean dietary pattern. MOD-Med: moderate-intake Mediterranean dietary pattern. Kcal/d: calories per day. Calories/kg BW: calories per kg body weight. Protein/kg BW: proteins per kg body weight. Numeric variables are represented as median (interquartile range). Categorical variables are represented as N (%).

Individuals adopting the MOD-MEDDP accounted for 67.2% of the non-frail group compared to 21.7% and 11%, for the HI-MEDDP and WDP, respectively. Nonetheless, in the univariate analysis, dietary patterns seemed to be associated with frailty status only in women. Women adopting the WDP accounted for 5% of the non-frail group compared to 17.1% of the frail group, and women adopting the MOD-MEDDP accounted for 63.1% of the non-frail group compared to 40% of the frail group.

Concerning nutrients, median caloric, carbohydrates, and protein intakes were higher in the non-frail compared to frail group, in the total population, and in men. Median g of protein/kg BW was found to be significantly higher in the non-frail group, only in the overall population.

The multivariate logistic regression analysis performed in the total sample (Table 5), included 327 individuals with complete set of data each, and fulfilling all criteria of inclusion. Within the total sample, in the first model, independent factors associated with frailty, included age above 75 years, female gender, and low level of education. When anthropometric and nutritional status parameters were added in the second model, factors associated with frailty were age above 75 years, WHTR > 0.718 and poor nutritional status compared to normal nutritional status. In the third model, when health-related parameters were added to the analysis, factors associated with frailty included age, WHTR > 0.718, poor nutritional status, polypharmacy, multimorbidity, and age-related conditions. In the final model, by adding dietary patterns, independent factors comprised age above 75 years, WHTR > 0.718, poor nutritional status, polypharmacy, age-related conditions, and WDP.

The multivariate association between dietary patterns and frailty is described in Table 6. In the overall sample, no association was observed between dietary patterns and frailty prevalence. After adjusting for main confounders, women adopting the WDP, compared to those adopting the MOD-MEDDP, exhibited a higher prevalence of frailty, in the first and second models, as well as in the fully adjusted model (odds ratio ((OR) 11.54, 95% confidence interval (CI) (2.02–65.85)). In men, similar results were observed: adopting a WDP was associated with a higher prevalence of frailty only in the fully adjusted model, ((OR) 6.63, 95% (CI) (1.82–24.21)), when compared to the MOD-MEDDP. Finally, the HI-MEDDP was not significantly associated with frailty prevalence, in the overall sample, nor in men compared with following a MOD-MEDDP.

Table 5. Binary logistic regression models of frail vs. non-frail for the total sample.

Associated Factors	Model 1	Model 2	Model 3	Model 4
	Sociodemographic Parameters			
Age > 75 years	3.667 (1.93–6.99)	3.55 (1.75–7.21)	2.91(1.42–5.94)	2.83(1.42–5.63)
Female gender	2.66 (1.33–5.29)	2.11 (0.99–4.49)		
Low Education level (<7 years of education)	2.19 (1.17–4.11)	1.96 (0.98–3.93)	1.93 (0.94–3.97)	
Living conditions (compared with living alone) with partner with others	0.64 (0.26–1.59) 1.14 (0.35–3.7)			
Marital status (married vs. other status)	1.95 (0.78–4.9)			
		Nutritional and Anthropometric Parameters		
WHTR>0.718		2.94 (1.27–6.76)	3.27 (1.56–6.83)	3.78 (1.71–8.33)
Poor nutritional status (malnutrition and at risk vs normal)		14.26 (4.64–43.81)	10.79 (3.29–35.35)	9.67 (3.1–30.18)
BMI (compared with BMI < 22 kg/m²) BMI (22–27) BMI (>27)		0.72 (0.16–3.25) 1.24 (0.52–2.98)		
			Health-Related Parameters	
Polypharmacy			2.74 (1.34–5.6)	4.42 (2.21–8.86)
Age related conditions			2.28 (1.03–5.03)	2.47 (1.17–5.24)
Multimorbidity			7.18 (0.92–56.03)	
				Dietary Patterns
MOD-MEDDP pattern WDP pattern HI-MEDDP pattern				1 2.97 (1.12–7.89) 2.27 (0.98–5.25)

Note: Bold values are statistically significant, $p < 0.05$.

Table 6. Multivariate associations between dietary patterns and frailty prevalence. Beirut 2021, N = 327.

	Dietary Patterns	Frail Individuals N (%) 53 (15)	Model 1 OR (95% CI)	p	Model 2 OR (95% CI)	p	Model 3 OR (95% CI)	p
				0.176		0.074		0.083
Total	MOD-MEDDP	28 (52.8)	1		1		1	
	WDP	9 (17)	2.25(0.91–5.53)	0.078	2.44 (0.93–6.43)	0.07	2.68 (0.98–7.29)	0.054
	HI-MEDDP	16 (30.2)	1.45 (0.7–2.98)	0.316	2.08 (0.96–4.54)	0.065	1.96 (0.86–4.45)	0.109
				0.482		0.735		0.011
Men	MOD-MEDDP	14 (77.8)	1		1		1	
	WDP	3 (16.7)	1.14 (0.29–4.53)	0.85	0.89 (0.18–4.39)	0.885	6.63 (1.82–24.21)	0.004
	HI-MEDDP	1 (5.6)	0.28 (0.03–2.35)	0.243	0.43 (0.05–3.62)	0.434	2.23 (0.93–5.32)	0.071
				0.027		0.013		0.013
Women	MOD-MEDDP	14 (40)	1		1		1	
	WDP	6 (17.1)	4.57 (1.25–16.76)	0.022	6.76 (1.56–29.22)	0.01	11.54 (2.02–65.85)	0.006
	HI-MEDDP	15 (42.9)	2.44 (1.02–5.79)	0.044	3.06 (1.15–8.15)	0.025	3.06 (0.97–9.62)	0.056

Model 1: model adjusted for age, gender, educational level. Model 2: model 1 further adjusted for nutritional status, and WHTR. Model 3: model 2 further adjusted for polypharmacy and age-related conditions.

4. Discussion

Our study aimed at describing the prevalence of frailty and its associated factors, including dietary patterns, in a national sample of community dwelling older Lebanese individuals. In this rural and urban low socioeconomic sample, the estimated prevalence of frailty was 15% on average, with 10% and 20% in men and women, respectively. In men, poor nutritional status and being older than 75 years were found to be associated with frailty. In women, in addition to these two factors, taking more than five drugs daily, having at least one age-related condition, having a WHTR > 0.718 and following a Westernized-type DP were found to be independently associated with frailty. In women, the HI-MEDDP showed a significant association with frailty prevalence after adjusting for age, educational level, nutritional status, and WHTR. However, this failed to be significant after further adjusting for polypharmacy and age-related conditions.

Our frailty prevalence can be compared to findings of a meta-analysis conducted in 2018, where pooled prevalence of frailty was 17.4% [42]. A Lebanese national study involving 1200 individuals reported a higher prevalence of frailty, at 36.4%, in an exclusively rural elderly population. In this previous study, 73% of the sample had a monthly income below the minimum wage, whereas in our studied sample, 57.8% had low or insufficient income [19]. The difference with our results can be explained by the variability in study design and tools used for the evaluation of frailty, as well as the heterogeneity between rural and urban settings. Rural areas, being usually poorer and more affected by urban migration of young adults, might witness a higher proportion of frail individuals. [45,54–56].

As shown in previous research, women are more often frail than men [54]. Our results also showed that a low educational level (less than 7 years) was associated with prevalence of frailty, particularly in women. As described in the Longitudinal Aging Study in Amsterdam, the impact of low educational level increased the odds of frailty almost three-fold and this association persisted throughout the 13 years of follow-up [57]. Health related parameters were also found to be associated with frailty, particularly in women; they were frailer if they were taking more than five drugs every day, suffered from two or more diseases, and had at least one age-related condition. These factors have been often linked to frailty in several settings [14,58–62].

WHTR was associated with frailty, in the multivariate analysis, suggesting a possible role of higher abdominal adiposity. Although low BMI is known to be associated with frailty, obesity is also considered as risk a factor of frailty [24]. A meta-analysis showed that overweight individuals (BMI between 25–30 kg/m^2) exhibited an increased risk of frailty by 20%, whereas obese (BMI $\geq$ 30), have an increased frailty risk of 90% [21]. In the longitudinal Doetinchem Study, a BMI < 23 kg/m^2 and $\geq$30 kg/m^2 was associated with higher incidence of frailty [25]. Similar results were found in the Japanese cohort with a lowest incidence of frailty at a BMI between 21.4 and 25.7 kg/m^2 [22]. As shown by Kim et al., the risk of frailty is higher in obese women, which is mediated by WHTR, but not in obese men [28]. In Spain, two cohort studies showed a parallel change of abdominal obesity and BMI to be associated with an increasing risk of frailty [63].

The level of malnutrition was identified as an independent risk factor associated with frailty, although our sample had a high proportion of obese. Our study showed that malnutrition was associated with a substantially increased prevalence of frailty in the total sample and in both gender groups. The relation between malnutrition and frailty was already clearly established in previous studies, and overweight and obesity often co-exist with frailty [21,22,27,28,63–65].

Among the three dietary patterns identified in our study, the WDP was associated with a higher prevalence of frailty, in both men and women, independently of major confounding factors. This pattern was characterized by a high median sugar intake particularly in in women, and the highest consumption among the three patterns in refined flour products. Several studies reported a link between sugar consumption and the risk of frailty. In the 5-year cohort Seniors-ENRICA study, a high consumption of added sugar, $\geq$ 36 g/day, compared to <15 g/day, was found to increase the odds of frailty by almost two-fold [66]. Furthermore, in the Nurses' Health Study, after adjustment for confounding factors, consumption of $\geq$2 servings of sugar-sweetened beverages per day compared to no consumption, increased the risk of frailty by almost 30% over a period of 22 years [67].

Healthy moderate DP and Mediterranean DP were often reported to be inversely associated with frailty [34,36,68,69]. Frailty risk was also found to be inversely associated with consumption of fruits and vegetables [70–72]. Our analysis showed that the Mediterranean dietary pattern with moderate intakes, represented by the MOD-MEDDP in our study, had the lowest prevalence of frailty. On the other hand, when HI-MEDDP group was compared to MOD-MEDDP in women, the predominance of obesity in this group, with a concomitant high fat intake (the highest among the 3 DPs) and a median protein intake of 0.9 g/kg BW, may have contributed to frailty in this subcategory. This could suggest that these conditions, regardless of the quality of fat and diet, could outweigh the beneficial effect of a Mediterranean diet on the prevalence of frailty. Previous reports suggested that protein intake between 1 and 1.5 g/kg BW were necessary for the prevention of frailty [29–32].

In summary, our study was the first to explore the association between frailty and specific dietary patterns extracted in a posteriori method, in adults over 60 years of age in Lebanon, using specifically validated questionnaires. Despite the difficulties in addressing this specific age group, we succeeded in shedding light on some findings specific to our Mediterranean older adult population. Age, age-related conditions, polypharmacy, and malnutrition, remain the main associated factors related to frailty in low socioeconomic settings. We also showed that malnutrition and abdominal obesity co-exist as risk factors for frailty. Most importantly, we demonstrated that a Westernized-type pattern with high sugar consumption, and to a lesser extent, a Mediterranean high caloric intake pattern, were also linked to frailty, and that a more moderate Mediterranean-like pattern was protective, especially in women. More efforts should target actions that improve modifiable factors to prevent or reverse frailty, such as eating patterns and diets that improve WHTR.

We note, however, some limitations concerning our results in relation to the low number of frail participants adopting the WDP; this consequently implies taking the present findings with caution.

Larger prospective studies are required to further investigate the impact of dietary patterns on risk of frailty with a special emphasis on WHTR.

In conclusion, WDP had the strongest association with frailty in this sample. MOD-MEDDP, in comparison to HI-MEDDP and WDP, was associated with the least prevalence of frailty. In this Mediterranean sample, a diet far from the traditional one appears as a key deleterious determinant of frailty.

Supplementary Materials: The following are available online at https://www.mdpi.com/article/10.3390/nu13072188/s1, Table S1: food groups and food items included in the cluster analysis, Table S2: consumption of predefined food categories according to dietary patterns for men and women separately, Table S3: nutritional characteristics of the dietary patterns.

Author Contributions: Conceptualization and methodology, N.Y., C.B.; validation, M.A., C.B., C.F.; formal analysis, C.Y. and N.Y.; data curation, N.Y.; writing—original draft preparation, N.Y.; review and editing, C.B., M.A., and C.F.; supervision, C.B.; project administration and funding acquisition, N.Y., M.A. All authors have read and agreed to the published version of the manuscript.

Funding: This research was funded by the Research Council of the Saint Joseph University of Beirut, grant number FPH66.

Institutional Review Board Statement: The study was conducted according to the guidelines of the Declaration of Helsinki, and approved by the Ethics Committee of SAINT JOSEPH UNIVERSITY (USJ 2016-99).

Informed Consent Statement: Informed consent was obtained from all subjects involved in the study.

Acknowledgments: We would like to thank Fernande Abou Haidar, Samar Sleilati, and Marie Elias from the Ministry of Social Affairs/Department of Family Affairs, and Rita Hayeck, & Rafic Baddoura from the National Commission for the Elderly, for their precious collaboration and support.

Conflicts of Interest: The authors declare no conflict of interest.

References

1. Fried, L.P.; Tangen, C.M.; Walston, J.; Newman, A.B.; Hirsch, C.; Gottdiener, J.; Seeman, T.; Tracy, R.; Kop, W.J.; Burke, G.; et al. Frailty in Older Adults: Evidence for a Phenotype. *J. Gerontol. A Biol. Sci. Med. Sci.* **2001**, *56*, M146–M157. [CrossRef]
2. Verlaan, S.; Ligthart-Melis, G.C.; Wijers, S.L.J.; Cederholm, T.; Maier, A.B.; de van der Schueren, M.A.E. High Prevalence of Physical Frailty Among Community-Dwelling Malnourished Older Adults—A Systematic Review and Meta-Analysis. *J. Am. Med. Dir. Assoc.* **2017**, *18*, 374–382. [CrossRef]
3. Crow, R.S.; Lohman, M.C.; Pidgeon, D.; Bruce, M.L.; Bartels, S.J.; Batsis, J.A. Frailty Versus Stopping Elderly Accidents, Deaths and Injuries Initiative Fall Risk Score: Ability to Predict Future Falls. *J. Am. Geriatr. Soc.* **2018**, *66*, 577–583. [CrossRef]
4. Marques, A.; Queirós, C. Frailty, Sarcopenia and Falls. In *Fragility Fracture Nursing*; Hertz, K., Santy-Tomlinson, J., Eds.; Perspectives in Nursing Management and Care for Older Adults; Springer International Publishing: Cham, Switzerland, 2018; pp. 15–26. ISBN 978-3-319-76680-5.
5. Morley, J.E. The New Geriatric Giants. *Clin. Geriatr. Med.* **2017**, *33*, xi–xii. [CrossRef]
6. Kojima, G. Frailty as a Predictor of Disabilities among Community-Dwelling Older People: A Systematic Review and Meta-Analysis. *Disabil. Rehabil.* **2017**, *39*, 1897–1908. [CrossRef]
7. Nwagwu, V.C.; Cigolle, C.; Suh, T. Reducing Frailty to Promote Healthy Aging. *Clin. Geriatr. Med.* **2020**, *36*, 613–630. [CrossRef]
8. Lorenzo-López, L.; López-López, R.; Maseda, A.; Buján, A.; Rodríguez-Villamil, J.L.; Millán-Calenti, J.C. Changes in Frailty Status in a Community-Dwelling Cohort of Older Adults: The VERISAÚDE Study. *Maturitas* **2019**, *119*, 54–60. [CrossRef]
9. Zamudio-Rodríguez, A.; Letenneur, L.; Féart, C.; Avila-Funes, J.A.; Amieva, H.; Pérès, K. The Disability Process: Is There a Place for Frailty? *Age Ageing* **2020**, *49*, 764–770. [CrossRef] [PubMed]
10. Fried, L.P.; Cohen, A.A.; Xue, Q.-L.; Walston, J.; Bandeen-Roche, K.; Varadhan, R. The Physical Frailty Syndrome as a Transition from Homeostatic Symphony to Cacophony. *Nat. Aging* **2021**, *1*, 36–46. [CrossRef]
11. Kojima, G.; Walters, K.; Iliffe, S.; Taniguchi, Y.; Tamiya, N. Kojima Gotaro Marital Status and Risk of Physical Frailty: A Systematic Review and Meta-Analysis. *J. Am. Med. Dir. Assoc.* **2020**, *21*, 322–330. [CrossRef] [PubMed]
12. Kingston, A.; Davies, K.; Collerton, J.; Robinson, L.; Duncan, R.; Kirkwood, T.B.L.; Jagger, C. The Enduring Effect of Education-Socioeconomic Differences in Disability Trajectories from Age 85 Years in the Newcastle 85+ Study. *Arch. Gerontol. Geriatr.* **2015**, *60*, 405–411. [CrossRef] [PubMed]
13. Soysal, P.; Veronese, N.; Thompson, T.; Kahl, K.G.; Fernandes, B.S.; Prina, A.M.; Solmi, M.; Schofield, P.; Koyanagi, A.; Tseng, P.T.; et al. Pinar Soysal Relationship between Depression and Frailty in Older Adults: A Systematic Review and Meta-Analysis. *Ageing Res. Rev.* **2017**, *36*, 78–87. [CrossRef] [PubMed]
14. Gutiérrez-Valencia, M.; Izquierdo, M.; Cesari, M.; Casas-Herrero, Á.; Inzitari, M.; Martínez-Velilla, N. The Relationship between Frailty and Polypharmacy in Older People: A Systematic Review: Frailty and Polypharmacy: A Systematic Review. *Br. J. Clin. Pharmacol.* **2018**, *84*, 1432–1444. [CrossRef]
15. Lorenzo-López, L.; Maseda, A.; de Labra, C.; Regueiro-Folgueira, L.; Rodríguez-Villamil, J.L.; Millán-Calenti, J.C. Nutritional Determinants of Frailty in Older Adults: A Systematic Review. *BMC Geriatr.* **2017**, *17*, 108. [CrossRef]
16. Hubbard, R.E. Sex Differences in Frailty. *Frailty Aging* **2015**, *41*, 41–53. [CrossRef]
17. Zhang, Q.; Guo, H.; Gu, H.; Zhao, X. Gender-Associated Factors for Frailty and Their Impact on Hospitalization and Mortality among Community-Dwelling Older Adults: A Cross-Sectional Population-Based Study. *PeerJ* **2018**, *6*, e4326. [CrossRef] [PubMed]
18. Ofori-Asenso, R.; Chin, K.L.; Mazidi, M.; Zomer, E.; Ilomaki, J.; Zullo, A.R.; Gasevic, D.; Ademi, Z.; Korhonen, M.J.; LoGiudice, D.; et al. Global Incidence of Frailty and Prefrailty Among Community-Dwelling Older Adults. *JAMA Netw. Open* **2019**, *2*. [CrossRef]
19. Boulos, C.; Salameh, P.; Barberger-Gateau, P. Malnutrition and Frailty in Community Dwelling Older Adults Living in a Rural Setting. *Clin. Nutr.* **2016**, *35*, 138–143. [CrossRef]
20. Kizilarslanoglu, M.C.; Sumer, F.; Kuyumcu, M.E. Malnutrition Increases Frailty among Older Adults: How? *Clin. Nutr.* **2016**, *35*, 979. [CrossRef]
21. Amiri, S.; Behnezhad, S.; Hasani, J. Amiri Sohrab Body Mass Index and Risk of Frailty in Older Adults: A Systematic Review and Meta-Analysis. *Obes. Med.* **2020**, *18*, 100196. [CrossRef]
22. Watanabe, D.; Yoshida, T.; Watanabe, Y.; Yamada, Y.; Kimura, M. A U-Shaped Relationship between the Prevalence of Frailty and Body Mass Index in Community-Dwelling Japanese Older Adults: The Kyoto–Kameoka Study. *J. Clin. Med.* **2020**, *9*, 1367. [CrossRef]
23. Crow, R.S.; Petersen, C.L.; Cook, S.B.; Stevens, C.J.; Titus, A.J.; Mackenzie, T.A.; Batsis, J.A. Weight Change in Older Adults and Risk of Frailty. *J. Frailty Aging.* **2020**, *9*, 74–81.
24. Tabue-Teguo, M.; Pérès, K.; Simo, N.; Le Goff, M.; Perez Zepeda, M.U.; Féart, C.; Dartigues, J.-F.; Amieva, H.; Cesari, M. Gait Speed and Body Mass Index: Results from the AMI Study. *PLoS ONE* **2020**, *15*, e0229979. [CrossRef]
25. Rietman, M.L.; van der A, D.L.; van Oostrom, S.H.; Picavet, H.S.J.; Dollé, M.E.T.; van Steeg, H.; Verschuren, W.M.M.; Spijkerman, A.M.W. The Association Between BMI and Different Frailty Domains: A U-Shaped Curve? *J. Nutr. Health Aging* **2018**, *22*, 8–15. [CrossRef] [PubMed]
26. Easton, J.F.; Stephens, C.R.; Román-Sicilia, H.; Cesari, M.; Pérez-Zepeda, M.U. Anthropometric Measurements and Mortality in Frail Older Adults. *Exp. Gerontol.* **2018**, *110*, 61–66. [CrossRef] [PubMed]
27. Krakauer, N.Y.; Krakauer, J.C. Association of Body Shape Index (ABSI) with Hand Grip Strength. *Int. J. Environ. Res. Public Health* **2020**, *17*, 6797. [CrossRef] [PubMed]

28. Kim, M.; Lee, Y.; Kim, E.-Y.; Park, Y. Mediating Effect of Waist: Height Ratio on the Association between BMI and Frailty: The Korean Frailty and Aging Cohort Study. Available online: https://www.cambridge.org/core/journals/british-journal-of-nutrition/article/mediating-effect-of-waistheight-ratio-on-the-association-between-bmi-and-frailty-the-korean-frailty-and-aging-cohort-study/CCF95088B753D1ED366C8C436D963F3F (accessed on 17 October 2020).
29. Coelho-Júnior, H.; Rodrigues, B.; Uchida, M.; Marzetti, E. Low Protein Intake Is Associated with Frailty in Older Adults: A Systematic Review and Meta-Analysis of Observational Studies. *Nutrients* **2018**, *10*, 1334. [CrossRef] [PubMed]
30. Sandoval-Insausti, H.; Pérez-Tasigchana, R.F.; López-García, E.; García-Esquinas, E.; Rodríguez-Artalejo, F.; Guallar-Castillón, P. Macronutrients Intake and Incident Frailty in Older Adults: A Prospective Cohort Study. *J. Gerontol. Ser. A* **2016**, *71*, 1329–1334. [CrossRef] [PubMed]
31. Nanri, H.; Yamada, Y.; Yoshida, T.; Okabe, Y.; Nozawa, Y.; Itoi, A.; Yoshimura, E.; Watanabe, Y.; Yamaguchi, M.; Yokoyama, K.; et al. Sex Difference in the Association Between Protein Intake and Frailty: Assessed Using the Kihon Checklist Indexes Among Older Adults. *J. Am. Med. Dir. Assoc.* **2018**, *19*, 801–805. [CrossRef]
32. Rahi, B.; Colombet, Z.; Gonzalez-Colaço Harmand, M.; Dartigues, J.-F.; Boirie, Y.; Letenneur, L.; Feart, C. Higher Protein but Not Energy Intake Is Associated With a Lower Prevalence of Frailty Among Community-Dwelling Older Adults in the French Three-City Cohort. *J. Am. Med. Dir. Assoc.* **2016**, *17*, 672.e7–672.e11. [CrossRef] [PubMed]
33. Rashidi Pour Fard, N.; Amirabdollahian, F.; Haghighatdoost, F. Dietary Patterns and Frailty: A Systematic Review and Meta-Analysis. *Nutr. Rev.* **2019**, *77*, 498–513. [CrossRef] [PubMed]
34. Kojima, G.; Avgerinou, C.; Iliffe, S.; Walters, K. Adherence to Mediterranean Diet Reduces Incident Frailty Risk: Systematic Review and Meta-Analysis. *J. Am. Geriatr. Soc.* **2018**, *66*, 783–788. [CrossRef]
35. Bollwein, J.; Diekmann, R.; Kaiser, M.J.; Bauer, J.M.; Uter, W.; Sieber, C.C.; Volkert, D. Dietary Quality Is Related to Frailty in Community-Dwelling Older Adults. *J. Gerontol. Ser. A Biol. Sci. Med. Sci.* **2013**, *68*, 483–489. [CrossRef] [PubMed]
36. Ntanasi, E.; Yannakoulia, M.; Kosmidis, M.-H.; Anastasiou, C.A.; Dardiotis, E.; Hadjigeorgiou, G.; Sakka, P.; Scarmeas, N. Adherence to Mediterranean Diet and Frailty. *J. Am. Med. Dir. Assoc.* **2018**, *19*, 315–322.e2. [CrossRef] [PubMed]
37. Machón, M.; Mateo-Abad, M.; Vrotsou, K.; Zupiria, X.; Güell, C.; Rico, L.; Vergara, I. Dietary Patterns and Their Relationship with Frailty in Functionally Independent Older Adults. *Nutrients* **2018**, *10*, 406. [CrossRef]
38. Parsons, T.J.; Papachristou, E.; Atkins, J.L.; Papacosta, O.; Ash, S.; Lennon, L.T.; Whincup, P.H.; Ramsay, S.E.; Wannamethee, S.G. Physical Frailty in Older Men: Prospective Associations with Diet Quality and Patterns. *Age Ageing* **2019**, *48*, 355–360. [CrossRef]
39. de Haas, S.C.M.; de Jonge, E.A.L.; Voortman, T.; Graaff, J.S.; Franco, O.H.; Ikram, M.A.; Rivadeneira, F.; Kiefte-de Jong, J.C.; Schoufour, J.D. Dietary Patterns and Changes in Frailty Status: The Rotterdam Study. *Eur. J. Nutr.* **2018**, *57*, 2365–2375. [CrossRef]
40. Pilleron, S.; Ajana, S.; Jutand, M.-A.; Helmer, C.; Dartigues, J.-F.; Samieri, C.; Féart, C. Dietary Patterns and 12-Year Risk of Frailty: Results From the Three-City Bordeaux Study. *J. Am. Med. Dir. Assoc.* **2017**, *18*, 169–175. [CrossRef]
41. Ghosh, T.S.; Rampelli, S.; Jeffery, I.B.; Santoro, A.; Neto, M.; Capri, M.; Giampieri, E.; Jennings, A.; Candela, M.; Turroni, S.; et al. Mediterranean Diet Intervention Alters the Gut Microbiome in Older People Reducing Frailty and Improving Health Status: The NU-AGE 1-Year Dietary Intervention across Five European Countries. *Gut* **2020**, *69*, 1218–1228. [CrossRef]
42. Siriwardhana, D.D.; Hardoon, S.; Rait, G.; Weerasinghe, M.C.; Walters, K.R. Prevalence of Frailty and Prefrailty among Community-Dwelling Older Adults in Low-Income and Middle-Income Countries: A Systematic Review and Meta-Analysis. *BMJ Open* **2018**, *8*, e018195. [CrossRef] [PubMed]
43. El Zoghbi, M.; Boulos, C.; Awada, S.; Rachidi, S.; All Hajje, A.; Bawab, W.; Saleh, N.; Salameh, P. Prevalence of Malnutrition and Its Correlates in Older Adults Living in Long Stay Institutions Situated in Beirut, Lebanon. *J. Res. Health Sci.* **2013**, *14*, 11–17. [CrossRef]
44. El-Hayeck, R.; Baddoura, R.; Wehbé, A.; Bassil, N.; Koussa, S.; Khaled, K.; Richa, S.; Khoury, R.; Alameddine, A.; Sellal, F. An Arabic Version of the Mini-Mental State Examination for the Lebanese Population: Reliability, Validity, and Normative Data. *J. Alzheimer's Dis.* **2019**, *71*, 525–540. [CrossRef]
45. Living Conditions of Households 2007 | UNDP in Lebanon. Available online: https://www.lb.undp.org/content/lebanon/en/home/library/poverty/living-conditions-of-households-2007.html (accessed on 13 October 2020).
46. Maillet, D.; Matharan, F.; Clésiau, H.; Bailon, O.; Peres, K.; Amieva, H.; Belin, C. TNI-93: A New Memory Test for Dementia Detection in Illiterate and Low-Educated Patients. *Arch. Clin. Neuropsychol. Off. J. Natl. Acad. Neuropsychol.* **2016**, *31*. [CrossRef] [PubMed]
47. Morley, J.E.; Malmstrom, T.K.; Miller, D.K. A Simple Frailty Questionnaire (FRAIL) Predicts Outcomes in Middle Aged African Americans. *J. Nutr. Health Aging* **2012**, *16*, 601–608. [CrossRef] [PubMed]
48. Folstein, M.F.; Folstein, S.E.; McHugh, P.R. "Mini-Mental State": A Practical Method for Grading the Cognitive State of Patients for the Clinician. *J. Psychiatr. Res.* **1975**, *12*, 189–198. [CrossRef]
49. Lipschitz, D.A. Screening for Nutritional Status in the Elderly. *Prim. Care* **1994**, *21*, 55–67. [CrossRef]
50. Ambagtsheer, R.; Visvanathan, R.; Cesari, M.; Yu, S.; Archibald, M.; Schultz, T.; Karnon, J.; Kitson, A.; Beilby, J. Feasibility, Acceptability and Diagnostic Test Accuracy of Frailty Screening Instruments in Community-Dwelling Older People within the Australian General Practice Setting: A Study Protocol for a Cross-Sectional Study. *BMJ Open* **2017**, *7*, e016663. [CrossRef]
51. Topolski, T.D.; LoGerfo, J.; Patrick, D.L.; Williams, B.; Patrick, M.M.B. The Rapid Assessment of Physical Activity (RAPA) Among Older Adults. *Prev. Chronic Dis.* **2006**, *3*, 8.
52. Guigoz, Y. The Mini Nutritional Assessment (MNA) review of the literature—What does it tell us? *J. Nutr. Health Aging* **2006**, *10*, 466.

53. U.S. Department of Health and Human Services and U.S. Department of Agriculture. 2015–2020 Dietary Guidelines for Americans. 8th Edition. December 2015. Available online: http://health.gov/dietaryguidelines/2015/guidelines/ (accessed on 25 June 2021).
54. Gray, W.K.; Richardson, J.; McGuire, J.; Dewhurst, F.; Elder, V.; Weeks, J.; Walker, R.W.; Dotchin, C.L. Frailty Screening in Low- and Middle-Income Countries: A Systematic Review. *J. Am. Geriatr. Soc.* **2016**, *64*, 806–823. [CrossRef] [PubMed]
55. Sibai, A.M.; Sen, K.; Baydoun, M.; Saxena, P. Population Ageing in Lebanon: Current Status, Future Prospects and Implications for Policy. *Bull. World Health Organ.* **2004**, *82*, 219–225.
56. United Nations, Department of Economic and Social Affairs, Population Division. *World Population Prospects 2019, Volume II: Demographic Profiles (ST/ESA/SER.A/427)*; United Nations: San Francisco, CA, USA, 2019.
57. Hoogendijk, E.O.; van Hout, H.P.J.; Heymans, M.W.; van der Horst, H.E.; Frijters, D.H.M.; Broese van Groenou, M.I.; Deeg, D.J.H.; Huisman, M. Explaining the Association between Educational Level and Frailty in Older Adults: Results from a 13-Year Longitudinal Study in the Netherlands. *Ann. Epidemiol.* **2014**, *24*, 538–544.e2. [CrossRef] [PubMed]
58. Veronese, N.; Stubbs, B.; Noale, M.; Solmi, M.; Pilotto, A.; Vaona, A.; Demurtas, J.; Mueller, C.; Huntley, J.; Crepaldi, G.; et al. Polypharmacy Is Associated With Higher Frailty Risk in Older People: An 8-Year Longitudinal Cohort Study. *J. Am. Med. Dir. Assoc.* **2018**, *18*, 624–628. [CrossRef] [PubMed]
59. Hakeem, F.F.; Bernabé, E.; Sabbah, W. Association between Oral Health and Frailty: A Systematic Review of Longitudinal Studies. *Gerodontology* **2019**, *36*, 205–215. [CrossRef] [PubMed]
60. Ensrud, K.E.; Blackwell, T.L.; Redline, S.; Ancoli-Israel, S.; Paudel, M.L.; Cawthon, P.M.; Dam, T.-T.L.; Barrett-Connor, E.; Leung, P.C.; Stone, K.L. Sleep Disturbances and Frailty Status in Older Community-Dwelling Men. *J. Am. Geriatr. Soc.* **2009**, *57*, 2085–2093. [CrossRef] [PubMed]
61. Kamil, R.J.; Li, L.; Lin, F.R. Association of Hearing Impairment and Frailty in Older Adults. *J. Am. Geriatr. Soc.* **2014**, *62*, 1186–1188. [CrossRef] [PubMed]
62. Swenor, B.K.; Lee, M.J.; Tian, J.; Varadaraj, V.; Bandeen-Roche, K. Visual Impairment and Frailty: Examining an Understudied Relationship. *J. Gerontol. A Biol. Sci. Med. Sci.* **2020**, *75*, 596–602. [CrossRef] [PubMed]
63. García-Esquinas, E.; José García-García, F.; León-Muñoz, L.M.; Carnicero, J.A.; Guallar-Castillón, P.; Gonzalez-Colaço Harmand, M.; López-García, E.; Alonso-Bouzón, C.; Rodríguez-Mañas, L.; Rodríguez-Artalejo, F. Obesity, Fat Distribution, and Risk of Frailty in Two Population-Based Cohorts of Older Adults in Spain. *Obesity* **2015**, *23*, 847–855. [CrossRef]
64. Bollwein, J.; Volkert, D.; Diekmann, R.; Kaiser, M.J.; Uter, W.; Vidal, K.; Sieber, C.C.; Bauer, J.M. Nutritional Status According to the Mini Nutritional Assessment (MNA®) and Frailty in Community Dwelling Older Persons: A Close Relationship. *J. Nutr. Health Aging* **2013**, *17*, 351–356. [CrossRef]
65. Chang, S.-F. Frailty Is a Major Related Factor for at Risk of Malnutrition in Community-Dwelling Older Adults: Frail Assessment for Nutrition. *J. Nurs. Scholarsh.* **2017**, *49*, 63–72. [CrossRef]
66. Laclaustra, M.; Rodriguez-Artalejo, F.; Guallar-Castillon, P.; Banegas, J.R.; Graciani, A.; Garcia-Esquinas, E.; Ordovas, J.; Lopez-Garcia, E. Prospective Association between Added Sugars and Frailty in Older Adults. *Am. J. Clin. Nutr.* **2018**, *107*, 772–779. [CrossRef]
67. Struijk, E.A.; Rodríguez-Artalejo, F.; Fung, T.T.; Willett, W.C.; Hu, F.B.; Lopez-Garcia, E. Sweetened Beverages and Risk of Frailty among Older Women in the Nurses' Health Study: A Cohort Study. *PLoS Med.* **2020**, *17*, e1003453. [CrossRef]
68. Feart, C. Nutrition and Frailty: Current Knowledge. *Prog. Neuro-Psychopharmacol. Biol. Psychiatry* **2019**, *95*, 109703. [CrossRef] [PubMed]
69. Barrea, L.; Muscogiuri, G.; Di Somma, C.; Tramontano, G.; De Luca, V.; Illario, M.; Colao, A.; Savastano, S. Association between Mediterranean Diet and Hand Grip Strength in Older Adult Women. *Clin. Nutr.* **2019**, *38*, 721–729. [CrossRef]
70. Fung, T.T.; Struijk, E.A.; Rodriguez-Artalejo, F.; Willett, W.C.; Lopez-Garcia, E. Fruit and Vegetable Intake and Risk of Frailty in Women 60 Years Old or Older. *Am. J. Clin. Nutr.* **2020**, *112*, 1540–1546. [CrossRef]
71. Kojima, G.; Avgerinou, C.; Iliffe, S.; Jivraj, S.; Sekiguchi, K.; Walters, K. Fruit and Vegetable Consumption and Frailty: A Systematic Review. *J. Nutr. Health Aging* **2018**, *22*, 1010–1017. [CrossRef]
72. Garcia-Esquinas, E.; Rahi, B.; Peres, K.; Colpo, M.; Dartigues, J.-F.; Bandinelli, S.; Feart, C.; Rodriguez-Artalejo, F. Consumption of Fruit and Vegetables and Risk of Frailty: A Dose-Response Analysis of 3 Prospective Cohorts of Community-Dwelling Older Adults. *Am. J. Clin. Nutr.* **2016**, *104*, 132–142. [CrossRef]

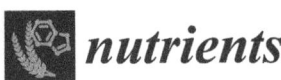

Review

Whole-Grain Intake in the Mediterranean Diet and a Low Protein to Carbohydrates Ratio Can Help to Reduce Mortality from Cardiovascular Disease, Slow Down the Progression of Aging, and to Improve Lifespan: A Review

Cristiano Capurso

Department of Medical and Surgical Sciences, University of Foggia, Viale Pinto 1, 71122 Foggia, Italy; cristiano.capurso@unifg.it

Citation: Capurso, C. Whole-Grain Intake in the Mediterranean Diet and a Low Protein to Carbohydrates Ratio Can Help to Reduce Mortality from Cardiovascular Disease, Slow Down the Progression of Aging, and to Improve Lifespan: A Review. *Nutrients* 2021, *13*, 2540. https://doi.org/10.3390/nu13082540

Academic Editor: Camillo Ricordi

Received: 16 June 2021
Accepted: 23 July 2021
Published: 25 July 2021

Publisher's Note: MDPI stays neutral with regard to jurisdictional claims in published maps and institutional affiliations.

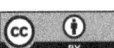

Copyright: © 2021 by the author. Licensee MDPI, Basel, Switzerland. This article is an open access article distributed under the terms and conditions of the Creative Commons Attribution (CC BY) license (https://creativecommons.org/licenses/by/4.0/).

Abstract: Increase in the aging population is a phenomenon all over the world. Maintaining good functional ability, good mental health, and cognitive function in the absence of severe disease and physical disability define successful aging. A healthy lifestyle in middle age predisposes successful aging. Longevity is the result of a multifactorial phenomenon, which involves feeding. Diets that emphasize fruit and vegetables, whole grains rather than refined grains, low-fat dairy, lean meats, fish, legumes, and nuts are inversely associated with mortality or to a lower risk of becoming frail among elderly subjects. A regular physical activity and a regular intake of whole grain derivatives together with the optimization of the protein/carbohydrate ratio in the diet, where the ratio is significantly less than 1 such as in the Mediterranean diet and the Okinawan diet, reduces the risk of developing aging-related diseases and increases healthy life expectancy. The purpose of our review was to analyze cohort and case-control studies that investigated the effects of cereals in the diet, especially whole grains and derivatives as well as the effects of a diet with a low protein–carbohydrate ratio on the progression of aging, mortality, and lifespan.

Keywords: aging; frailty; lifespan; diet; carbohydrates; whole grain; protein

1. Introduction

According to the World Health Organization, population aging is a global phenomenon rapidly evolving worldwide. By 2030, the number of people aged 60 and over in the world is projected to grow from 901 million to 1.4 billion, or 56%. It is expected that by 2050, the global population of people over 65 will amount to about 2.1 billion people, more than double compared to 2015. In addition, it is estimated that by 2050, the over eighty-year-olds throughout the world will be around 434 million, or more than three times compared to 2015, when they reached 125 million. The rapid aging of the population can be observed above all in emerging economy countries. In fact, over the next 15 years, the elderly population will grow more rapidly in Latin America and the Caribbean with an expected increase of 71%, followed by Asia (66%), Africa (64%), Oceania (47%), North America (41%), and Europe (23%) [1]. This means that while European countries have had more than 150 years to adjust to an increase of up to 20% in the proportion of the population over 65, countries like Brazil, China, and India will have less than 20 years to adapt to a similar one. The population as of 1 January 2018 in the European Union (EU) was estimated to be 512.4 million. People over 65 years old amounted to 19.7%, an increase of 2.6% compared to 10 years earlier. The percentage of people aged over 80 is expected to at least double by 2100 to 14.6% of the entire EU population [2].

It is also true that many elderly people maintain good autonomy and live life with a good level of well-being. These subjects, despite the presence of one or more diseases, however, do not have serious illnesses or physical disabilities; they have good mental health, preserved cognitive functions, maintain a good level of physical activity levels and in some cases, are engaged in social and productive activities [3,4]. All these conditions define successful aging.

It is known that a healthy life in middle age predisposes successful success. This includes a healthy diet with adequate caloric intake to the state of health and physical activity, smoking cessation, and taking moderate amounts of alcohol, preferably with meals. The traditional Mediterranean diet (MD) is characterized by a high intake of foods of plant origin (fruit, vegetables, whole-meal bread, beans, nuts, and seeds) and fresh fruit; extra virgin olive oil is the main dietary source of fat.

Traditional MD has long been recognized as a highly healthy dietary pattern. High adherence to traditional MD leads to a significant reduction in mortality and a reduced risk of developing cardiovascular disease and cancer as well as a reduced risk of developing chronic disease and disability in later life. The main source of complex carbohydrates is made up of cereals and their derivatives (bread, pasta, rice); these provide 55–60% of the total caloric intake and are placed at the bottom of the food pyramid [5–15].

Another health diet model other than MD is the traditional Okinawan diet [16]. This is also characterized by a low overall caloric intake, high consumption of vegetables, high consumption of legumes (mainly soybeans), moderate consumption of fish, especially in coastal areas, in any case, by the low consumption of meat, especially lean pork. Characteristic of traditional Okinawa is also a low consumption of dairy products, a high intake of mono- and polyunsaturated fats, with a low omega 6:3 ratio, the consumption of low glycemic index carbohydrates with a high intake of fiber, and a moderate consumption of alcohol. Figure 1 compares the composition of the MD and the Okinawan diets.

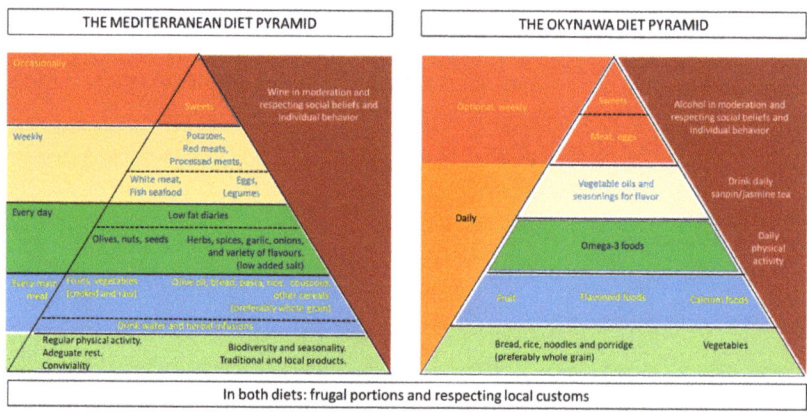

Figure 1. Mediterranean diet and Okinawan diet pyramids.

The purpose of our review was to analyze both cohort and case-control studies that investigated, on one hand, the effects of cereals, of whole grains (WG), and derivatives in the diet, on the other, the effects of a diet with low protein–carbohydrate ratio on aging progression, mortality, and lifespan.

2. Cereals

Cereals (from Ceres, the Roman goddess of crops and fields) have been the staple food for most people around the world since ancient times. Cereals, especially when consumed as WG [17], are a healthy source of carbohydrates, fiber, and bioactive peptides with anticancer, antioxidant, and antithrombotic effects [18]. In traditional MD [19], grains provide up to 47–50% of the daily calorie intake. The cereals and derivatives mainly consumed in MD are wheat, spelled, oats, rye, barley, and, to a lesser extent, rice and maize. Table 1 summarizes the nutritional properties of all the above cereals.

Table 1. Nutritional properties of cereals.

	Wheat (Variety Hard, Red Winter)	Spelt (Uncooked)	Oats	Rye	Barley (Raw and Pearled)	Rice (Unenriched White Rice)	Maize (Sweetcorn, Yellow, Raw)
Energy (KJ)	1368	1415	1628	1414	1473	1498	1506
Protein (g)	12.61	14.57	16.89	10.34	9.91	6.5	3.27
Global fats (g)	1.54	2.43	6.9	1.63	1.16	0.52	1.35
Global saturated fatty acids (g)	0.269	0.406	1.217	0.197	0.244	0.140	0.325
Global monounsaturated fatty acids (g)	0.2	0.445	2.178	0.208	0.149	0.161	0.432
Polysaturated fatty acids (g)	0.627	1.258	2.535	0.767	0.560	0.138	0.487
Carbohydrates (g)	71.18	70.19	66.27	75.86	77.72	79.15	18.7
Sugars (g)	0.41	6.82	0	0.98	0.80	0	6.26
Dietary fibers (g)	12.2	10.7	10.6	15.1	15.6	0	2
Vitamin A IU	9	10	0	11	22	0	187
Thiamine (B1) (mg; % DV)	0.383; 33%	0.364; 32%	0.763; 66%	0.316; 26%	1.191;16%	0.07; 6%	0.155; 13%
Riboflavin (B2) (mg; % DV)	0.115; 10%	0.113; 9%	0.139; 12%	0.251; 19%	0;0%	0.048; 4%	0.055; 4%
Niacin (B3) (mg; % DV)	5.464; 36%	6.843; 46%	0.961; 6%	4.27; 27%	4.604;29%	1600; 10%	1.77; 11%
Pantothenic acid (B5) (mg; % DV)	0.954; 19%	1.068; 11%	1.349; 27%	1.456; 29%	0.282;6%	1287; 26%	0.717; 14%
Vitamin B6 (mg; % DV)	0.3; 23%	0.230; 18%	0.120; 9%	0.294; 23%	0.260;20%	0.171; 13%	0.093; 7%
Folate (B9) (µg; % DV)	38; 10%	45; 11%	56; 5%	38; 10%	23;6%	6; 1.5%	42; 11%
Vitamin B12 (µg; % DV)	0; 0%	0; 0%	0; 0%	0; 0%	0;0%	0; 0%	0; 0%
Vitamin E (mg; % DV)	1.01; 7%	0.79; 5%	0; 0%	0.85; 6%	0.02;0%	0; 0%	0.07; 0%
Vitamin K (µg; % DV)	1.9; 2%	3.6; 3%	0; 0%	5.9; 5%	2.2;2%	0; 0%	0.3; 0%
Calcium (mg; % DV)	29; 3%	27; 3%	54; 5.58%	24; 2.48%	29;2%	1; 0.08%	2; 0.2%
Iron (mg; % DV)	3.19; 25%	4.44; 34%	5; 38%	2.63; 15%	2.5;14%	0.2; 1%	0.52; 3%
Magnesium (mg; % DV)	126; 35%	136; 38%	177; 50%	110; 28%	79;20%	8; 2%	37; 9%
Manganese (mg; % DV)	3.985; 190%	3; 143%	4.9; 233%	2.577; 112%	1.322;57%	0.357; 16%	0.163; 7%
Phosphorus (mg; % DV)	288; 41%	401; 57%	523; 75%	332; 47%	221;32%	33; 5%	89; 13%
Potassium (mg; % DV)	363; 8%	388; 8%	429; 9%	510; 11%	280;6%	26; 1%	270; 6%
Selenium (µg; % DV)	70.7; 129%	11.7; 17%	Not reported	13.9; 25%	37.7;69%	0; 0%	0.6; 1%
Sodium (mg; % DV)	2; 0.13%	8; 0.53%	2; 0.13%	2; 0.13%	9;0%	0; 0%	15; 1%
Zinc (mg; % DV)	2.65; 28%	3.28; 35%	4; 42%	2.65; 28%	2.13;19%	0.4; 4%	0.46; 4%

2.1. Wheat

Wheat (Triticum aestivum, Triticum durum) is a cereal of ancient culture, whose area of origin is located between the Mediterranean Sea, the Black Sea, and the Caspian Sea, and is currently cultivated all over the world [20]. Wheat has a protein content of 13–14%, higher than that of the other main cereals and staple foods; therefore, it is the main plant source of protein in human nutrition worldwide. A total of 100 g of wheat provides 327 calories; wheat is also an important source of dietary fiber, niacin, several B vitamins, and other dietary minerals. Furthermore, 75–80% of total wheat protein is made up of gluten [21].

2.1.1. Starch and Protein

Starch, on average, is approximately 80% of the dry weight of the endosperm and consists of a mixture of two polymers, amylose and amylopectin, in a ratio of about 1:3. The protein content of wheat has wider variations than the starch content [22]. An analysis from the World Wheat Collection, after comparing 212,600 germplasm lines, showed a wide variability of the protein content, with a range from 7 to 22% of protein on dry weight [23]. Similarly, the result of the comparison analysis between 150 lines of wheat grown under the same agronomic conditions, as part of the HEALTHGRAIN program, highlighted a variation in the protein content of wheat from 12.9 to 19.9% with regard to wholemeal flours and from 10.3 to 19.0% for white flours [24] More than half of the total protein content of the wheat grain, as already stated above, is made up of gluten, in a measure directly proportional to the total protein content [25].

2.1.2. Wheat Fibers and Cell Wall Polysaccharides

According to the 2009 Codex definition [26], dietary fiber (DF) is a "... carbohydrate polymer with a degree of polymerization (DP) not lower than 3, which are neither digested nor absorbed in the small intestine ... "

The European Commission under Commission Directive 2008/100/EC [27], subsequently established under Regulation (EU) No. 1169/2011 of The European Parliament and of The Council [28], further defines DF. In this definition, all carbohydrates with a degree of polymerization (DP) ≥ 3 can be included in dietary fiber; of these, the most common in cereals are fructo-oligosaccharides.

Whole wheat is among the main sources of DF and mainly comprises non-starch polysaccharides (NSPs), which are derived from the cell walls. Most of the fibers are removed during grinding, as refined flour has an extremely low amount of fiber. The amount of fiber in whole wheat varies from 12 to 15% of the dry weight, mainly concentrated in the bran. The most common fiber of wheat bran, equal to about 70%, is arabinoxylan (Figure 2); this is composed of hemicellulose, and β-glucan (20%) as well as a small amount of cellulose (2%) and glucomannan (7%) [29]. Bran obtained from grinding includes a set of compounds that comprise up to 45–50% of cell wall material [30]. The pericarp is the main component and is composed of about 30% of cellulose, about 60% of arabinoxylan, and about 12% of lignin [31].

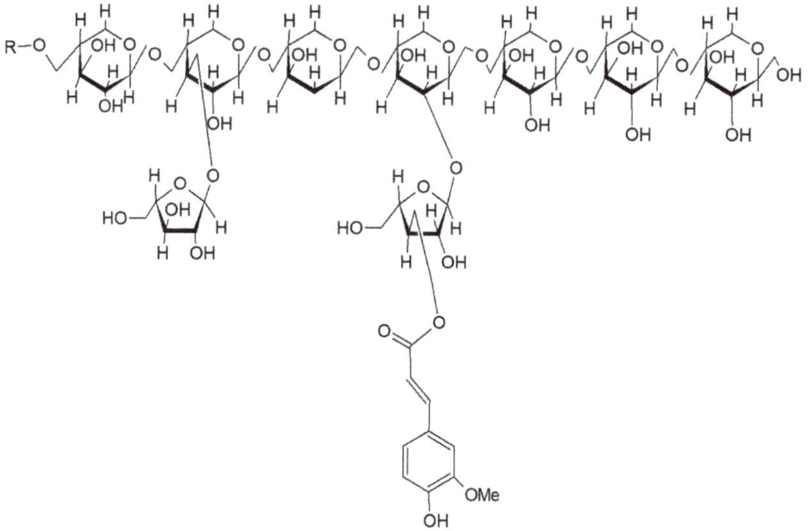

Figure 2. Arabinoxylan (drawn by ACD/ChemSketch).

2.1.3. Antioxidant Components and B Vitamins in Wheat

The grain of wheat contains numerous antioxidants, mainly concentrated in the bran and germ, parts absent in refined white wheat flour. The main antioxidants in the wheat grain are terpenoids (including vitamin E) and phenolic acids [21]. In the wheat grain, phenolic acids are mostly derivatives of hydroxycinnamic acid. In particular, these are dehydrodimers and dehydrotrimers of ferulic acid and synapic and p-coumaric acids [32]. In the outer layer of the bran, we find most of the phenolic acids, mostly bound through ester bonds, to the structural components of the cell wall. The highest shares of antioxidants are found in the outermost layer of the endosperm (i.e., the aleurone). Therefore, the antioxidant properties (i.e., the presence of relevant quantities of phenolic compounds) are directly correlated to the aleurone content of the wheat grain [33]. Among the polyphenols of wheat and other cereals, ferulic acid is the predominant. Other classes of antioxidants contained in wheat bran are flavonoids, carotenoids (mainly lutein), and lignans [34,35].

Wheat is an important source of the so-called "methyl donors", important cofactors in the methylation process, necessary for the synthesis of dopamine and serotonin as well as for the biosynthesis of melatonin and coenzyme Q10. The main component is betaine glycine, therefore, in smaller quantities, it is choline (precursor of betaine) and trigonellin (a structural analogue of betaine and choline). Concerning B group vitamins, wheat is a good source of thiamin (B1), riboflavin (B2), niacin (B3), pyridoxine (B6), and folate (B9) [21].

2.1.4. Health Effects

The health effects of wheat are due to the high content of numerous nutrients and fibers as well as proteins and minerals. Wheat, if consumed as whole wheat, is recommended in several daily portions in the nutrition of both children and adults in quantities equal to about one third of the total diet. For example, whole wheat is a common component found in breakfast cereals and is associated with a reduced risk for various pathologies. Thanks also to the high intake of insoluble fiber, whole wheat in the diet contributes to reducing the risk of coronary heart disease [CHD], stroke, cancer, and type 2 diabetes mellitus as well as helping to reduce mortality due to all causes [36,37].

2.2. Rye

Rye (Secale cereale) is part of the Graminaceae family (Triticeae), and is similar to barley (genus Hordeum) and wheat (Triticum). Rye is used for the production of flour, bread, crispbreads, beer, whiskey, vodka; it is also used as forage for animals [20].

2.2.1. Nutrition Properties

A 100 g serving of rye contains 338 calories and consists of carbohydrates (28%), proteins (20%), dietary fiber (54%), niacin (27%), pantothenic acid (29%), riboflavin (19%), thiamine (26%), vitamin B6 (23%), and minerals. [21].

Compared to wheat flour, rye flour has a lower gluten content, being rich in gliadin but low in glutenin. Although in small quantities, the gluten content makes rye a cereal unsuitable for consumption by people with celiac disease, non-celiac gluten sensitivity, or wheat allergy.

2.2.2. Health Effects

Thanks to the high content of non-cellulosic polysaccharides, rye is an excellent source of fiber, with an exceptionally high capacity to bind water, and which therefore quickly gives a feeling of fullness and satiety. For this reason, rye bread is a valuable aid in the weight loss diet.

2.2.3. Rye Bread and Glucose Metabolism

Juntunen et al. [38] evaluated, in a sample of 20 healthy, non-diabetic, postmenopausal women, the effect on insulin response after intake of refined wheat bread, endosperm rye bread, traditional whole-meal rye bread, and high-fiber rye bread. They measured blood glucose and insulinemia, glucose-dependent insulinotropic polypeptide (GIP), and glucagon-like peptide 1 (GLP-1). All these markers of insulin response were measured in blood samples taken at fasting (time 0) and respectively after 15, 30, 45, 60, 90, 120, 150 and 180 min from the consumption of the different types of bread. The authors demonstrated that post-prandial blood glucose values after the consumption of rye bread were not significantly different from the values measured after the consumption of refined white wheat bread. In contrast, the blood values of insulin, GIP, and C-peptide after the consumption of rye bread were significantly lower than the values obtained after the consumption of wheat bread ($p < 0.001$). Furthermore, plasma GLP-1 values after consumption of rye bread were not significantly different from those obtained after consumption of the other breads, except at 150 and 180 min ($p = 0.012$). The authors also demonstrated that the lower insulin response after eating rye bread cannot simply be explained by the higher amount of fiber contained in rye bread. Micrographic examination revealed differences in the structure of refined wheat bread, rye endosperm bread, high fiber rye bread, and traditional rye bread. For example, in wheat bread, gluten proteins formed a continuous matrix in which the starch grains were dispersed. On the other hand, in the rye bread, the starch grains were more swollen and the amylose was partially leached. The starch granules were well packaged and formed a continuous matrix. It was clear, therefore, that the softness and porosity of refined wheat bread and the hardness of rye bread were based on these differences in their structure.

Nordlund et al. [39] subsequently confirmed these data. They analyzed the mechanical, structural, and biochemical properties of various types of rye and wheat bread as well as the particle size of the breads after gastric digestion in in vitro and in vivo glycemic and insulin responses on a sample of 29 volunteers. Therefore, 10 different types of bread from ten different flours were packaged, with 10 different characteristics of composition and consistency, namely: refined wheat, whole rye, whole rye (commercial), whole rye + bran, refined rye, refined rye (flat), refined rye + gluten (flat), rye/whole wheat, wheat/whole wheat, and refined wheat + fermented bran. A sourdough baking process was used for baking rye breads, while a straight dough baking process was used for baking wheat breads. Upon microscopic observation, both 100% wholemeal rye flour bread and sourdough refined rye flour bread had a higher number of digestive particles larger than 2 or 3 mm in size, meaning that they appeared less "disintegrated" "compared to wheat flour bread. Microstructural examination of the digestive particles of sourdough rye bread also showed more aggregated and less degraded starch granules than refined wheat bread. The postprandial insulin response produced from 100% rye flour bread by the sourdough method was significantly lower than the insulin response produced by refined wheat flour bread ($p = 0.001$). From principal component analysis (PCA), the authors confirmed that the insulin response was inversely related to the larger digestive particle size obtained after in vitro digestion, the number of soluble fibers, and the sourdough process. That is, the larger starch particles obtained after gastric digestion of bread from wholemeal rye flour were associated with a reduced postprandial insulin response. This mechanism, likely in synergy with fiber and WG, explains the reduction in the risk of diabetes obtained with the consumption of rye bread in the diet.

More recently, Rojas-Bonzi et al. [40] conducted a study on pigs with a catheterized portal vein fed on wheat bread and wholemeal rye bread to analyze the kinetics of the in vitro digestion of breads by varying the dietary fiber content and composition, thus comparing the results obtained with the data of a previous in vivo study [41]. Five varieties of bread were analyzed: white wheat bread (WWB), whole grain rye bread (WRB), and whole grain rye bread with kernels (WRBK), which were commercial breads; in addition, two varieties of experimental breads (i.e., specially prepared for the study: concentrated wheat Arabinoxylan (AXB) and concentrated wheat β-glucan (BGB)). As expected, WWB had the highest total starch content (711 g/kg dry matter, DM), while the starch content was lowest in all high DF content breads (588, 608, 514, 612 g/kg DM, respectively). Total DF was low in the WWB (77 g/kg DM) and high in all high DF breads (209, 220, 212, 199 g/kg DM, respectively). Total DFs were lowest in WWB (77 g/kg DM) and highest in all high-DF breads (209, 220, 212, 199 g/kg DM, respectively). Of course, the characteristics of the total and soluble DFs varied considerably between the loaves. The BGB had a high content of total and soluble β-glucan (52 and 40 g/kg DM), while the WRB, WRBK, and AXB had a high content of total and soluble arabinoxylan (76 and 36, 77 and 37, 78 and 66 g/kg DM, respectively). The highest percentage value of starch hydrolysis in vitro was observed from time 0 and within the first 5 min and subsequently decreased. The highest rate of hydrolysis during the first 5 min was observed in WWB (13.9% starch/min), followed by WRB (10.4% starch/min), WRBK (8.7% starch/min), and finally from AXB and BGB (7.4–8.5% starch/min). In order to be able to compare the data obtained in vitro with the in vivo data, the measurement of portal glucose values was reported by the authors as a percentage of hydrolyzed starch (absorbed starch) per 100 g of dry starch (ingested starch). After the first 15 min, the highest values were observed in the WWB, the lowest values for the WRB and WRBK, and intermediate values for the AXB and BGB ($p < 0.05$). The authors explained the extremely high rate of hydrolysis of the WWB with a porous physical structure of white wheat flour, which makes the readily degradable bread. The quantity of DF, both naturally present in the cell walls (WRB, WRBK) and added (AXB, BGB), delays its digestion in vitro, extending the hydrolysis time in the first 5 min. The greatest effect was observed in the BGB, probably due to the increased viscosity of the BGB compared to other types of bread. The reduced in vitro digestion rate within the first 5 min of arabinoxylan compared to b-glucan is due to its more branched structure. Arabinoxylan is also less sensitive to the change in acidity during the passage from the stomach to the small intestine, unlike b-glucan. The authors therefore confirmed the results already obtained by Juntunen et al. [38], or that the processing of white wheat bread gives it a more porous structure to rye bread, which has a more compact structure. The inclusion of unrefined grains in bread has also been proven to be an efficient way to regulate starch hydrolysis: the insoluble fibrous network surrounds the starch, forming a real physical barrier against amylases, limiting its gelatinization. The viscous nature of soluble DFs further increases the viscosity of the digestive bolus, limiting its diffusion and delaying the absorption of glucose through intestinal cells.

2.3. Spelt (Triticum Spelta)

Spelt (Triticum spelta), is a species of wheat that has been cultivated since ancient times. It originated as a natural hybridization of a domesticated tetraploid wheat and a wild goat grass Aegilops tauschii.

In the twentieth century, spelt was almost completely replaced by wheat flour bread, but it has become popular again in recent years, thanks to the spread of organic agriculture. Spelt is very disease resistant and also grows in poor growing conditions such as wet and cold soils or at high altitudes, and requires less fertilizer. Furthermore, it does not require any chemical treatment of the hulled seeds used for sowing, thanks to the protection provided by the hull [20].

Nutrients

A 100 g of raw spelt provides 338 calories. It is composed of about 70% carbohydrates, of which 11% is dietary fiber, and is low in fat. Spelt has a good protein content; it is also a terrific source of dietary fiber, B vitamins including niacin and of a wide variety of dietary minerals including manganese and phosphorus [21]. The comparison between nine samples of hulled spelt and five of soft winter wheat [42] showed a higher average quantity of total lipids and unsaturated fatty acids, with a lower tocopherol content, both in whole spelt and in spelt from grinds, compared to wheat. This suggests that the higher lipid content of spelt might not be related to a higher proportion of germs. The proportions of flour and bran after grinding were similar in spelt and wheat; the content of ash, copper, iron, zinc, magnesium, and phosphorus was higher in the samples of spelt, particularly in fine bran rich in aleurone and in the coarse bran. The phosphorus content was higher, while the phytic acid content was lower in spelt than in fine wheat bran. This could suggest that spelt has either a higher endogenous phytase activity or a lower phytic acid content than wheat.

Compared to hard red winter wheat, spelt has lower insoluble polymeric proteins, which contribute to the swelling capacity of the gluten. Spelt also has higher gliadins, which have the opposite effects, and higher values of soluble polymeric proteins. It follows that the gluten in spelt is less elastic and more extensible than wheat gluten, resulting in the typical weaker spelt dough [43].

2.4. Oats

Oat (Avena sativa, the best known species of the Avena genus), unlike other varieties of cereals and pseudocereals, is cultivated for their seed, known by the same name, usually in the plural. Oats are commonly eaten rolled or ground as oatmeal or as fine oatmeal and consumed primarily as porridge, but are also used as an ingredient for making cakes, cookies, and bread. Oats are also an ingredient in breakfast cereals, particularly in muesli. In the United Kingdom, oats are used for the production of beer. A popular refreshment throughout Latin America is a characteristic cold, sweet drink made from ground oats and milk [20].

2.4.1. Nutrients

A 100 g of oats provide 389 calories. Oats are made up of about 66% carbohydrates, 11% dietary fiber, 4% beta-glucans, 7% fat, and 17% protein. Oats are also an excellent source of B vitamins and minerals, particularly manganese [21].

After corn, oats have the highest lipid content of most other cereals of over 10% compared to 2–3% for wheat. Furthermore, oats are the only cereal containing a globulin, avenaline, as the main storage protein (around 80%). Compared to gluten, zein, and prolamins, the most typical cereal proteins, globulins, are characterized by their solubility in diluted saline solution. Avenin, a prolamine, is the minor protein of oats. In nutritional qualities, oat proteins are almost equivalent to soy proteins, which in turn are equivalent in nutritional quality to proteins in meat, milk, and eggs, according to research by the World Health Organization. A skinless oat grain (semolina) has a protein content ranging from 12 to 24%, the highest among cereals. Some pure oat cultivars (oats not contaminated by other gluten-containing grains) can be a safe food in a gluten-free diet, which requires knowledge of the varieties of oats used in foods. Oats contain about 11% fiber, most of which is composed of b-glucans, indigestible polysaccharides found naturally in cereals as well as in barley, yeast, bacteria, algae, and fungi [14,20]. Oats, particularly the more "ancient" varieties, contain more soluble fibers than common western varieties, which induce a slowdown in digestion with a consequent greater feeling of satiety and reduced appetite [44,45].

It has been shown that dietary benefits from whole oats are associated with an improved control of cardio-metabolic risk factors by reducing blood lipids and blood glucose. Eating oat-based foods, either as whole grains or as bread, porridge, or soaking oats in milk, has been shown to allow for better glycemic control [46–51].

2.4.2. Oat Beta-Glucan

Oat beta-glucan is made up of mixed-bonded polysaccharides. This means that the bonds between the D-glucose or D-glucopyranosyl units are beta-1, 3 or beta-1, 4 bonds. This type of beta-glucan is also defined as a mixed bond $(1 \rightarrow 3)$, $(1 \rightarrow 4)$-beta-D-glucan (Figure 3). These bonds $(1 \rightarrow 3)$ break the uniform structure of the beta-D-glucan molecule and make it soluble and flexible. In comparison, the cellulose indigestible polysaccharide, which is also a beta-glucan, is not soluble because of its $(1 \rightarrow 4)$-beta-D-bonds. The percentages of beta-glucan vary in the various products based on whole oats such as oat bran (range 5.5–23.0%), oat flakes (about 4%), and oat flour integral (about 4%). Oats also contain some insoluble fibers including lignin, cellulose, and hemicellulose [20]. Beta-glucans are known to have cholesterol-lowering properties as they increase the excretion of bile acids, with a consequent reduction in blood cholesterol [52]. This cholesterol-lowering effect of beta-glucans has allowed oats to be classified as a health food [53].

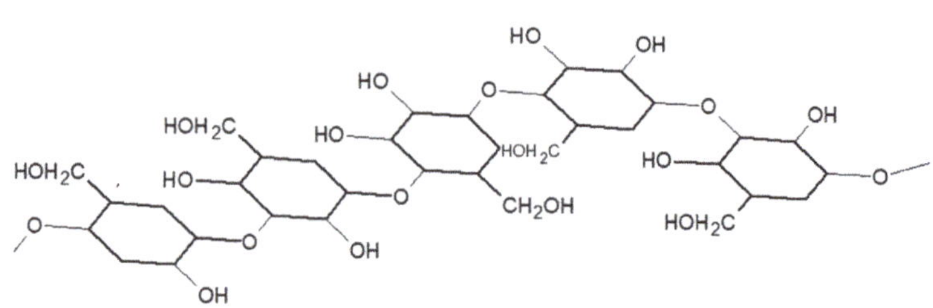

Figure 3. Beta-D-glucan (drawn by ACD/ChemSketch).

2.5. Rice

Rice is the seed of the monocotyledonous flowering plants Oryza glaberrima (African rice) or Oryza sativa (Asian rice). It is the most consumed cereal by the human population in the world and is the basis of Asian cuisine. It is the staple food for about half of the world's population and is grown in almost every country in the world. It is the agricultural product with the highest world production (741.5 million tons recorded in 2014), after sugar cane (1.9 billion tons) and corn (1.0 billion tons). There are many varieties of rice, and culinary preferences tend to vary regionally.

Nutrients

The nutritional value of rice depends on several factors. First of all, it varies according to the rice strain, that is white rice, brown rice, red rice, or black rice, which have a different percentage of distribution in different regions of the world [54]. After that, the nutritional value of rice depends on the nutrient quality of the soil in which it is grown, if and how it is polished or processed, and if and how it is enriched and how it is prepared before consumption [55].

A 100 g serving of unenriched white rice provides an average of 360 calories, distributed between carbohydrates, proteins, fats, and fibers. Rice is also a good source of B vitamins and several dietary minerals including manganese. Raw white rice contains 66% carbohydrates, mostly starch, 11% dietary fibers, 4% beta-glucans, 7% fats, and 17% proteins. Cooked unenriched white rice is composed of 68% water, 28% carbohydrates, 13% protein, and fat in minimal quantity (less than 1%). Cooked short-grain white rice provides the same food energy and contains moderate amounts of B vitamins, iron, and manganese (10–17% of daily value, DV) per 100-g serving [21].

Starch and proteins, as main components of rice grains, accumulate in specific organelles called amyloplasts and protein bodies, respectively, in the endosperm cells and in the aleurone layer. Endosperm cells contain many amyloplasts with multiple starch grains and protein bodies with glutellin (protein body II) and prolamine (protein body I), which are storage proteins. On the other hand, the cells in the aleurone layer contain another type of protein body called grain aleurone, with non-storage proteins and small amyloplasts. The protein content of rice grains is of course lower than meat (15–25%) and cheese (20%), but is higher than dairy milk (3.3%) and yoghurt (4.3%). About 6–7% of polished rice and about 13% of rice bran is protein [56].

Amino acid score, in combination with protein digestibility, which refers to how well a given protein is digested, is the method used to determine if a protein is complete (i.e., whether it contains an adequate proportion of each of the nine essential amino acids necessary in the human diet). Together with the amino acid score, the digestibility of proteins determines the values for Protein Digestibility-Corrected Amino Acid Score (PDCAAS) and Digestible Indispensable Amino Acid Score (DIAAS). DIAAS was proposed in March 2013 by the FAO to replace the PDCAAS. DIAAS provides a more accurate measure of the number of amino acids absorbed by the body or the contribution of the protein to the needs of amino acids and nitrogen in humans, as it estimates the digestibility of amino acids at the end of the small intestine. PDCAAS, already adopted by the FAO in 1993 as a method for determining the quality of proteins is based on an estimate of crude protein digestibility determined over the total digestive tract, and values stated using this method generally overestimate the number of amino acids absorbed [57]. Compared with casein, which has a DIAAS of 101, rice has a DIASS of 47, whereas wheat has a DIASS of 48, oat has a DIASS of 57, and corn (Maize) has a DIASS of 36 [58]. If instead we take into consideration the PDCAAS, rice bran protein has a PDCAAS of 0.90, whereas casein has a PDCASS of 1.00, and rice endosperm protein has a PDCAAS of 0.63 [59]

2.6. Maize (Corn)

Maize, also known as corn, is a large grass plant already domesticated by the native populations of Mexico about 10,000 years ago. The word corn derives from the term "mahiz", with which the indigenous Taino people of the Caribbean and Florida called the plant, later transliterated into Spanish. In the United States, Canada, Australia, and New Zealand, the term mainly refers to maize with the term "corn", derived from the shortening of the expression "Indian corn", which mainly refers to maize, which is the staple cereal of Native Americans [20].

2.6.1. Nutrients

A 100 g serving of uncooked corn kernels provide 86 calories; it contains 3.27 g of proteins, 18.7 g of carbohydrates, 2 g of fibers, 6.26 g of sugars, and 1.35 g of fats, of which 26% of saturated fatty acids, 39% of polyunsaturated fatty acids, and 35% of monounsaturated fatty acids. Raw maize is a good source of group B vitamins, particularly niacin (11% of DV), riboflavin (4% of DV), thiamine (13% of DV), and vitamin B6 (7% of DV). Raw maize is also a good source of several dietary minerals, especially copper (6% of DV), iron (3% of DV), magnesium (9% of DV), manganese (7% of DV), phosphorus (13% of DV), potassium (6% of DV), zinc (4% of DV), selenium (1% of DV), and sodium (1% of DV) [21].

2.6.2. Maize Oil

Corn oil (corn oil, CO) is obtained by extraction from the corn germ. It is mainly used in the kitchen, thanks to its high smoking temperature, which makes corn oil suitable for frying. It is also a staple ingredient in margarine production. It is also used as an excipient in the pharmaceutical industry [20].

A total of 100 g of maize oil contains 13% of saturated fatty acids, of which 82% is palmitic acid (C 16:0) and 14% is stearic acid (C 18:0); 28% of monounsaturated fatty acids, of which 99% is oleic acid (C 18:1); and 55% of polyunsaturated fatty acids, of which 98% is linoleic acid (C 18:2), and 2% is omega-3 linolenic acid (C 18:3) [21,60].

2.6.3. Corn Oil vs. Extra-Virgin Olive Oil

Unlike CO, whose production takes place through the solvent extraction of the oil from the grain after the separation of the corn germ with fragmentation or centrifugation, the production of olive oil takes place essentially by mechanical pressing of the drupe. A 100 g serving of extra virgin olive oil (EVOO) provides 884 calories. Almost 98% of the total weight of EVOO is represented by fatty acids, which constitute the saponifiable fraction of olive oil. The fatty acid content of EVOO consists of 75% monounsaturated fatty acids (mostly oleic acid), 11% polyunsaturated fatty acids (mostly linoleic acid), and 14% saturated fatty acids (mostly palmitic acid) [20,21]. The remaining 2% of the total weight of EVOO is represented by the unsaponifiable fraction. The stability and flavor of olive oil are given by the components of the unsaponifiable fraction.

The unsaponifiable fraction is divided into the non-polar, non-water-soluble, solvent-extractable fraction after saponification of the oil, which contains squalene and other triterpenes, sterols, tocopherol (mainly alpha-tocopherol, or vitamin E), and pigments, and the polar fraction, water-soluble, which contains phenolic compounds, or polyphenols.

Polyphenols make up 18–37% of the unsaponifiable fraction of EVOO; these are responsible for most of the health benefits associated with taking EVOO. It is a heterogeneous group of molecules with important properties that are both organoleptic and nutritional [21]. Extra virgin olive oil has an average concentration of phenolic compounds of about 230 mg/kg [61], with a concentration of polyphenols ranging from 50 to 800 mg/kg [62,63]. The absorption efficiency of olive oil polyphenols in humans has been evaluated around 55–66 mmol% [64]. Tyrosol and hydroxytyrosol are two of the most important phenols in olive oil. Hydroxytyrosol is present in olive oil in the form of ester with elenolic acid to form oleuropein; the absorption in humans is dose-dependent, related to the phenolic content of olive oil [65].

2.6.4. Poly- and Monounsaturated Fatty Acids, Serum Cholesterol Levels and Cardiovascular Disease

A meta-analysis by Mensink et al. [66] showed that under isocaloric, metabolic ward conditions, when carbohydrates in the diet were replaced by fatty acids, HDL increased and triglycerides decreased, while LDL increased. In addition, if polyunsaturated fats replace saturated fats, then a more marked decrease in serum LDL and triglyceride levels was observed. Authors also showed that replacing saturated fatty acids with unsaturated fatty acids increased the ratio of HDL to LDL cholesterol, thus obtaining the most favorable lipoprotein risk profile for CHD. Substitution of saturated fatty acids with carbohydrates had no favorable effect on the CHD risk profile.

Subsequently, Maki et al. [67], in their randomized, double-blind, controlled-feeding trial, showed that CO reduced total cholesterol (TC), low-density lipoprotein cholesterol (LDL), very low-density lipoprotein cholesterol (VLDL), non-high-density lipoprotein cholesterol (non-HDL), and ApoB concentration to a greater extent compared with EVOO intake (CO compared with EVOO intake: TC = -0.37 vs. 0.02 mmol/L, $p > 0.001$; LDL = -0.36 vs. -0.08 mmol/L, $p > 0.001$; VLDL = -0.03 vs. 0.04 mmol/L, $p > 0.001$; non-HDL = -0.39 vs. -0.04 mmol/L, $p > 0.001$). ApoB, an indicator of circulating small and dense, and therefore highly atherogenic, LDL, was lowered largely by CO, compared to EVOO intake (-9.0 vs. -2.5 mg/dL, $p > 0.001$). HDL-C concentration did not differ significantly between CO vs. EVOO intake (0.02 vs. 0.05 mmol/L, $p = 0.112$), but ApoA1, which is the major protein component of HDL particles in plasma, increased more with EVOO compared with CO intake (4.6 vs. 0.7 mg/dL, $p = 0.016$).

The Nurses' Health Study [68] prospectively investigated the association between different types of dietary fat intake and the risk of coronary heart disease in a 14-year follow-up in a cohort of 80,082 women, aged between 34 and 59 years of age, without a history of CHD, stroke, cancer, hypercholesterolemia, or diabetes. The authors demonstrated that a 5% increase in energy intake from saturated fat was associated with a 17% increase, although not statistically significant in the relative risk (RR) of CHD (RR = 1.17; 95% CI = 0.97–1.41; $p = 0.10$) compared to the equivalent energy intake from carbohydrates. The authors also demonstrated that for each 2% increase in energy intake from trans-unsaturated fats, a significant 93% increase in the risk of CHD was associated (RR = 1.93; 95% CI = 1.43–2.61; $p = 0.001$). Finally, the authors demonstrated that while for each 5% increase in energy intake from monounsaturated fats, there was a non-statistically significant 19% decrease in the risk of CHD (RR = 0.81; 95% CI = 0.65–1.00; $p = 0.05$); with each 5% increase in energy intake from polyunsaturated fats, there was a significant 38% reduction in the risk of CHD (RR = 0.62; 95% CI = 0.46–0.85; $p < 0.003$). The authors also showed that replacing 5% energy from saturated fat with unsaturated fat resulted in a 42% reduction in CHD risk (95% CI = 0.23–0.56; $p < 0.001$), while replacing 2% of energy from trans unsaturated fat with un-hydrogenated, unsaturated fats was associated with a 53% decrease of the risk of CHD (95% CI = 0.34–67; $p < 0.001$). The authors concluded by confirming that the replacement of saturated fats (SF) and trans-unsaturated fats in the diet with non-hydrogenated monounsaturated and polyunsaturated fats favorably alters the lipid profile, but that reducing overall fat intake has little effect.

W. C. Willett [69] confirmed these data in a subsequent review by concluding that trans-unsaturated fatty acids in hydrogenated vegetable oils have obvious negative effects and should be eliminated. He also stated that a further reduction in CHD rates is possible if saturated fats are replaced by a combination of poly- and monounsaturated fats and the benefits of polyunsaturated fats appear stronger.

A subsequent pooled analysis of 11 cohort studies by Jakobsen et al. [70] confirmed the effects of the polyunsaturated fatty acids. The authors showed a significant association between PUFA replacement and reduced risk of coronary events (HR: 0.87; 95% CI: 0.77, 0.97) and a significant association between PUFA replacement and reduced risk of mortality for CHD (HR: 0.74; 95% CI: 0.61, 0.89). In conclusion, the authors stated that, rather than increasing the consumption of MUFA or carbohydrates, increasing the consumption of

PUFA in place of saturated fatty acids (SFA) could significantly prevent coronary heart disease among middle-aged women and men and among the elderly.

Lai et al. [71] investigated the associations between de novo lipogenesis (DNL)-related fatty acids (FA) with total mortality and specific cause mortality including cardiovascular disease (CVD), CHD, and stroke, analyzing the data from the Cardiovascular Health Study (CHS) [72], measured at three time points over 13 years. Surprisingly, they found a direct association between higher oleic acid levels (18: 1n-9) and a high risk (hazard risk, HR) of all-cause mortality (HR = 1.56, 95% CI = 1.35–1.80, $p < 0.001$) including CVD and non-CVD mortality (HR = 1.48, 95% CI = 1.21–1.82, $p < 0.001$; HR = 1.50, CI = 95% 1.28–1.75, $p < 0.001$, respectively). They also found an association between higher oleic acid levels and fatal and non-fatal CVD, fatal and non-fatal CHD, fatal and non-fatal stroke (HR = 1.33, 95% CI = 1.12–1.57, $p < 0.001$; HR = 1.23, 95% CI = 1.01–1.48, $p = 0.008$; HR = 1.34, 95% CI = 1.02–1.75, $p = 0.005$, respectively).

Results of a meta-analysis by Borges et al. [73], which included five cohort studies and one matched case-control study, involving 23,518 subjects, showed that the risk (odds ratio, OR) of CHD was lower with higher circulating docosahexaenoic acid (DHA) levels (OR = 0.85; 95% CI = 0.76–0.95), but was not associated with stroke risk (OR = 0.95; 95% CI = 0.89–1.02; risk of stroke was lower with higher circulating linoleic acid (LA) levels (OR = 0.82; 95% CI = 0.75–0.90), but was not associated with CHD (OR = 1.01; 95% CI = 0.87–1.18); circulating MUFA were associated with higher CHD risk of stroke (OR = 1.22; 95% CI = 1.03–1.44) and CHD (OR = 1.36; 95% CI = 1.15–1.61). SFA was not related both with increased CHD risk (OR = 0.94; 95% CI = 0.82–1.09) and with stroke risk (OR = 0.94; 95% CI = 0.79–1.11).

Finally, Lee et al. [74] studied the associations between plasma AF levels with the risk of incident heart failure (HF) by analyzing data from CHS. They showed that plasma habitual levels and changes in the levels of palmitic acid (16:0) were associated with higher risk of HF (HR = 1.17, 95% CI 1.00–1.36; HR = 1.26 95% CI 1.03–1.55, respectively); plasma habitual levels of 7-hexadecenoic acid (16:1n-9) were not associated with risk of HF (HR = 1.05, 95% CI 0.92–1.18), but changes in levels were associated with a higher risk of HF (HR = 1.36, 95% CI 1.13–1.62); plasma habitual levels of vaccenic acid (18:1n-7) were not associated with risk of HF (HR = 1.06, 95% CI 0.92–1.22), but changes in levels were associated with a higher risk of HF (HR = 1.43, 95% CI 1.18–1.72); habitual levels and changes in levels of myristic acid (14:0) (HR = 0.90, 95% CI = 0.77–1.05; HR = 1.11, 95% CI = 0.91–1.36, respectively), palmitoleic acid (16:1n-7) (HR = 1.01, 95% CI = 0.88–1.16; HR = 1.06, 95% CI = 0.87–1.28, respectively), stearic acid (18:0) (HR = 0.94, 95% CI = 0.81–1.09; HR = 0.94, 95% CI = 0.76–1.15, respectively), and oleic acid (18:1n-9) (HR = 1.13, 95% CI = 0.98–1.30; HR = 1.13, 95% CI = 0.93–1.37, respectively) were not associated with HF risk,

Despite these conflicting results, the advice to replace saturated fats with polyunsaturated fats in the diet remains a cornerstone of international guidelines for reducing the risk of CHD.

On the other hand, it would be overly simplistic to say that replacing SFAs with MUFA (oleic or linoleic acid) or PUFA may be sufficient in reducing the risk of CVD or mortality risk. The benefits of taking MUFAs are observed when they are associated with the concomitant intake of polyphenols and other natural antioxidants, contained, for example, in EVOO. In fact, there is no evidence to suggest that simply replacing SFA with MUFA reduces the risk of CVD or mortality. Similarly, the benefits of daily intake of PUFA-n3 are attributable to PUFAs, but above all where they are associated, similarly to MUFAs, with the intake of polyphenols or other natural antioxidants, and as part of a healthy diet such as the traditional Mediterranean diet. All the above-mentioned studies are shown in Table 2.

Table 2. Poly- and monounsaturated fatty acids, serum cholesterol levels, and CVD.

Author and Year of Publication	Study Design	Duration of Study	Sample Size	Lipoprotein Levels and CVD
Mensink, 1992 [66]	Meta-analysis of 27 case-control studies	14–91 days	682 subjects, 474 men and 208 women	**Carbohydrates in the diet replaced isocaloricalry by saturated fatty acids:** Increase HDL cholesterol ($p < 0.001$), LDL cholesterol ($p < 0.001$), Total Cholesterol ($p < 0.001$); lower triglycerides ($p < 0.001$). **Carbohydrates in the diet replaced isocaloricalry by monounsaturated fatty acids:** Increase HDL cholesterol ($p < 0.001$); no effects on LDL cholesterol ($p = 0.114$), Total Cholesterol ($p = 0.342$); lower triglycerides ($p < 0.001$). **Carbohydrates in the diet replaced isocaloricalry by polyunsaturated fatty acids:** Increase HDL cholesterol ($p = 0.002$), LDL cholesterol ($p = 0.002$), Total Cholesterol ($p < 0.001$), triglycerides ($p < 0.001$).
Maki, 2017 [67]	Randomized, double-blind, crossover trial	21-day treatment (54 g per day of CO or EVOO) 21-day washout	54 volunteers, men and women	**CO intake vs. EVOO intake:** Total cholesterol = −0.37 vs. 0.02 mmol/L ($p > 0.001$); LDL = −0.36 vs. −0.08 mmol/L ($p > 0.001$); VLDL = −0.03 vs. 0.04 mmol/L ($p > 0.001$); non-HDL = −0.39 vs. −0.04 mmol/L ($p > 0.001$). ApoB = −9.0 vs. −2.5 mg/dl ($p > 0.001$). HDL = 0.02 vs. 0.05 mmol/L ($p = 0.112$). **EVOO intake vs. CO intake:** ApoA1 = 4.6 vs. 0.7 mg/dl ($p = 0.016$).
Hu, 1997 [68] Willet, 2012 [69]	Prospective Cohort Study	Follow-up: 14 years	80,082 women, from the cohort of the Nurses' Health Study	**CHD Risk for each 5% increase in energy intake from saturated fats:** RR = 1.17; 95% CI = 0.97–1.41; $p = 0.10$. **CHD Risk for each 2% increase in energy intake from trans-unsaturated fats:** RR = 1.93; 95% CI = 1.43–2.61; $p = 0.001$) **CHD Risk for each 5% increase in energy intake from monounsaturated fats:** RR = 0.81; 95% CI = 0.65–1.00; $p = 0.05$). **CHD Risk for each 5% increase in energy intake from polyunsaturated fats:** RR = 0.62; 95% CI = 0.46–0.85; $p < 0.003$. **CHD Risk by replacing 5% energy from saturated fat with unsaturated fat:** RR = 0.58; 95% CI = 0.23–0.56; $p < 0.001$) **CHD Risk by replacing 2% of energy from trans unsaturated fat with un-hydrogenated, unsaturated fats:** RR = 0.47; 95% CI = 0.34–0.67; $p < 0.001$.
Jakobsen, 2009 [70]	Meta-analysis of prospective cohort studies	Follow-up: 4 to 10 years	344,696 subjects from 11 American and European studies included in the Pooling Project of Cohort Studies on Diet and Coronary Disease	**CHD Risk by replacing 5% of energy from SFA with MUFA or PUFA or carbohydrates (CHs):** MUFAs vs. SFAs: HR = 1.19; 95% CI = 1.00–1.42. PUFAs vs. SFAs: HR = 0.87; 95% CI = 0.77–0.97. CHs vs. SFAs: HR = 1.07; 95% CI = 1.01–1.14. **Coronary deaths Risk by replacing 5% of energy from SFA with MUFA or PUFA or carbohydrates (CHs):** MUFAs vs. SFAs: HR = 1.01; 95% CI = 0.73–1.41. PUFAs vs. SFAs: HR = 0.74; 95% CI = 0.61–0.89. CHs vs. SFAs: HR = 0.96; 95% CI = 0.82–1.13.

Table 2. Cont.

Author and Year of Publication	Study Design	Duration of Study	Sample Size	Lipoprotein Levels and CVD
Lai, 2019 [71]	Prospective Cohort Study	Follow-up: 22 years	3869 subjects from the cohort of the Cardiovascular Health Study (CHS)	**Palmitic acid (16:0) and risk of mortality** All-cause mortality: HR = 1.35; 95% CI = 1.17–1.56; $p < 0.001$. CVD mortality: HR = 1.44; 95% CI = 1.18–1.76; $p < 0.001$. Non-CVD mortality: HR = 1.36; 95% CI = 1.16–1.59; $p < 0.001$. **Palmitoleic acid (16:1n-7) and risk of mortality** All-cause mortality: HR = 1.40; 95% CI = 1.21–1.62; $p < 0.001$. CVD mortality: HR = 1.42; 95% CI = 1.15–1.76; $p = 0.001$. Non-CVD mortality: HR = 1.30; 95% CI = 1.12–1.52; $p = 0.001$ **Stearic acid (18:0) and risk of mortality** All-cause mortality: HR = 0.76; 95% CI = 0.66–0.88; $p < 0.001$. CVD mortality: HR = 0.77; 95% CI = 0.62–0.94; $p = 0.003$. Non-CVD mortality: HR = 0.72; 95% CI = 0.62–0.84; $p < 0.001$ **Oleic acid (18:1n-9) and risk of mortality** All-cause mortality: HR = 1.56; 95% CI = 1.35–1.80; $p < 0.001$. CVD mortality: HR = 1.48; 95% CI = 1.21–1.82; $p < 0.001$. Non-CVD mortality: HR = 1.50 95% CI = 1.28–1.75; $p < 0.001$. **Palmitic acid (16:0) and risk of incident CVD** Fatal and non-fatal CVD: HR = 1.20; 95% CI = 1.01–1.43; $p = 0.029$. Fatal and non-fatal CHD: HR = 1.13; 95% CI = 0.93–1.38; $p = 0.287$. Fatal and non-fatal Stroke: HR = 1.26; 95% CI = 0.96–1.66; $p = 0.028$. **Palmitoleic acid (16:1n-7) and risk of incident CVD** Fatal and non-fatal CVD: HR = 1.28; 95% CI = 1.07–1.53; $p = 0.012$. Fatal and non-fatal CHD: HR = 1.07; 95% CI = 0.88–1.31; $p = 0.506$. Fatal and non-fatal Stroke: HR = 1.38; 95% CI = 1.05–1.83; $p = 0.038$. **Stearic acid (18:0) and risk of incident CVD** Fatal and non-fatal CVD: HR = 0.82; 95% CI = 0.69–0.97; $p = 0.003$. Fatal and non-fatal CHD: HR = 0.93; 95% CI = 0.77–1.13; $p = 0.266$. Fatal and non-fatal Stroke: HR = 0.77; 95% CI = 0.59–1.00; $p = 0.013$. **Oleic acid (18:1n-9) and risk of incident CVD** Fatal and non-fatal CVD: HR = 1.33; 95% CI = 1.12–1.57; $p < 0.001$. Fatal and non-fatal CHD: HR = 1.23; 95% CI = 1.01–1.48; $p = 0.008$. Fatal and non-fatal Stroke: HR = 1.34; 95% CI = 1.02–1.75; $p = 0.005$.
Borges, 2020 [73]	Meta-analysis of prospective cohort and case-control studies	Follow-up: 10 to 25 years	23,518 subjects from 5 cohort studies and 1 case-control study, from the UCL-LSHTM-Edinburgh-Bristol (UCLEB) Consortium	**DHA and risk for CHD** OR = 0.85; 95% CI = 0.76–0.95 **LA and risk for CHD** OR = 1.01; 95% CI = 0.87–1.18 **MUFA and risk for CHD** OR = 1.36; 95% CI = 1.15–1.61 **SFA and risk for CHD** OR = 0.94; 95% CI = 0.82–1.09 **DHA and risk for Stroke** OR = 0.95; 95% CI = 0.89–1.02 **LA and risk for Stroke** OR = 0.82; 95% CI = 0.75–0.90 **MUFA and risk for Stroke** OR = 1.22; 95% CI = 1.03–1.44 **SFA and risk for Stroke** OR = 0.94; 95% CI = 0.79–1.11
Lee, 2020 [74]	Prospective Cohort Study	Follow-up: 22 years	4249 subjects from the cohort of the Cardiovascular Health Study (CHS)	**Habitual levels of plasma fatty acids and risk of incident HF** palmitic acid: HR = 1.17, 95% CI 1.00–1.36; 7-hexadecenoic acid: HR = 1.05, 95% CI 0.92–1.18; vaccenic acid: HR = 1.06, 95% CI 0.92–1.22; but changes in levels were associated with a higher risk of HF (HR = 1.43, 95% CI 1.18–1.72); myristic acid: HR = 0.90, 95% CI = 0.77–1.05; palmitoleic acid: HR = 1.01, 95% CI = 0.88–1.16; stearic acid: HR = 0.94, 95% CI = 0.81–1.09; oleic acid: HR = 1.13, 95% CI = 0.98–1.30; **Change in serial levels of plasma fatty acids and risk of incident HF** palmitic acid: HR = 1.26 95% CI 1.03–1.55; 7-hexadecenoic acid: HR = 1.36, 95% CI 1.13–1.62; vaccenic acid: HR = 1.43, 95% CI 1.18–1.72; myristic acid: HR = 1.11, 95% CI = 0.91–1.36; palmitoleic acid: HR = 1.06, 95% CI = 0.87–1.28; stearic acid: HR = 0.94, 95% CI = 0.76–1.15; oleic acid: HR = 1.13, 95% CI = 0.93–1.37.

CO: corn oil; EVOO: extra virgin olive oil; CHD: coronary heart disease; LA: linoleic acid; HF: heart failure

2.7. Barley

Barley (Hordeum vulgare) is a cereal grain that is grown in temperate climates worldwide. It is one of the oldest cultivated cereals, originally in the Fertile Crescent area of the Middle East and Egypt. Barley is used commonly as animal fodder. Concerning human nutrition, two types of barley are commonly found: hulled barley, which requires a long cooking time and preventive soaking, and pearl barley, which undergoes a refining process (similar to whitening rice) to remove the outermost part. This can be used without prior soaking and cooking time is shorter. Barley is used for the preparation of soups and stews and also for cooking barley bread. From the coarse ground, coarse semolina is obtained, suitable for typical North African dishes similar to couscous. Roasted in the oven at temperatures around 170–180 °C, and very finely ground until obtaining a powder similar to flour, and freeze-dried, it is used to quickly prepare drinks by adding hot water or milk or used as a substitute for coffee. Roasted fine flours are also obtained from the roasting of barley and are used in the preparation of sweets or pastries. Barley grains are commonly made into malt as a source of fermentable material for beer and distilled beverages, like whisky.

2.7.1. Nutrients

A 100 g of barley provides 352 calories. Barley is made up of about 28% carbohydrates, 57% dietary fiber, 2% fat, and 20% protein. Barley is also a good source of B vitamins and minerals including copper, iron, magnesium, manganese, phosphorus, selenium, and zinc [21].

2.7.2. Barley β-Glucan

B-glucan constitutes approximatively 75% of dry weight of endosperm cell walls, and arabinoxylan constitutes 25% [75]. The percentages of beta-glucan content in the barley grain vary according to the different polymorphisms of the genes that encode the corresponding synthase and endohydrolase enzymes [76]. Barley β-glucans also have cholesterol-lowering properties [77,78], however, lower than oats [79]. In addition, it is known that β-glucans from barley reduce post-prandial glycemic response with lowering blood glucose. This effect is due not because of the high viscosity of the β-glucans, but rather to the direct inhibition of the activities of glucose transporters and intestinal brush border enzymes [80,81]. More evidence has shown that β-glucans exert their beneficial effects on lipid and glucose metabolism and reduce CVD risk by the increase in colonic microbial population and activity, particularly favoring the increase in Lactobacillus over Bacteroidetes spp, yielding short-chain fatty acids as end products [48,82]. In animal models, these health benefits, on microbial gut flora, are also associated with an increase in lifespan and better locomotor activity, muscle coordination, and balancing activity [83].

3. Diet Pattern and Risk of Frailty and Mortality

It is now known that fruits and vegetables, in addition to the intake of whole grains, monounsaturated and omega-3 fatty acids, and moderate amounts of alcohol are fundamental elements of a cardioprotective diet [84]. Furthermore, it is known that a prevalent consumption of fruit, vegetables, and WG, even in a dietary model different from traditional MD, is protective (i.e., associated with a reduced risk of frailty) [85].

Lo et al. [86] analyzed data from the Nutrition and Health Survey in Taiwan. They showed that elderly subjects in the higher tertile of the dietary pattern score (i.e., with a high consumption of fruit, nuts and seeds, tea, vegetables, WG, omega-3-rich deep-sea fish, and shellfish and milk as protein-rich foods) had a reduced risk (Odds Ratio, OR) of frailty (OR = 0.12, 95% CI 0.02–0.76, p = 0.019) or pre-frailty (OR = 0.40, 95% CI 0.19–0.83, p = 0.015).

Following the studies by Ancel Keys, MD has been proposed as a model of healthy eating, associated with a reduced risk of developing cardiovascular and metabolic diseases [5]. Subsequently, Trichopoulou et al. showed that high adhesion to MD was associated with a reduction in the risk of total mortality [6,87].

Subsequently, the PREDIMED study [8,9,88] demonstrated that high-risk CVD subjects who followed an MD pattern, in which monounsaturated and antioxidant fatty acids came from taking EVOO, or alternatively taking omega-3 fatty acids from nut consumption, had a reduced risk of acute myocardial infarction, stroke, or death from CVD (MD with EVOO: HR = 0.70, 95% CI: 0.53–0.91, p = 0.009; MD with nuts: HR = 0.70, 95% CI: 0.53–0.94, p = 0.02), but not of total mortality (MD with EVOO: HR = 0.81, 95% CI: 0.63–1.05, p = 0.11; MD with nuts: HR = 0.95, 95% CI: 0.73–1.23, p = 0.68).

A meta-analysis [10] that involved 1,574,299 subjects followed for a time period of 3–18 years found a significant direct association between higher adherence to MD, improved health status, and reduced mortality risk (Rate Risk, RR) (RR = 0.91, 95% CI 0.89–0.94; $p < 0.0001$), particularly in mortality due to CHD (RR = 0.91, 95% CI: 0.87–0.95, $p < 0.0001$) and cancer (RR = 0.94; 95% CI: 0.92–0.96; $p < 0.0001$).

Another meta-analysis by the same authors [11] also showed a significant association between higher MD adherence, improved health and quality of life, and reduced overall mortality (RR = 0.92, CI 95%: 0.90–0.94, $p < 0.00001$). In particular, the authors showed a significant reduction in mortality from CHD (RR = 0.90; 95% CI: 0.87–0.93; $p < 0.00001$) or from cancer (RR = 0.94; 95% CI: 0.92–0.96; $p < 0.00001$).

Kromhout et al. [89] confirmed the association between a higher adherence to a dietary model with the characteristics of MD with a reduction in CHD mortality ($r = -0.91$). The authors further highlighted the protective role in the diet of cereals ($r = -0.52$), vegetables ($r = -0.52$), and legumes ($r = -0.62$) as well as the intake of a moderate amount of alcohol ($r = -0.54$).

Subsequently, Zaslavsky et al. [90] analyzed a sample of 10,431 women aged 65–84 years from the Women's Health Initiative Observational Study [91,92] with complete frailty according to Fried's criteria [93]. MD pattern adherence was assessed using the alternative MD (aMed) index [6,94], which considered the intake of fruit, vegetables, nuts, legumes, WG, fish, ratio of monounsaturated to saturated fat, red and processed meats, and alcohol. The authors further showed the association between a higher intake of vegetables, nuts, and WG with a significant reduction in mortality risk (HR = 0.91, 95% CI: 0.84–0.99, p = 0.02; HR = 0.87, 95% CI: 0.80–0.94, $p < 0.001$; HR = 0.83, 95% CI: 0.77–0.90, $p < 0.001$, respectively). The relative contribution of these components to the reduction of mortality risk, obtained by subtracting each component from the aMed Index, was respectively 21% (vegetables), 42% (nuts) and 57% (WG).

More recently, Campanella et al. [95] performed a survival analysis involving 4896 subjects from Castellana Grotte and Putignano (Apulia, Italy) included in the MICOL study [96] and in the NUTRIHEP study [97], respectively. The relative Mediterranean scoring system (rMED) [98] was used to measure adherence to MD. The rMED considers the intake of fruit (excluding fruit juices), vegetables (excluding potatoes), legumes, cereals, fresh fish, olive oil, meat and dairy products, and alcohol. The authors noted that higher MD adherence was directly correlated with longer lifespan. In particular, among subjects with greater adherence to MD at the baseline, the mean time to death was estimated to be postponed from 6.21 to 8.28 years compared to subjects with lower MD adherence.

The protective effect of the MD [99] are certainly due to the lipid-lowering effect, protection against oxidative stress, inflammation, and platelet aggregation, modification of hormones and growth factors involved in the pathogenesis of cancer, inhibition of nutrient sensing pathways by specific amino acid restriction, and gut microbiota-mediated production of metabolites influencing metabolic health. Specifically, the moderate energy restriction provided by the high consumption of fiber-rich energy-poor plant foods and the specific restriction of sulfur compounds, branch-chain amino acids, and saturated fatty acids, characteristics of the MD, play a prominent role in mediating the beneficial effects on the health and longevity of this dietary model. In addition, the intestinal microbiome, which is actively involved in the processing of many plant foods rich in fiber as well as several vitamins and phytochemicals, plays a vital role in maintaining both metabolic and molecular health.

Hernaez et al. [100] reported the results of a study conducted on a subsample of 296 subjects at high cardiovascular risk, extracted from the cohort of the PREDIMED study [8,9]. The authors confirmed the beneficial effects of the intake of EVOO, nuts, legumes, WG, and fish. Mostly, they showed that increase for one year in the intake of these cardioprotective foods was linked to an improvement in HDL biological functions. In particular, increase in daily intake of 10 g of EVOO and 25 g of whole grain was associated with increment in cholesterol efflux capacity, in other words, the capacity of HDL to pick up cholesterol (+0.7%, $p = 0.026$; +0.6%, $p = 0.017$, respectively). Increase in daily intake of 30 g of nuts and 25 g of legumes and 25 g of fresh fish was linked to increment in the activity of paraoxonase-1, a key HDL-bound antioxidant enzyme (+12.2%, $p = 0.049$; +11.7%, $p = 0.043$; +3.9%, $p = 0.030$, respectively). Increase in legumes and fish consumption was also related to decreases in the activity of cholesteryl ester transfer protein, pro-atherogenic when excessively active (−4.8%, $p = 0.028$; −1.6%, $p = 0.021$, respectively).

The above evidence reaffirms a fundamental concept, namely, that it is not the single nutrient or the single antioxidant that is effective in reducing mortality, nor the risk of frailty, but the set of nutrients in the diet. Another key point is that diet is not intended as an effective therapy or as something to be taken for a defined time. In contrast, the diet should be understood as a diet to be practiced for life and in the context of a healthy lifestyle, as observed, for example, in populations following the traditional MD or the Okinawa diet.

All the above-mentioned studies are shown in Table 3.

Table 3. Diet pattern and risk of frailty, cardiovascular risk, and mortality.

Author and Year of Publication	Study Design	Duration of Study	Sample Size	Risk of Frailty and Mortality
Lo, 2017 [86]	Cross-sectional study	3 years	923 subjects aged 65 years and older from the cohort of Nutrition and Health Survey in Taiwan (NAHSIT)	Associations between tertiles of dietary pattern score and frailty according Fried criteria: OR = 0.12 (95% CI = 0.02–0.76; $p = 0.019$) for tertile 3 of dietary pattern score. Associations between tertiles of dietary pattern score and pre-frailty according Fried criteria: OR = 0.40 (95% CI = 0.19–0.83; $p = 0.015$) for tertile 3 of dietary pattern scores.
Trichopoulou, 2003 [6]	Population-based, prospective study	Median duration of follow-up: 3.7 years	8895 men and 13,148 women	All-cause death: HR = 0.75 (95% CI 0.64–0.87) for a Two-Point Increase in the Mediterranean-Diet Score Death from CHD (coronary heart disease): HR = 0.67 (95% CI 0.47–0.94) for a Two-Point Increase in the Mediterranean-Diet Score Death from cancer: HR = 0.76 (95% CI 0.59–0.98) for a Two-Point Increase in the Mediterranean-Diet Score
Estruch, 2018 [9]	Parallel-group, multicenter, randomized trial	Median duration of follow-up: 4.8 years	1050 men and 1493 women with MD(Mediterranean-Diet) with EVOO(extra virgin olive oil) 1128 men and 1326 women with MD with nuts 987 men and 1463 women with Control Diet	Myocardial infarction: HR = 0.82 (95% CI 0.52–1.30) for MD with EVOO vs. Control Diet HR = 0.76 (95% CI 0.47–1.25) for MD with Nuts vs. Control Diet Stroke: HR = 0.65 (95% CI 0.44–0.95) for MD with EVOO vs. Control Diet HR = 0.54 (95% CI 0.35–0.82) for MD with Nuts vs. Control Diet Death from CVD: HR = 0.62 (95% CI 0.36–1.06) for MD with EVOO vs. Control Diet HR = 1.02 (95% CI 0.63–1.67) for MD with Nuts vs. Control Diet All-cause death: HR = 0.90 (95% CI 0.69–1.18) for MD with EVOO vs. Control Diet HR = 1.12 (95% CI 0.86–1.47) for MD with Nuts vs. Control Diet

Table 3. Cont.

Author and Year of Publication	Study Design	Duration of Study	Sample Size	Risk of Frailty and Mortality
Sofi, 2008 [10]	Meta-analysis of prospective cohort studies	Follow-up time range: from 3.7 to 18 years	1,574,299 subjects from 12 studies	**Mortality from CVD:** RR = 0.91 (95% CI 0.87–0.95) **All-cause mortality:** RR = 0.91 (95% CI 0.89–0.94) **Mortality from cancer:** RR = 0.94 (95% CI 0.92–0.96) **Incidence of Parkinson's disease and Alzheimer's disease:** RR = 0.87 (95% CI 0.80–0.96)
Sofi, 2010 [11]	Meta-analysis of prospective cohort studies	Follow-up time range: from 4 to 20 years	508,393 subjects from 7 studies	**Mortality from CVD:** RR = 0.90 (95% CI 0.87–0.93) **All-cause mortality:** RR = 0.92 (95% CI 0.90–0.94) **Mortality from cancer:** RR = 0.94 (95% CI 0.92–0.96) **Incidence of neurodegenerative disease:** RR = 0.87 (95% CI 0.81–0.94)
Kromhout, 2018 [89]	Prospective Cohort Study	Follow-up time: 50-years	12,763 subjects from 16 cohorts of the Seven Countries Study.	**Mortality from CVD:** Inverse correlation between consumption of cereals, vegetables, legumes, and alcohol and long-term CHD mortality rates ($r = -0.52$ to -0.62) Direct correlation between consumption of hard fat plus sweet products, animal foods except fish, and long-term CHD mortality rates ($r = 0.68$ to 0.84)
Zaslavsky, 2018 [90]	Prospective Cohort Study	Mean follow-up: 12.4 years	10,431 women aged 65–84 year from the cohorts of the Women's Health Initiative Observational Study	**Associations between of dietary pattern and mortality:** HR = 0.91, 95% CI: 0.84–0.99, $p = 0.02$, for high intake of vegetables; HR = 0.87, 95% CI: 0.80–0.94, $p < 0.001$, for high intake of nuts; HR = 0.83, 95% CI: 0.77–0.90, $p < 0.001$, for high intake of whole grains.
Campanella, 2020 [95]	Prospective Cohort Study	Median follow-up time: 12.82, 12.91 and 12.84 years for high, medium and low rMED subjects	5152 subjects from the cohorts of MICOL/PANEL and NUTRIHEP Study (2851 from MICOL/PANEL; 2301 from NUTRIHEP)	**Associations between of dietary pattern and mortality:** Direct correlation between higher adherence to the MD at baseline and mortality. Higher adherence to the MD at baseline was related to a lifespan 6.21 and 8.28 years longer.
Hernaez, 2019 [100]	Parallel-group, multicenter, randomized trial	Follow-up time: 1 year.	296 subjects from the cohort of the PREDIMED Study	**Association among food groups and improvements in HDL functions:** Increments in cholesterol efflux capacity: +0.7% ($p = 0.026$) for increase in daily intake of 10 g of EVOO; +0.6% ($p = 0.017$) for increase in daily intake of 25 g of WG; −1.1% ($p = 0.010$) for increase in daily intake of 25 g of fish. Increments in PON1(Paraoxonase 1) activity: +12.2% ($p = 0.049$) for increase in daily intake of 30 g of nuts; +11.7% ($p = 0.043$) for increase in daily intake of 25 g of legume; +3.9% ($p = 0.030$) for increase in daily intake of 25 g of fish. Decreases in CETP(cholesteryl ester transfer protein) activity: −4.8% ($p = 0.028$) for increase in daily intake of 25 g of legume; −1.6%, ($p = 0.021$) for increase in daily intake of 25 g of fish.

4. Whole Grains Intake, Cardiovascular Risk Factors, and Body Weight

According to the HEALTHGRAIN Consortium definition [101], whole grain (WG) means "the intact, ground, cracked or flaked kernel after the removal of inedible parts such as the hull and husk. The principal anatomical components, as the starchy endosperm, germ, and bran, are present in the same relative proportions, as they exist in the intact kernel. Small losses of components, that is, less than 2% of the grain/10% of the bran, that occur through processing methods consistent with safety and quality are allowed".

Maras et al. [102] analyzed data from the Baltimore Longitudinal Study on Aging [103] and identified the main sources of WG as breakfast cereals (57.5%), multi-grain and whole wheat bread (16.5%), corn chips snack type (4.2%), popcorn (3.8%), and rye bread (3.6%).

Sette et al. [104] calculated whole grain intakes in an Italian sample of 2830 adults and older adults and of 440 children and adolescents from the INRAN-SCAI 2005–06 Study. The main source of total WG intake among adults and older adults were bread (46%), biscuits (20%), savory fine bakery products (15%), breakfast cereals (7%), and wheat and other cereals (6%).

Subsequently, Ruggiero et al. [105] calculated WG intakes in a different Italian sample of 2830 adults and older adults and of 440 children and adolescents from the Italian Nutrition & Health Survey (INHES) Study. In this study, the major food sources of WG among adults and older adults were bread (53.3%), biscuits (27.4%), pasta (13.1%), breakfast cereals (4.8%), and soups (1.3%). Figure 4 summarizes the different intake of whole grain among U.S. and Italian populations.

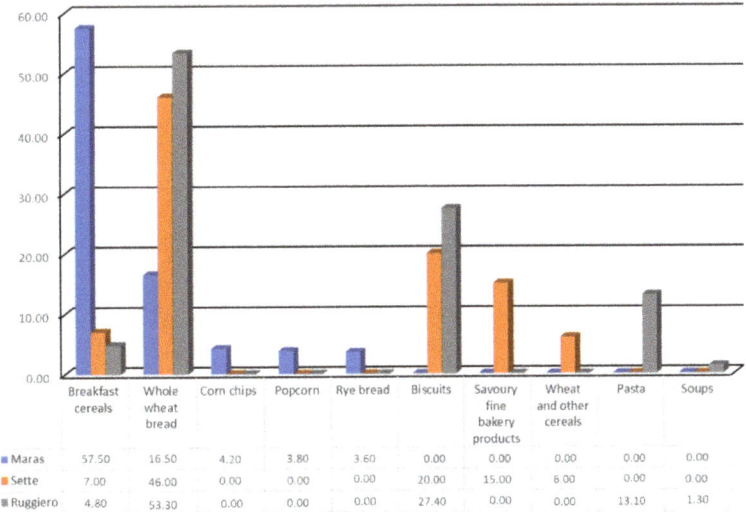

Figure 4. Intake of whole grain: U.S. vs. Italian population. Adapted from Ruggiero et al. [105].

There is now growing epidemiological evidence that WG exerts beneficial effects on human health, especially concerning the metabolic profile [106]. In particular, the consumption of WG has been associated with a reduction in cardiovascular risk factors such as postprandial insulin, blood lipid profile, and finally, the intestinal microbiome [107–109], as summarized in Figure 5.

Kelly et al. [110] conducted a systematic review to evaluate the effect of WG diets on total cardiovascular mortality, cardiovascular events, and cardiovascular risk factors (blood lipids, blood pressure). Nine randomized clinical trials (RCTs) published from 2008 to 2014 were included involving 1414 subjects. All included studies reported the effect of WG on major CVD risk factors such as body weight, blood lipids, and blood pressure. The authors did not find any study that clearly reported any effect of WG diets on total cardiovascular mortality or on cardiovascular events (i.e., total myocardial infarction, unstable angina, coronary artery bypass graft surgery, percutaneous transluminal coronary angioplasty, total stroke). Furthermore, the authors specified that all studies involved primary prevention populations and had an unclear or high risk of bias, and no studies had a duration of intervention greater than 16 weeks.

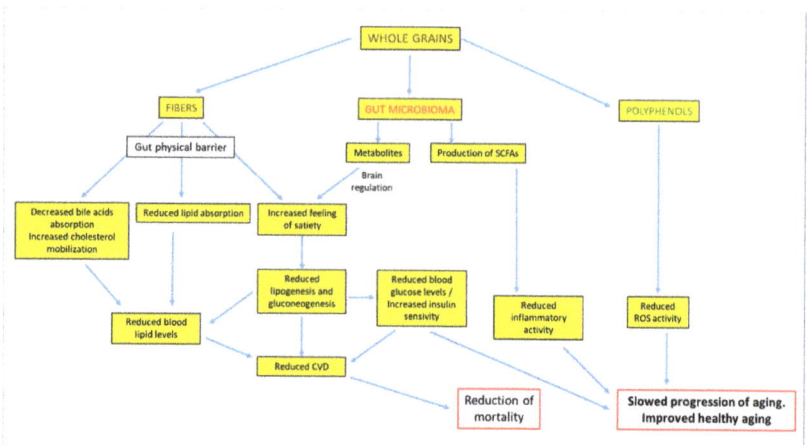

Figure 5. WG(whole grain)'s main mechanisms in reducing mortality and slowing aging.

Kirwan et al. [111] reported the results of a double-blind randomized case-control study conducted in a sample of 40 men and women aged <50 years, with no known history of CVD but who were overweight or frankly obese to compare the effects on body composition and metabolism of a diet containing WG versus an energy diet with refined grains. Each group followed the two diets for eight weeks; a washout period of 10 weeks was interposed between the two diets. The authors described an improvement in diastolic blood pressure (DBP) among overweight and obese adults that was >3 times greater at the end of the feeding period with the WG diet compared to the period of consumption of refined grains (−5.8 mm Hg, 95% CI: −7.7–−4.0 mm Hg; −1.6 mm Hg, 95% CI: −4.4–1.3 mm Hg; p = 0.01, respectively). Regarding systolic blood pressure (SBP), the authors did not observe any significant differences in the magnitude of reduction between WG diet and refined-grain diet group (p = 0.80). In addition, the authors observed a lower decrease in plasma adiponectin levels after the whole-grain diet compared with the control diet (−0.1 µg/mL, 95% CI: −0.9–0.7; −1.4 µg/mL, 95% CI: −2.6–−0.3, p = 0.05, respectively). The preserved total circulating adiponectin concentrations were related to the concentration of circulating adiponectin (r = 0.35, p = 0.04).

Subsequently, Marventano et al. [112] performed a meta-analysis including 41 RCTs to evaluate the effect of WG-containing foods on glycemic control and insulin sensitivity in healthy individuals in the short-, medium-, and long-term by analyzing changes from baseline fasting blood glucose and insulin levels and insulin levels by measuring the area under the curve (iAUC). The authors showed that WG foods induced a significant reduction in the post-prandial values of the glucose iAUC and of insulin iAUC at 120 min by −29.71 mmol min/L and by −2.01 nmol min/L, respectively. They concluded by stating that in healthy subjects, the consumption of WG foods improved postprandial glycemia, insulin response as well as insulin and glucose homeostasis compared to the consumption of refined grain derivatives. The authors suggested, as a possible mechanism that could explain these effects of WG, both the slower digestion rate and the action produced by the microbiome in the large intestine through the fermentation of resistant fibers and starches, with the consequent production of short-chain fatty acids (SCFAs). These short-chain fatty acids, once in the liver, would improve glucose homeostasis and insulin sensitivity by increasing glucose oxidation, the reduction of fatty acid release, and by augmenting insulin clearance [113].

In addition, Musa-Veloso et al. [114] conducted a meta-analysis on 20 full-text articles with the aim of evaluating the effects induced by the consumption of WG wheat, WG rice, or WG rye on postprandial glycemia by comparing the glycemic values after the consumption of the same refined grains. They reported that a significant reduction in blood glucose AUC was observed only after consumption of WG rice compared to white rice (−40.5 mmol/L × min; 95% C =−59.6−−21, 3; $p < 0.001$). In contrast, no significant change in blood glucose AUC was reported, either after the consumption of whole wheat, compared to white wheat, or after the consumption of whole-meal rye compared to refined rye (−6.7 mmol/L × min, 95% CI = −25.1–11.7, $p = 0.477$; −5.5 mmol/L × min; 95% CI = −24.8–13.8; $p = 0.576$, respectively).

Kirø et al. [115] analyzed data from the Diet, Cancer, and Health cohort study [116]. They reported a reduction in the risk of type 2 diabetes of 11% for men and 7% for women, for each increase in consumption of WG (mainly rye) of 16 g/day (HR = 0.89, CI 95% = 0.87, 0.91; HR = 0.93, 95% CI = 0.91. 0.96, respectively). The highest quartile group of WG consumption had a reduction in the risk of type 2 diabetes of 34% for men and 22% for women (HR = 0.66, 95% CI: 0.60–0.72, $p < 0.0001$; HR = 0.78, 95% CI: 0.70–0.86, $p < 0.0001$, respectively). The authors also observed a reduced risk of 12% type 2 diabetes mellitus for men and 7% for women for every increase in the consumption of WG products (mainly rye bread) 50 g/day (HR = 0.88, 95% CI = 0.86–0.90; HR = 0.93, 95% CI = 0.90–0.96, respectively). In addition, a 37% reduction in the risk of type 2 diabetes mellitus for men and 20% for women was observed in the highest quartile group of consumption of WG products (HR = 0.63, CI 95%: 0.58–0.69, $p < 0.0001$; HR = 0.80, 95% CI: 0.72–0.88, $p < 0.0001$, respectively).

Maki et al. [117] performed a meta-regression analysis of cross-sectional data from 12 observational studies involving 136,834 subjects, and a meta-analysis of nine RCTs (WG versus controls) that involved 973 subjects to examine the relationship of WG intake with body weight; they also qualitatively reviewed six prospective cohort publications. The meta-regression analysis from cross-sectional studies indicated a significant inverse correlation between WG intake and body mass index (BMI) ($r = −0.526$, $p = 0.0001$). The review of the results of the qualitative analysis from the prospective cohort studies, with a follow-up period from five to 20 years, showed an inverse correlation between WG consumption and body weight change. Meta-analysis of RCTs, with a length from 12 to 16 weeks, did not show any significant difference in weight change (standardized mean difference = −0.049 Kg; 95% CI = −0.388–0.199; $p = 0.698$).

The discordant results are easily explained by the short duration of some of the studies. Twelve or even 16 weeks is too short a period to observe a significant reduction in cardiovascular events and mortality. The most significant results were observed in long-term prospective studies. This further reinforces the key concept that the intake of WGs should not be compared to taking a drug therapy, which in any case has effects in the short- and medium-term. The intake of WG in the diet must be contextualized, and the above evidence confirms it as part of a healthy diet.

All studies are summarized in Table 4.

Table 4. Whole grains(WG) intake, cardiovascular risk factors and body weight.

Author and Year of Publication	Study Design	Duration of Study	Sample Size	Effect of WG Intake on Cardiovascular Risk Factors and Body Weight
Kelly, 2017 [110]	Meta-analysis of RCTs	Duration of studies: 12 to 16 weeks	1414 subjects from 9 RCTs	**Total CVD mortality and CVD events:** Authors did not find any studies that reported significative effects of WG foods on total cardiovascular mortality or cardiovascular events. **CVD risk factors (mean difference, MD; 95% CI):** Body weight change (kg) = (MD −0.41; 95% CI = −1.04–0.23); BMI = (MD −0.12; 95% CI = −0.24–0.01); Total cholesterol (mmol/L) = (MD 0.07; 95% CI = −0.07–0.21); LDL cholesterol (mmol/L) = (MD 0.06; 95% CI = −0.05–0.16); HDL cholesterol (mmol/L) = (MD −0.02; 95% CI = −0.05–0.01); Triglycerides (mmol/L) = (MD 0.03; 95% CI = −0.08–0.13); SBP(systolic blood pressure) (mmHg) (MD 0.04; 95% CI = −1.67–1.75); DBP(diastolic blood pressure) (mmHg) (MD 0.16; 95% CI = −0.89–1.21).

Table 4. Cont.

Author and Year of Publication	Study Design	Duration of Study	Sample Size	Effect of WG Intake on Cardiovascular Risk Factors and Body Weight
Kirwan, 2016 [111]	Double-blind, randomized, controlled crossover study	Duration of study: 8 weeks, with a 10 weeks washout period between diets	33 overweight or obese men and women.	Body weight: No significant difference between WG vs. control diets. SBP: No significant difference between WG vs. control diets ($p = 0.80$). DBP: WG vs. control diet = (-5.8 mm Hg (95% CI = 27.7–24.0) vs. -1.6 mm Hg (95% CI = 24.4–1.3 mm Hg), $p = 0.01$. Total Cholesterol and LDL Cholesterol: No significant difference between WG vs. control diets HbA1c (glycated hemoglobin): WG diet significantly lowered HbA1c ($p = 0.04$) FPI (fasting plasma insulin): WG diet significantly lowered FPI ($p = 0.02$) Adiponectin: WG vs. control diet = -0.1 mg/mL (95% CI = -0.9–0.7) vs. -1.4 mg/mL (95% CI = -2.6–-0.3), $p = 0.05$.
Marventano, 2017 [112]	Meta-analysis of RCTs	Where available, AUC(area under the curve) values range from 0 to 240 min	206 subjects from 14 RCTs	Changes from baseline in glucose iAUC values at 120 min (MD; 95% CI): MD = -29.71 mmol $\times$ min/L; 95% CI = -43.57–-15.85 Changes from baseline in insulin iAUC values at 120min (MD; 95% CI): MD = -2.01 nmol $\times$ min/L; 95% CI = -2.88–-1.14
Musa-Veloso, 2018 [114]	Meta-analysis of RCTs	Where available, AUC values range from 0 to 120 min	274 subjects from 20 RCTs	Postprandial blood glucose AUC of WG vs. refined wheat, rice, or rye: WG vs. white wheat: AUC = -6.7 mmol/L $\times$ min; 95% CI = -25.1–11.7; $p = 0.477$. WG vs. endosperm rye: AUC = -5.5 mmol/L $\times$ min; 95% CI = -24.8–13.8; $p = 0.576$. WG vs. white rice: AUC = -40.5 mmol/L $\times$ min; 95% CI = -59.6–-21.3; $p < 0.001$.
Kirø, 2018 [115]	Prospective Cohort Study	Median follow-up: 15 years	55,565 subjects (26,251 men, 29,214 women) from the Diet, Cancer, and Health Cohort	Increment of 16 g/day of WG intake and risk of type 2 diabetes: Men: HR = 0.89, 95% CI = 0.87, 0.91 Women: HR = 0.93, 95% CI = 0.91, 0.96 Highest vs. lowest quartile of WG intake and risk of type 2 diabetes: Men: HR = 0.66, 95% CI: 0.60–0.72, $p < 0.0001$ Women: HR = 0.78, 95% CI: 0.70–0.86, $p < 0.0001$ Increment of 50 g/day of WG intake and risk of type 2 diabetes: Men: HR = 0.88, 95% CI = 0.86–0.90 Women: HR = HR = 0.93, 95% CI = 0.90–0.96 Highest vs. lowest quartile of WG intake and risk of type 2 diabetes: Men: HR = 0.63, 95% CI: 0.58–0.69, $p < 0.0001$ Women: HR = 0.80, 95% CI: 0.72–0.88, $p < 0.0001$
Maki, 2019 [117]	Meta-analysis of observational studies and RCTs	Mean duration of 3 prospective cohort studies: 8 years. Mean duration of 9 cross-sectional studies: 5 years. Mean duration of 9 RCTs: 90 days	136,834 subjects from 12 observational studies (3 prospective cohort studies and 9 cross-sectional studies) and 973 subjects from 9 RCTs	Meta-Regression Analysis from Cross-Sectional Studies: Inverse correlation between WG consumption and BMI (r = -0.526, $p = 0.0001$) Qualitative Analysis from Prospective Cohort Studies: Inverse association between WG consumption and weight change, with a follow-up period from 5 to 20 years Meta-Regression of RCTs: No significant difference between WG consumption and weight change (standardized MD = -0.049 Kg; 95% CI = -0.388–0.199; $p = 0.698$)

5. Whole Grains Intake and Reduction of Mortality

Accumulating evidence indicates that high intake of WG decreases the risks of mortality from all causes, CVD, and cancer in the general population.

Ma et al. [118] conducted a meta-analysis of prospective cohort studies involving 843,749 subjects and 101,282 deaths to quantify the association between WG intake and all-cause mortality. They showed that high WG intake was associated with a reduction of 18% for all-cause mortality risk (RR = 0.82, 95% CI = 0.78–0.87). In addition, the authors reported a 7% reduction in the risk of mortality from all causes for each increment of 16 g/day of WG consumption (RR = 0.93, 95% CI = 0.89 to 0.97).

A subsequent interesting meta-analysis by Zong et al. [119] involving 786,076 subjects with 97,867 total deaths confirmed the association between WG intake and reduction in mortality. The authors showed that a high WG intake was associated with a significative reduction in total mortality, CVD mortality, and cancer mortality (RR = 0.84, 95% CI = 0.80–0.88, $p < 0.001$; RR = 0.82, 95% CI = 0.79–0.85, $p < 0.001$; RR = 0.88, 95% CI = 0.83–0.94, $p < 0.001$, respectively). The authors also estimated that each serving/day increase in WG intake was associated to a reduction of 7% for total mortality (RR = 0.93, 95% CI = 0.92–

0.94), 9% for CVD mortality (RR = 0.91, 95% CI = 0.90–0.93), and 5% for cancer mortality (RR = 0.95, 95% CI = 0.94–0.96).

The meta-analysis by Wei et al. [120] involving 816,599 subjects with 89,251 all-cause deaths, 23,280 CVD deaths, and 35,189 cancer deaths obtained similar results. The authors found that a high WG intake was associated with a signification reduction in risk (summary relative risk, SRR) for total mortality, CVD mortality, and cancer mortality (SRR = 0.87, 95% CI = 0.84–0.90; SRR = 0.81, 95% CI = 0.75–0.89; SRR = 0.89, 95% CI = 0.82–0.96, respectively). The dose-response analysis showed a reduction in overall mortality risk of 19% as well as a reduction of CVD mortality risk and cancer mortality risk of 26% and 9%, respectively (SRR = 0.81, 95% CI = 0.76–0.85; SRR = 0.74, 95% CI = 0.66–0.83; SRR = 0.91, 95% CI = 0.84–0.98), for every three servings/day increase in WG consumption.

Furthermore, a meta-analysis conducted by Aune et al. [36] confirmed the association between WG intake and reduction of mortality. The meta-analysis was performed on 45 prospective studies involving 245,012 to 705,253 participants with 7068 cases of coronary heart disease, 2337 cases of stroke, 26,243 cases of cardiovascular disease, 34,346 deaths from cancer, and 100,726 all cause deaths. In their study, the authors found that a high WG intake was associated with a signification reduction in CHD (RR = 0.79, 95% CI = 0.73–0.86), stroke (RR = 0.87, 95% CI = 0.72–1.05), and CVD (RR = 0.84, 95% CI = 0.80–0.87). The authors also reported a reduction in the risk of CHD, stroke, and CVD respectively of 19% (RR = 0.81, 95% CI = 0.75–0.87), 12% (RR = 0.88, 95% CI = 0.75–1.03), and 22% (RR = 0.78, 95% CI = 0.73–0.85) for each increase of 90 g/day (three servings/day) of the consumption of WG. In addition, the authors estimated that a high WG intake was associated with a signification reduction in mortality risk for CHD (RR = 0.65, 95% CI = 0.52–0.83), stroke (RR = 0.85, 95% CI = 0.64–1.13), CVD (RR = 0.81, 95% CI = 0.75–0.87), cancer (RR = 0.89, 95% CI = 0.82–0.96), and mortality for all-cause (RR = 0.82, 95% CI = 0.77–0.88). In particular, a reduced risk of coronary heart disease, stroke, CVD, cancer and overall mortality was observed by 19% (RR = 0.81, 95% CI = 0.74–0.89), 14% (RR = 0.86, 95% CI = 0.74–0.99), 29% (RR = 0.71, 95% CI = 0.61–0.82), 15% (RR = 0, 85, 95% CI = 0.80–0.91), and 17% (RR = 0.83, 95% CI = 0.77–0.90), respectively, for each increase in consumption of 90 g/day (three portions/day) of WG.

Another meta-analysis performed by Benisi-Kohansal et al. [121] involving 2,282,603 participants from 20 prospective cohort studies further confirmed the association between WG intake and reduction in mortality. Authors found that higher consumption of WG was associated with a reduction in overall mortality (RR = 0.87; 95% CI = 0.84–0.91), CVD mortality (RR = 0.84; 95% CI = 0.78–0.89), and cancer mortality (RR = 0.94; 95% CI = 0.91, 0.98). The authors also estimated a reduction of overall mortality, CVD, and cancer mortality of 17% (SRR = 0.83; 95% CI = 0.79–0.88), 25% (SRR = 0, 75; 95% CI = 0.68–0.83) and 10% (SRR = 0.90; 95% CI = 0.83–0.98), respectively, for each additional three servings/day (90 g/day) of the consumption of WG.

A further confirmation of the beneficial effects of WG consumption on the reduction of overall mortality risk as well as CVD and cancer mortality risk was provided by Zhang et al. [122], which conducted a meta-analysis on 19 prospective cohort studies involving 1,041,692 subjects. The authors confirmed the relationship between a high intake of WG and the risk reduction of all-cause mortality (RR = 0.84; 95% CI = 0.81–0.88). The authors also confirmed that higher WG consumption was related with a reduction in mortality risk for both CVD (RR = 0.83; 95% CI = 0.79–0.86) and for cancer (RR = 0.94; 95% CI = 0.87–1.01). After performing the dose-response analysis, the author estimated that each serving/day intake of whole grain could reduce the overall mortality by 9% (RR = 0.91; 95% CI = 0.90–0.93), CVD mortality by 14% (RR = 0.86; 95% CI = 0.83–0.89), and cancer mortality by 3% (RR = 0.97; 95% CI = 0.95–0.99).

This latest evidence on the reduction in total cardiovascular mortality and even of mortality from neoplastic disease obtained from long-term perspective studies, further confirms the key concept that the benefits of taking WG cannot be interpreted as the beneficial effect of an isolated nutrient, but must be contextualized as part of a healthy diet in a healthy lifestyle. All studies are reported in Table 5.

Table 5. Whole grains(WG) intake and reduction of mortality.

Author and Year of Publication	Study Design	Duration of Study	Sample Size	Highest vs. Lowest Whole Grains Intake and Reduction of Mortality
Ma, 2016 [118]	Meta-analysis of prospective cohort studies	Median follow-up time: 5.9 to 26 years	809,901 subjects (99,224 deaths) from 10 prospective cohort studies	WG intake and all-cause mortality: RR = 0.82; 95% CI = 0.78–0.87 Increment of 1 serving/day of WG intake and all-cause mortality risk: RR = 0.93; 95% CI = 0.89–0.97
Zong, 2016 [119]	Meta-analysis of prospective cohort studies	Median follow-up time: 6 to 28 years	786,076 subjects (97,867 deaths) form 14 prospective cohort studies	WG intake and all-cause death: RR = 0.84; 95% CI = 0.80–0.88; $p < 0.001$ WG intake and death from CVD: RR = 0.82; 95% CI = 0.79–0.85; $p < 0.001$ WG intake and death from cancer: RR = 0.88; 95% CI = 0.83–0.94; $p < 0.001$ Increment of 1 serving/day of WG intake and total mortality risk: RR = 0.93; 95% CI = 0.92–0.94 Increment of 1 serving/day of WG intake and CVD mortality risk: RR = 0.91; 95% CI = 0.90–0.93 Increment of 1 serving/day of WG intake and cancer mortality risk: RR = 0.95; 95% CI = 0.94–0.96
Wei, 2016 [120]	Meta-analysis of prospective cohort studies	Median follow-up time: 14 years (range: 5.5–26 years)	816,599 subjects (89,251 deaths) form 11 prospective cohort studies	WG intake and all-cause death: SRR = 0.87; 95% CI = 0.84–0.90 WG intake and death from CVD: SRR = 0.81; 95% CI = 0.75–0.89 WG intake and death from cancer: SRR = 0.89; 95% CI = 0.82–0.96 Increment of 3 serving/day of WG intake and total mortality risk: SRR = 0.81; 95% CI = 0.76–0.85 Increment of 3 serving/day of WG intake and CVD mortality risk: SRR = 0.74; 95% CI = 0.66–0.83 Increment of 3 serving/day of WG intake and cancer mortality risk: SRR = 0.91; 95% CI = 0.84–0.98
Aune, 2016 [36]	Meta-analysis of prospective cohort studies	Follow-up time range: 3–26 years	245,012 to 705,253 subjects (34,346 deaths from cancer; 100,726 deaths from any cause) from 45 prospective studies	WG intake and death from CHD: RR = 0.65; 95% CI = 0.52–0.83 WG intake and death from Stroke: RR = 0.85; 95% CI = 0.64–1.13 WG intake and death from CVD: RR = 0.81; 95% CI = 0.75–0.87 WG intake and death from cancer: RR = 0.89; 95% CI = 0.82–0.96 WG intake and all-cause death: RR = 0.82; 95% CI = 0.77–0.88 Increment of 3 serving/day of WG intake and total CHD mortality risk: RR = 0.81; 95% CI = 0.74–0.89 Increment of 3 serving/day of WG intake and Stroke mortality risk: RR = 0.86; 95% CI = 0.74–0.99 Increment of 3 serving/day of WG intake and CVD mortality risk: RR = 0.71; 95% CI = 0.61–0.82 Increment of 3 serving/day of WG intake and cancer mortality risk: RR = 0.85; 95% CI = 0.80–0.91 Increment of 3 serving/day of WG intake and all-cause mortality risk: RR = 0.83; 95% CI = 0.77–0.90
Benisi-Kohansal, 2016 [121]	Meta-analysis of prospective cohort studies	Follow-up time range: 5.5–26 years	2,282,603 subjects from 20 prospective cohort studies	WG intake and all-cause death: RR = 0.87; 95% CI = 0.84–0.91 WG intake and death from CVD: RR = 0.84; 95% CI = 0.78–0.89 WG intake and death from cancer: RR = 0.94; 95% CI = 0.91, 0.98 Increment of 3 serving/day of WG intake and total all-cause mortality risk: SRR = 0.83; 95% CI = 0.79–0.88 Increment of 3 serving/day of WG intake and CVD mortality risk: SRR = 0.75; 95% CI = 0.68–0.83 Increment of 3 serving/day of WG intake and cancer mortality risk: SRR = 0.90; 95% CI = 0.83–0.98
Zhang, 2018 [122]	Meta-analysis of prospective cohort studies	Follow-up time range: 4–26 years	1,041,692 subjects (96,710 deaths) from 19 prospective cohort studies	WG intake and all-cause death: RR = 0.84; 95% CI = 0.81–0.88 WG intake and death from CVD: RR = 0.83; 95% CI = 0.79–0.86 WG intake and death from cancer: RR = 0.94; 95% CI = 0.87–1.01 Increment of 1 serving/day of WG intake and total all-cause mortality risk: RR = 0.91; 95% CI = 0.90–0.93 Increment of 1 serving/day of WG intake and CVD mortality risk: RR = 0.86; 95% CI = 0.83–0.89 Increment of 1 serving/day of WG intake and cancer mortality risk: RR = 0.97; 95% CI = 0.95–0.99

It is therefore evident that a high intake of WG, vegetables, fruits, nuts, and coffee is associated with a reduced risk of mortality whereas a high intake of red and processed meat is related to a higher mortality risk. High-quality diets such as MD are associated with a reduced risk of all-cause mortality [123].

Few studies relate the effects of a diet high in fibers on gastrointestinal function, glycemic or lipid metabolism, or on body weight [124]. Gopinath et al. [125] examined the relationship between total dietary carbohydrate intake, glycemic index (GI), glycemic load (GL), and fiber intake, with the state of successful aging [3,4] and with mortality risk, for a follow-up period of 10 years in a cohort of 1609 adults from The Blue Mountains Eye Study [126]. The authors showed that higher intake of total fiber, and particularly vegetable fibers and fruit fibers, was associated with greater odds of successful aging (OR = 1.79, 95% CI = 1.13–2.84; OR = 1.26, 95% CI = 0.83–1.91; OR = 1.81, 95% CI = 1.15–2.83, respectively).

Nevertheless, there have been a small number of studies examining the effect of WG on outcomes other than cardio-metabolic function or gastro-enteric function, or glycemic or lipid metabolism, or body weight. For example, there are very few studies analyzing the effect of WG in the diet on aging.

In this regard, Foscolou et al. [127] conducted an interesting study on a sample of 3349 elderly subjects from the ATTICA study and from the MEDIS study [36,128], both aimed to assess the association between WG intake with the diet and successful aging, and evaluated with the successful aging index (SAI) [129]. By applying the linear regression models, the authors observed a significant association between low vs. high intake of WG and SAI (b ± SE = −0.278 ± 0.091, p = 0.002). They did not observe any significant association between low vs. moderate WG intake and SAI (b ± SE = 0.010 ± 0.083, p = 0.901), and between moderate vs. high WG intake and SAI (b ± SE = −0.178 ± 0.095, p = 0.062).

6. Reduction of Protein to Carbohydrates Ratio Influence Aging and Lifespan

There is a consensus among gerontology researchers that dietary interventions can slow down aging, that is, prevent or delay the onset of numerous age-related chronic diseases [130–132]. The study of the relationship between nutrition and healthy aging has increasingly become a subject of great interest. Caloric restriction (CR), avoiding malnutrition, is the most studied dietary intervention known to extend life in many organisms [133–135]. To date, CR has been the focus of most non-genetic nutritional interventions. CR has been shown to improve several markers of health [136,137]. Fasting is the most extreme of the CR interventions, which requires the complete elimination of nutrients. Indeed, one of the more evaluated forms of fasting in both rodent and human studies is intermittent fasting [IF]. IF reduces body weight, body fat, and particularly abdominal fat, plasma insulin concentrations in both men and women, and reduces blood pressure, improving insulin sensitivity and lipid profile [138–140].

As reported by de Cabo and Mattson [141], cells exposed to fasting produce an adaptive stress response that leads to an increased expression of the antioxidant defenses, DNA repair, and control of protein quality, mitochondrial biogenesis, and autophagy, and down-regulation of inflammation. In particular, the cell in intermittent fasting regimen showed a better and stronger resistance to a wide range of potentially harmful insults that involve metabolic, oxidative, ionic, traumatic, and proteotoxic stress. The protective effects of intermittent fasting are mediated by the stimulation of autophagy and mitophagy and by the inhibition of the mTOR (mammal target of rapamycin) protein synthesis pathway [142]. These responses allow cells to remove damaged proteins and mitochondria from oxidation and to recycle the molecular constituents not damaged by temporarily reducing the overall protein synthesis to conserve energy and molecular resources. In humans, intermittent fasting interventions induce health benefits than can largely be attributed to simply reducing caloric intake. These benefits are due to the loss of fat mass, and consequently to the decrease in fasting insulin levels and to the increase in insulin sensitivity, resulting in a decrease of insulin resistance, dyslipidemia, hypertension, and a pro-inflammatory state typical of advanced age. Nevertheless, the IF needs medical supervision as it may cause serious adverse effects in patients with extremely low BMI or between the frail and elderly patients [132].

Further evidence has suggested that macronutrient balance, rather than simple calorie restriction, plays a more important role in extending lifespan [143–145]. That is, modulating protein and carbohydrate intake, rather than simplistically reducing the entire energy intake, may offer a more feasible nutritional intervention in humans [146]. That is, it has become clear that specific nutrients and nutritional balance (i.e., the result of interactions between nutrients) play an important role in the biology of aging.

The "Geometric Framework for Nutrition" (GNF) [147,148] is a method developed in nutritional ecology with the purpose of understanding the nutritional interactions of animals with their environments by explicitly distinguishing the roles of calories, individual nutrients, and nutrient balance. In this model, the nutritional requirements of an animal can be schematized in a two-dimensional or three-dimensional Cartesian space, called the nutrient space. The axes that define this space each represent a functionally important food component, for example, proteins, carbohydrates, and fats. The intake target (IT) represents the balance and quantity of functional nutrients for regulatory mechanisms (e.g., proteins and carbohydrates). The animal can reach the IT if appropriate foods are available. As shown in Figure 6, foods are represented by radials or nutritional tracks (T), which are projected into the space between nutrients according to angles determined by the ratio of the nutrients they contain. The animal can reach its target state by selecting Food 1, which is nutritionally balanced with respect to its target, or by mixing its intake with nutritionally complementary foods (Food 2 and Food 3). Therefore, when on the T1, the animal is unbalanced toward Food 2, that is, off course with respect to its target; however, it can get closer to the target by approaching Food 3, then passing into T2, and a further passage to Food 2 brings it closer to its nutrition target.

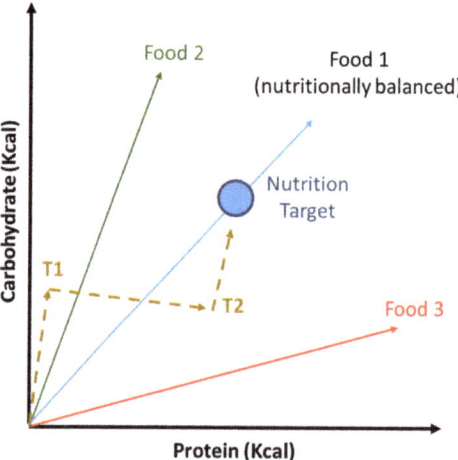

Figure 6. Dietary imbalance in nutritional geometry. Adapted from Raubenheimer et al. [148].

In this regard, basic research studies conducted on Drosophila have shown that longevity was maximal when the diet included a 1:16 ratio of proteins to carbohydrates, while reproductive capacity, measured in insects through egg production, was maximum with a ratio of proteins and carbohydrates between 1:2 and 1:4. This increased lifespan observed with a low-protein diet was attributed to a reduction in initial mortality and a delayed acceleration of age-dependent mortality [149,150]. Further studies conducted on male decorated crickets have confirmed that a low protein and high carbohydrate diet could induce higher immune functions and consequently lower mortality [151]. Similar results were observed in studies conducted on Gasterosteus aculeatus, or stickleback fish, where a significant increase in lifespan was observed in fish with a diet with a lower protein content than carbohydrates, as opposed to an increased reproductive capacity observed in a diet higher in protein than carbohydrates [152].

Evidence showed that these models of a low protein, high carbohydrate diet would induce a reduced TOR signaling [145,153]. In this regard, Senior et al. [154] examined data from the Solon-Biet study [145] to evaluate how the macronutrient content in the diet could influence life expectancy and mortality in a sample of mice. They showed that the mouse's self-selected diet, which was composed of 22% protein, 47% carbohydrate, and 31% fat, with a protein–carbohydrate ratio lower than one, was associated with a long-life expectancy, low mortality in early and middle age, and high mortality in old age. In contrast, a diet rich in proteins or fats relative to carbohydrates produces low life expectancy with high mortality rates across all age classes.

There are no studies on humans that have applied nutritional geometry. However, the great longevity of populations from Sardinia in Italy or from Okinawa in Japan is well known as is the generally low mortality of the populations of the Mediterranean basin who follow a traditional Mediterranean diet [6,7,16]. The explanation for this high life expectancy lies in traditional eating habits, both in the Mediterranean diet and in the Okinawan diet, which are rich in carbohydrates taken with cereals (wheat or rice) or its derivatives and with low protein content, with a protein/carbohydrate ratio for both diets of about 1:10 [155].

Regarding protein intake, Pedersen et al. [156] conducted an interesting review that aimed to assess the health effects of protein intake in healthy adults. The 64 papers that were included in the study were classified according to the grade of evidence as "convincing", "probable", "suggestive", or "inconclusive". The authors assessed as "suggestive" the evidence regarding the increased risk of all-cause mortality in relation to a low carbohydrates high protein (LCHP) diet, where total protein intake of at least 20–23% of total energy; they also assessed as "suggestive" the evidence concerning relations between vegetable protein intake and low risk of cardiovascular mortality.

With regard to the carbohydrates, it is known that molecules are essential for many cellular processes, mainly for the production of energy, after having been converted into glucose by the cells. Furthermore, high blood glucose levels are known to be responsible for the progression of chronic diseases such as diabetes mellitus. More importantly, glucose is one of the most studied nutrient molecules, influencing lifespan in various model organisms. For example, diets enriched with glucose reduce lifespan in Caenorhabditis elegans by inhibiting the insulin/IGF-1 (IIS) signaling pathway. Diets enriched with glucose act by inhibiting DAF-16/FOXO, HSF-1, and SKN-1/nuclear factor erythroid-related factor (NRF), which regulate the expression of several target genes in the IIS pathway. Treatments with high glucose content also produce negative effects of aging on human endothelial progenitor cells (EPCs) and fibroblasts. In these human cells, elevated glucose treatment accelerates various aging-related phenotypes through the activation of the p38 mitogen-activated protein kinase (MAPK). High-glucose treatments induce downregulation of sirtuins; this leads to a reduction in FOXO activity and accelerates cellular senescence. In these glucose-rich conditions, we observed in the EPC some cellular aging phenotypes such as increased levels of b-gal staining SA, reduced cell proliferation, irregular morphology, and increased levels of ROS [150].

Regarding the relation between dietary carbohydrate intake and mortality, Seidelmann [157] conducted a prospective cohort study aimed at investigating the association of carbohydrate intake with mortality and residual life span in a large cohort of adults from the risk of community atherosclerosis (ARIC), which involved 15,428 subjects with a 25-year follow-up. The authors also investigated whether the replacement of carbohydrates with animal or vegetable sources of fats and proteins changed the observed associations. As a benefit of the study, they combined their findings with data from seven studies from North America, Europe, Asia, and multinationals involving 432,179 participants to contextualize all findings in a meta-analysis. The author showed that an increased risk of mortality was related to low carbohydrate consumption (low versus moderate carbohydrate consumption: HR = 1.20; 95% CI = 1.09–1.32; $p < 0.0001$) and high carbohydrate consumption (high versus moderate carbohydrate consumption: HR = 1.23; 95% CI = 1.11–1.36; $p < 0.0001$). After exploring the association between mortality and alternative source of fat and protein to carbohydrate intake, the authors found that increasing the protein and animal fat intake instead of carbohydrates was associated with a significantly increased mortality risk (HR = 1.18; 95% CI = 1.08–1.29; $p < 0.0001$). Alternatively, an increased intake of protein and vegetable fats instead of carbohydrates has been related to a significant reduction in mortality risk (HR = 0.82; 95% CI = 1.78–1.87; $p < 0.0001$). In conclusion, the authors stated that a diet with a low carbohydrate content, in which carbohydrates are replaced with fat and protein mainly of plant origin, might be associated with a higher life expectancy and a long-term approach could be considered to promote healthy aging. It would be simplistic, in fact, if we wanted to evaluate the effects of nutrition on aging and longevity, consider separately the intake of proteins or carbohydrates, or extrapolate from the context caloric intake total daily, for example, by simply reducing energy intake.

7. Discussion

The application of the GNF method to study the effects of macronutrients and caloric intake on aging and lifespan has allowed us to understand that not the single nutrient but the interaction between macronutrients affects age-related health and lifespan. Animal model studies, which applied the GNF method, have shown that a low-protein, high-carbohydrate diet increases lifespan in many species. These studies were performed using ad libitum feeding regimes, which considered the eating behavior in a not strictly organized environment (i.e., less artificial), which produces more reliable results, if we want to translate them into human populations. Food intake is recorded so that diet content and calorie and macronutrient intake can be assessed [158]. All these studies have shown that longer lifespans are generated by diets low in protein and high in carbohydrates (low protein high carbohydrates, LPHC diet) where the optimal ratio of protein and carbohydrates is about 1:10, with the protein content of diet about 10% or less. All these studies have also shown that simple reduced caloric intake has no effect or negative effect on lifespan, which is clearly in contrast to many previous studies on CR.

Although CR overall has shown established benefits for health and aging, this model is not readily feasible in practice in both humans and animals that have free access to food. In contrast, alternative dietary models such as the LPHC diet, which allow ad libitum access to food, are more likely to be feasible as health interventions. Comparing the results of LPHC diets with those of caloric restriction, we can find similarities such as the reduction of insulin and inactivation of mTOR, and differences, the most interesting of those concerning mitochondrial biogenesis between cellular mechanisms concerning aging and life span [159]. Interestingly, LPHC diets are associated with reduced mitochondrial number and reduced expression of the master regulator of mitochondrial biogenesis, peroxisome proliferator-activated receptor gamma coactivator 1-alpha [PGC-1α], unlike CR, where there is an increase in the number of mitochondria associated with a greater expression of PGC-1α.

The concept of "mythormesis" could explain the paradox that both LPHC and CR diets increase lifespan but induce opposite effects on mitochondria. After postulating that low levels of oxidative stress induce the activation of systemic defense mechanisms beneficial for aging such as the activation of endogenous antioxidant enzymes, LPHC diets can increase the production of hydrogen peroxide sufficiently to generate hormetic benefits without producing mitochondrial damage.

It is now an irrefutable fact that a healthy lifestyle during a younger age, which includes consuming healthy foods in an amount appropriate to both health and physical activity, smoking cessation, and even taking moderate amounts of alcohol, prepares for successful aging. It is also an irrefutable fact that one of the main factors in increasing the average life span in the last two centuries has been the improvement in the nutritional status of the population. In contrast, a poor-quality diet is still the main risk factor of mortality, but above all, of disability in older age, even in developed and wealthy nations [160].

The most recent evidence has shown that diets that are rich in low glycemic index carbohydrates, combined with low amounts of proteins, are optimal to determine a longer and healthier life expectancy. In addition, diets that combine high amounts of refined, starch rich, high glycemic index carbohydrates with high contents of animal-derived proteins and fats determine a higher mortality rate, especially from CVD [161–164].

Dietary patterns that demonstrated greater adherence to diets that emphasized fruit and vegetables, WG rather than refined grains, low-fat dairy, lean meats, legumes, and nuts were inversely associated with mortality [165,166]. We already know that adherence to a diet pattern such as the traditional MD [6] was associated with a reduction in overall mortality, coronary heart disease, and cardiovascular disease. An overall high-quality diet that emphasizes a high consumption of polyunsaturated and monounsaturated fatty acids, raw vegetables, dairy, legumes, low-fat lean meats fat, fresh fish, bread (especially whole-grain bread), and wine in moderation, has been inversely associated with overall mortality, especially in the elderly [167,168]. In addition, a healthy diet of high quality can increase the number of years without disease and without disabilities [169]. Evidence also suggests that higher adherence to a dietary pattern that includes mainly legumes, fruit, vegetables, cereals, bread, olive oil, and dairy products, more occasionally meat, fish, and seafood, is associated with lower risk of becoming frail in old age [170]. In contrast, an eating style characterized by a high consumption of refined cereals has been associated with a greater risk of total mortality, especially mortality from major CVD [171].

Concerning protein intake, an established dietary bias is that older people need to obtain more protein with their diet, even though they are not malnourished. The main objective of this advice is to first prevent sarcopenia, then to maintain a good state of health, which allows for the prevention of malnutrition, improving wound healing and faster recovery from acute illness [167]. Instead, these recommendations are in contrast with the results of basic research on animal models and with the results of observational studies on population cohorts, which on the contrary have shown that a low-protein, high-carbohydrate diet (LPHC) can delay aging and extend lifespan [123,133,142,159,172].

Residents of the Japanese island of Okinawa and people living in the central-eastern mountainous area of the Italian island of Sardinia [173,174], although so distant, share a unique characteristic: both populations show one of the highest concentrations of centenarians in the world, whose ages have been carefully validated. Several factors contribute to the exceptional longevity of these populations. Among these are a moderate caloric intake that is never excessive, a high quality of food, constant physical activity, and genetic predisposition.

Regarding centenarians in Okinawa, their dietary energy intake comes from 85% carbohydrates and only 9% from proteins. [175]. Furthermore, the ratio of proteins to carbohydrates is extremely low [1:10], like what has been discovered to optimize lifespan in aging studies in animal models [159].

Concerning Sardinian centenarians [174], the consumption of sourdough bread, which is prepared from WG with a microbial yeast containing lactobacilli called "mother yeast", with chemical and physical characteristics quite different from bread bought from the ovens, and a plant soup called "minestrone" containing fresh vegetables (onions, fennel, carrots, celery) and legumes (beans, broad beans, peas) is very widespread. Honey was generally used as a sweetener. Meat consumption does not exceed 2–4 portions per month. As for the consumption of dairy products, these people make extensive use of ricotta (whey cheese and dry curd), both goat and sheep, rather than mature cheese, and a local fresh sour cheese called "casu axedu" in the local dialect, which is rich in lactobacilli.

Indeed, the consumption of sourdough bread is very widespread in the traditional MD in southern Italy. This type of bread can reduce blood glucose and postprandial insulin levels by 25%, thus being able to preserve the function of pancreatic insulin-secreting cells and prevent obesity and diabetes [176].

Other predisposing health promoting factors between both people from Sardinia and from Okinawa are physical activity, low stress levels, and strong community support. We have already stated [177] that the benefits of MD should not be simply attributed to the high content of fiber, antioxidants, and proteins of vegetable origin. Nevertheless, it should be reiterated that the benefits of MD should be considered as part of a cultural context where food, together with the convivial aspect, is part of a "Mediterranean" lifestyle [178,179].

8. Conclusions

Longevity is the result of a multifactorial phenomenon that also involves nutrition. Among the main causes of the increase in lifespan in the last two centuries, we certainly recognize that the improvement in the nutritional status [180–182], while paradoxically an energy-intensive diet but of low nutritional quality widespread in the last century in developed countries, represents the main risk factor for mortality and disability [160]. Many studies have shown that a higher consumption of proteins and fats is related to a reduction in life expectancy, while high intake of low glycemic index carbohydrates from WG might play a protective role. Indeed, evidence shows that regular WG intake reduces the risks of cardiovascular disease and stroke, hypertension, metabolic syndrome, and diabetes as well as several forms of cancer [183]. Furthermore, more recent evidence shows that, instead of simply reducing overall calorie intake, ad libitum access to foods as part of a low-protein, high-carbohydrate diet extends lifespan. In conclusion, a high healthy life expectancy is the result of several factors. The most important undoubtedly include a healthy lifestyle with continuous physical activity, abstention from smoking, and intake of moderate quantities of alcohol, combined with a healthy diet in close symbiosis with lifestyle. In particular, optimizing caloric intake in relation to physical activity and age-related changes in metabolism, regular intake of whole-grain derivatives, together with the optimization of the protein/carbohydrate ratio in the diet, where the ratio is significantly lower than 1 such as in the traditional MD and the Okinawa diet, increases healthy life expectancy by reducing the risk of developing CVD and aging-related diseases.

Funding: This research received no external funding.

Acknowledgments: This review paper was endorsed by the "Fondazione Dieta Mediterranea, Ostuni, Italy" https://www.fondazionedietamediterranea.it/ (Accessed date: 1 June 2021).

Conflicts of Interest: The author declares no conflict of interest.

References

1. United Nations, Department of Economic and Social Affairs, Population Division. World Population Ageing 2015 (ST/ESA/SER.A/390). Available online: https://www.un.org/en/development/desa/population/publications/pdf/ageing/WPA2015_Report.pdf (accessed on 1 August 2020).
2. Eurostat. Population Structure and Ageing. Available online: https://ec.europa.eu/eurostat/statistics-explained/index.php/Population_structure_and_ageing#The_share_of_elderly_people_continues_to_increase (accessed on 1 August 2020).
3. Rowe, J.W.; Kahn, R.L. Human aging: Usual and successful. *Science* **1987**, *237*, 143–149. [CrossRef] [PubMed]
4. Rowe, J.W.; Kahn, R.L. Successful Aging. *Gerontologist* **1997**, *37*, 433–440. [CrossRef]
5. Keys, A.B. *Seven Countries: A Multivariate Analysis of Death and Coronary Heart Disease*; Harvard University Press: Cambridge, MA, USA, 1980; ISBN 9780674497887.
6. Trichopoulou, A.; Costacou, T.; Bamia, C.; Trichopoulos, D. Adherence to a Mediterranean Diet and Survival in a Greek Population. *N. Engl. J. Med.* **2003**, *348*, 2599–2608. [CrossRef]
7. Trichopoulou, A. Diet and overall survival in the elderly. *BMJ* **1995**, *311*, 1457–1460. [CrossRef] [PubMed]
8. Estruch, R.; Ros, E.; Salas-Salvadó, J.; Covas, M.-I.; Corella, D.; Arós, F.; Gómez-Gracia, E.; Ruiz-Gutiérrez, V.; Fiol, M.; Lapetra, J.; et al. Primary Prevention of Cardiovascular Disease with a Mediterranean Diet. *N. Engl. J. Med.* **2013**, *368*, 1279–1290. [CrossRef]
9. Estruch, R.; Ros, E.; Salas-Salvadó, J.; Covas, M.I.; Corella, D.; Arós, F.; Gómez-Gracia, E.; Ruiz-Gutiérrez, V.; Fiol, M.; Lapetra, J.; et al. Primary Prevention of Cardiovascular Disease with a Mediterranean Diet Supplemented with Extra-Virgin Olive Oil or Nuts. *N. Engl. J. Med.* **2018**, *378*, e34. [CrossRef]
10. Sofi, F.; Cesari, F.; Abbate, R.; Gensini, G.F.; Casini, A. Adherence to Mediterranean diet and health status: Meta-analysis. *BMJ* **2008**, *337*, a1344. [CrossRef]
11. Sofi, F.; Abbate, R.; Gensini, G.F.; Casini, A. Accruing evidence on benefits of adherence to the Mediterranean diet on health: An updated systematic review and meta-analysis. *Am. J. Clin. Nutr.* **2010**, *92*, 1189–1196. [CrossRef]

12. Akbaraly, T.; Sabia, S.; Hagger-Johnson, G.; Tabak, A.; Shipley, M.J.; Jokela, M.; Brunner, E.; Hamer, M.; Batty, G.; Singh-Manoux, A.; et al. Does Overall Diet in Midlife Predict Future Aging Phenotypes? A Cohort Study. *Am. J. Med.* **2013**, *126*, 411–419.e3. [CrossRef] [PubMed]
13. Samieri, C.; Sun, Q.; Townsend, M.K.; Chiuve, S.E.; Okereke, O.I.; Willett, W.C.; Stampfer, M.; Grodstein, F. The association between dietary patterns at midlife and health in aging: An observational study. *Ann. Intern. Med.* **2013**, *159*, 584–591. [CrossRef]
14. Brites, C. Cereals in the context of the Mediterranean Diet. In *Dimensions of Mediterranean Diet: World cultural Heritage*; Universidade do Algarve: Faro, Portugal, 2015; pp. 181–195. ISBN 978-989-8472-74-8.
15. Fundación Dieta Mediterránea. 2010. Available online: https://dietamediterranea.com (accessed on 30 August 2020).
16. Willcox, D.C.; Scapagnini, G.; Willcox, B.J. Healthy aging diets other than the Mediterranean: A focus on the Okinawan diet. *Mech. Ageing Dev.* **2014**, *136–137*, 148–162. [CrossRef] [PubMed]
17. Forum, O.B.O.T.H.; Ross, A.B.; van der Kamp, J.-W.; King, R.; Lê, K.-A.; Mejborn, H.; Seal, C.J.; Thielecke, F. Perspective: A Definition for Whole-Grain Food Products—Recommendations from the Healthgrain Forum. *Adv. Nutr.* **2017**, *8*, 525–531. [CrossRef]
18. Cavazos, A.; De Mejia, E.G. Identification of Bioactive Peptides from Cereal Storage Proteins and Their Potential Role in Prevention of Chronic Diseases. *Compr. Rev. Food Sci. Food Saf.* **2013**, *12*, 364–380. [CrossRef]
19. Solfrizzi, V.; Panza, F.; Torres, F.; Mastroianni, F.; Del Parigi, A.; Venezia, A.; Capurso, A. High monounsaturated fatty acids intake protects against age-related cognitive decline. *Neurology* **1999**, *52*, 1563. [CrossRef]
20. Capurso, A.; Crepaldi, G.; Capurso, C. *Benefits of the Mediterranean Diet in the Elderly Patient, Practical Issues in Geriatrics*; Springer: Berlin/Heidelberg, Germany, 2018; Chapter 8; pp. 139–172.
21. NutritionValue.Org. Available online: https://www.nutritionvalue.org (accessed on 15 October 2020).
22. Peter, R. Natural Variation in Grain Composition of Wheat and Related Cereals. *J. Agric. Food Chem.* **2013**, *61*, 8295–8303.
23. Vogel, K.P.; Johnson, V.A.; Mattern, P.J. Protein and Lysine Content of Grain, Endosperm, and Bran of Wheats from the USDA World Wheat Collection 1. *Crop. Sci.* **1976**, *16*, 655–660. [CrossRef]
24. Rakszegi, M.; Boros, D.; Kuti, C.; Láng, L.; Bedo, Z.; Shewry, P.R. Composition and End-Use Quality of 150 Wheat Lines Selected for the HEALTHGRAIN Diversity Screen. *J. Agric. Food Chem.* **2008**, *56*, 9750–9757. [CrossRef] [PubMed]
25. Shewry, P.R. Genetics of wheat gluten proteins. *Adv Genet.* **2003**, *49*, 111–184.
26. Philips, G.O. An introduction: Evolution and finalisation of the regulatory definition of dietary fibre. *Food Hydrocolloids* **2011**, *25*, 139–143. [CrossRef]
27. Official Journal of the European Union, 29 October 2008; L 285 (51): 9. Available online: https://eur-lex.europa.eu/legal-content/EN/TXT/PDF/?uri=OJ:L:2008:285:FULL&from=PL (accessed on 1 June 2021).
28. Official Journal of the European Union, 22 November 2011; L 304 (54): 18. Available online: https://eur-lex.europa.eu/legal-content/EN/TXT/PDF/?uri=OJ:L:2011:304:FULL&from=FR (accessed on 1 June 2021).
29. Jmares, D.; Stone, B. Studies on Wheat Endosperm I. Chemical Composition and Ultrastructure of the Cell Walls. *Aust. J. Biol. Sci.* **1973**, *26*, 793. [CrossRef]
30. Barron, C.; Surget, A.; Rouau, X. Relative amounts of tissues in mature wheat (Triticum aestivum L.) grain and their carbohydrate and phenolic acid composition. *J. Cereal Sci.* **2007**, *45*, 88–96. [CrossRef]
31. Stone, B. Carbohydrates. In *Wheat: Chemistry and Technology*, 4th ed.; Khan, K., Shewry, P.R., Eds.; AACC: St. Paul, MN, USA, 2009; pp. 299–362.
32. Laddomada, B.; Caretto, S.; Mita, G. Wheat Bran Phenolic Acids: Bioavailability and Stability in Whole Wheat-Based Foods. *Molecules* **2015**, *20*, 15666–15685. [CrossRef] [PubMed]
33. Anson, N.M.; Berg, R.V.D.; Havenaar, R.; Bast, A.; Haenen, G. Ferulic Acid from Aleurone Determines the Antioxidant Potency of Wheat Grain (Triticum aestivumL.). *J. Agric. Food Chem.* **2008**, *56*, 5589–5594. [CrossRef]
34. Adom, K.K.; Sorrells, A.M.E.; Liu, R.H. Phytochemicals and Antioxidant Activity of Milled Fractions of Different Wheat Varieties. *J. Agric. Food Chem.* **2005**, *53*, 2297–2306. [CrossRef]
35. Qu, H.; Madl, R.L.; Takemoto, D.J.; Baybutt, R.C.; Wang, W. Lignans Are Involved in the Antitumor Activity of Wheat Bran in Colon Cancer SW480 Cells. *J. Nutr.* **2005**, *135*, 598–602. [CrossRef]
36. Aune, D. Whole grain consumption and risk of cardiovascular disease, cancer, and all cause and cause specific mortality: Systematic review and dose-response meta-analysis of prospective studies. *Br. Med. J.* **2016**, *353*, i2716. [CrossRef]
37. American Heart Association. Whole Grains and Fiber. 2016. Available online: https://www.heart.org/en/healthy-living/healthy-eating/eat-smart/nutrition-basics/whole-grains-refined-grains-and-dietary-fiber (accessed on 1 June 2021).
38. Juntunen, K.S.; Laaksonen, D.; Autio, K.; Niskanen, L.K.; Holst, J.J.; Savolainen, K.; Liukkonen, K.-H.; Poutanen, K.S.; Mykkänen, H.M. Structural differences between rye and wheat breads but not total fiber content may explain the lower postprandial insulin response to rye bread. *Am. J. Clin. Nutr.* **2003**, *78*, 957–964. [CrossRef]
39. Nordlund, E.; Katina, K.; Mykkänen, H.; Poutanen, K. Distinct Characteristics of Rye and Wheat Breads Impact on Their in Vitro Gastric Disintegration and in Vivo Glucose and Insulin Responses. *Foods* **2016**, *5*, 24. [CrossRef] [PubMed]
40. Rojas-Bonzi, P.; Vangsøe, C.T.; Nielsen, K.L.; Lærke, H.N.; Hedemann, M.S.; Knudsen, K.E.B. The Relationship between In Vitro and In Vivo Starch Digestion Kinetics of Breads Varying in Dietary Fibre. *Foods* **2020**, *9*, 1337. [CrossRef]

41. Christensen, K.L.; Hedemann, M.S.; Lærke, H.N.; Jørgensen, H.; Mutt, S.J.; Herzig, K.-H.; Knudsen, K.E.B. Concentrated Arabinoxylan but Not Concentrated β-Glucan in Wheat Bread Has Similar Effects on Postprandial Insulin as Whole-Grain Rye in Porto-arterial Catheterized Pigs. *J. Agric. Food Chem.* **2013**, *61*, 7760–7768. [CrossRef]
42. Ruibal-Mendieta, N.L. Spelt (Triticum aestivum ssp. spelta) as a source of breadmaking flours and bran naturally en-riched in oleic acid and minerals but not phytic acid. *J. Agric. Food Chem.* **2005**, *53*, 2751–2759. [CrossRef] [PubMed]
43. Schober, T.J.; Bean, S.R.; Kuhn, M. Gluten proteins from spelt (Triticum aestivum ssp. spelta) cultivars: A rheological and size-exclusion high-performance liquid chromatography study. *J. Cereal Sci.* **2006**, *44*, 161–173. [CrossRef]
44. Gonzalez, J.T.; Stevenson, E.J. Postprandial glycemia and appetite sensations in response to porridge made with rolled and pinhead oats. *J. Am. Coll. Nutr.* **2012**, *31*, 111–116. [CrossRef]
45. Alyami, J.; Ladd, N.; Pritchard, S.E.; Hoad, C.; Sultan, A.A.; Spiller, R.C.; Gowland, P.A.; Macdonald, I.; Aithal, G.P.; Marciani, L.; et al. Glycaemic, gastrointestinal and appetite responses to breakfast porridges from ancient cereal grains: A MRI pilot study in healthy humans. *Food Res. Int.* **2019**, *118*, 49–57. [CrossRef]
46. Augustin, L.S.A.; Aas, A.-M.; Astrup, A.; Atkinson, F.S.; Baer-Sinnott, S.; Barclay, A.W.; Brand-Miller, J.C.; Brighenti, F.; Bullo, M.; Buyken, A.E.; et al. Dietary Fibre Consensus from the International Carbohydrate Quality Consortium (ICQC). *Nutrients* **2020**, *12*, 2553. [CrossRef]
47. Sievenpiper, J.L. Low-carbohydrate diets and cardiometabolic health: The importance of carbohydrate quality over quantity. *Nutr. Rev.* **2020**, *78*, 69–77. [CrossRef]
48. Tosh, S.M.; Bordenave, N. Emerging science on benefits of whole grain oat and barley and their soluble dietary fibers for heart health, glycemic response, and gut microbiota. *Nutr. Rev.* **2020**, *78*, 13–20. [CrossRef] [PubMed]
49. Bączek, N.; Jarmułowicz, A.; Wronkowska, M.; Haros, C.M. Assessment of the glycaemic index, content of bioactive compounds, and their in vitro bioaccessibility in oat-buckwheat breads. *Food Chem.* **2020**, *330*, 127199. [CrossRef] [PubMed]
50. Wolever, T.M.S.; Jones, P.J.H.; Jenkins, A.L.; Mollard, R.C.; Wang, H.; Johnston, A.; Johnson, J.; Chu, Y. Glycaemic and insulinaemic impact of oats soaked overnight in milk vs. cream of rice with and without sugar, nuts, and seeds: A randomized, controlled trial. *Eur. J. Clin. Nutr.* **2018**, *73*, 86–93. [CrossRef]
51. Åberg, S.; Mann, J.; Neumann, S.; Ross, A.B.; Reynolds, A.N. Whole-Grain Processing and Glycemic Control in Type 2 Diabetes: A Randomized Crossover Trial. *Diabetes Care* **2020**, *43*, 1717–1723. [CrossRef] [PubMed]
52. Whitehead, A.; Beck, E.J.; Tosh, S.; Wolever, T.M. Cholesterol-lowering effects of oat β-glucan: A meta-analysis of randomized controlled trials. *Am. J. Clin. Nutr.* **2014**, *100*, 1413–1421. [CrossRef]
53. Food Service Guidelines Federal Workgroup. *Food Service Guidelines for Federal Facilities*; U.S. Department of Health and Human Services: Washington, DC, USA, 2017.
54. *Guideline: Fortification of Rice with Vitamins and Minerals as a Public Health Strategy*; World Health Organization: Geneva, Switzerland, 2018; Licence: CC BY-NC-SA 3.0 IGO; ISBN 978-92-4-155029-1.
55. Bienvenido, O.J. *Rice in Human Nutrition*; Food and Agricultural Organization of the United Nations: Rome, Italy, 1993; ISSN 1014-3181.
56. Matsuda, T. Rice Flour: A Promising Food Material for Nutrition and Global Health. *J. Nutr. Sci. Vitaminol.* **2019**, *65*, S13–S17. [CrossRef]
57. FAO. *Food and Nutrition Paper 92. Dietary Protein Quality Evaluation in Human Nutrition*; Report of an FAO Expert Consultation; Food and Agricultural Organization of the United Nations: Rome, Italy, 2013; ISBN 9789251074176.
58. Herreman, L.; Nommensen, P.; Pennings, B.; Laus, M.C. Comprehensive overview of the quality of plant- and animal-sourced proteins based on the digestible indispensable amino acid score. *Food Sci. Nutr.* **2020**, *8*, 5379–5391. [CrossRef]
59. Sung-Wook, H. Nutritional quality of rice bran protein in comparison to animal and vegetable protein. *Food Chem.* **2015**, *172*, 766–769.
60. Barrera-Arellano, D.; Badan-Ribeiro, A.P.; Serna-Saldivar, S.O. Chapter 21—Corn Oil: Composition, Processing, and Utilization. *Corn*, 3rd ed.; AACC International Press: Washington, DC, USA, 2019; pp. 593–613. ISBN 9780128119716. [CrossRef]
61. Owen, R.; Giacosa, A.; Hull, W.; Haubner, R.; Spiegelhalder, B.; Bartsch, H. The antioxidant/anticancer potential of phenolic compounds isolated from olive oil. *Eur. J. Cancer* **2000**, *36*, 1235–1247. [CrossRef]
62. Perona, J.; Cabello-Moruno, R.; Ruiz-Gutiérrez, V. The role of virgin olive oil components in the modulation of endothelial function. *J. Nutr. Biochem.* **2006**, *17*, 429–445. [CrossRef] [PubMed]
63. Ouni, Y. Characterisation and quantification of phenolic compounds of extra-virgin olive oils according to their geo-graphical origin by a rapid and resolutive LC–ESI-TOF MS method. *Food Chem.* **2011**, *127*, 1263–1267. [CrossRef] [PubMed]
64. Vissers, M.N.; Zock, P.; Katan, M.B. Bioavailability and antioxidant effects of olive oil phenols in humans: A review. *Eur. J. Clin. Nutr.* **2004**, *58*, 955–965. [CrossRef] [PubMed]
65. Visioli, F.; Galli, C.; Bornet, F.; Mattei, A.; Patelli, R.; Galli, G.; Caruso, D. Olive oil phenolics are dose-dependently absorbed in humans. *FEBS Lett.* **2000**, *468*, 159–160. [CrossRef]
66. Mensink, R.P.; Katan, M.B. Effect of dietary fatty acids on serum lipids and lipoproteins. A meta-analysis of 27 trials. *Arter. Thromb. A J. Vasc. Biol.* **1992**, *12*, 911–919. [CrossRef]
67. Maki, K.C.; Lawless, A.L.; Kelley, K.M.; Kaden, V.N.; Geiger, C.J.; Palacios, O.M.; Dicklin, M.R. Corn oil intake favorably impacts lipoprotein cholesterol, apolipoprotein and lipoprotein particle levels compared with extra-virgin olive oil. *Eur. J. Clin. Nutr.* **2016**, *71*, 33–38. [CrossRef] [PubMed]

68. Hu, F.B.; Stampfer, M.J.; Manson, J.E.; Rimm, E.; Colditz, G.; Rosner, B.A.; Hennekens, C.H.; Willett, W.C. Dietary Fat Intake and the Risk of Coronary Heart Disease in Women. *N. Engl. J. Med.* **1997**, *337*, 1491–1499. [CrossRef]
69. Willett, W.C. Dietary fats and coronary heart disease. *J. Intern. Med.* **2012**, *272*, 13–24. [CrossRef]
70. Jakobsen, M.U.; O'Reilly, E.J.; Heitmann, B.L.; Pereira, M.; Bälter, K.; Fraser, G.; Goldbourt, U.; Hallmans, G.; Knekt, P.; Liu, S.; et al. Major types of dietary fat and risk of coronary heart disease: A pooled analysis of 11 cohort studies. *Am. J. Clin. Nutr.* **2009**, *89*, 1425–1432. [CrossRef]
71. Lai, H.; Otto, M.C.D.O.; Lee, Y.; Wu, J.; Song, X.; King, I.B.; Psaty, B.M.; Lemaitre, R.N.; McKnight, B.; Siscovick, D.S.; et al. Serial Plasma Phospholipid Fatty Acids in the De Novo Lipogenesis Pathway and Total Mortality, Cause-Specific Mortality, and Cardiovascular Diseases in the Cardiovascular Health Study. *J. Am. Heart Assoc.* **2019**, *8*, e012881. [CrossRef] [PubMed]
72. Fried, L.P.; Borhani, N.O.; Enright, P.; Furberg, C.D.; Gardin, J.M.; Kronmal, R.A.; Kuller, L.H.; Manolio, T.A.; Mittelmark, M.B.; Newman, A.B.; et al. The cardiovascular health study: Design and rationale. *Ann. Epidemiol.* **1991**, *1*, 263–276. [CrossRef]
73. Borges, M.C. Circulating Fatty Acids and Risk of Coronary Heart Disease and Stroke: Individual Participant Data Me-ta-Analysis in Up to 16 126 Participants. *J. Am. Heart Assoc.* **2020**, *9*, e013131. [CrossRef]
74. Lee, Y. Serial Biomarkers of De Novo Lipogenesis Fatty Acids and Incident Heart Failure in Older Adults: The Cardio-vascular Health Study. *J. Am. Heart Assoc.* **2020**, *9*, e014119. [CrossRef]
75. Fincher, G.B. Morphology and Chemical Composition of Barley Endosperm Cell Walls. *J. Inst. Brew.* **1975**, *81*, 116–122. [CrossRef]
76. Garcia-Gimenez, G. Barley grain (1,3;1,4)-β-glucan content: Effects of transcript and sequence variation in genes encod-ing the corresponding synthase and endohydrolase enzymes. *Sci. Rep.* **2019**, *9*, 17250. [CrossRef] [PubMed]
77. AbuMweis, S.S. b-glucan from barley and its lipid-lowering capacity: A meta-analysis of randomized, controlled trials. *Eur. J. Clin. Nutr.* **2010**, *64*, 1472–1480. [CrossRef]
78. Ho, H.V.T. A systematic review and meta-analysis of randomized controlled trials of the effect of barley β-glucan on LDL-C, non-HDL-C and apoB for cardiovascular disease risk reduction i-iv. *Eur. J. Clin. Nutr.* **2016**, *70*, 1239–1245. [CrossRef]
79. Hui, S.; Liu, K.; Lang, H.; Liu, Y.; Wang, X.; Zhu, X.; Doucette, S.; Yi, L.; Mi, M. Comparative effects of different whole grains and brans on blood lipid: A network meta-analysis. *Eur. J. Nutr.* **2019**, *58*, 2779–2787. [CrossRef]
80. EFSA NDA Panel (EFSA Panel on Nutrition, Novel Foods and Food Allergen). *Beta-glucans from oats and/or bar-ley in a ready-to-eat cereal manufactured via pressure cooking and reduction of blood-glucose rise after consumption: Evaluation of a health claim pursuant to Article 13(5) of Regulation (EC) No 1924/2006. EFSA J.* **2021**, *19*, e06493.
81. Malunga, L.N.; Ames, N.; Zhouyao, H.; Blewett, H.; Thandapilly, S.J. Beta-Glucan From Barley Attenuates Post-prandial Glycemic Response by Inhibiting the Activities of Glucose Transporters but Not Intestinal Brush Border Enzymes and Amylolysis of Starch. *Front. Nutr.* **2021**, *8*. [CrossRef] [PubMed]
82. Henrion, M.; Francey, C.; Lê, K.-A.; Lamothe, L. Cereal B-Glucans: The Impact of Processing and How It Affects Physiological Responses. *Nutrients* **2019**, *11*, 1729. [CrossRef]
83. Shimizu, C.; Wakita, Y.; Kihara, M.; Kobayashi, N.; Tsuchiya, Y.; Nabeshima, T. Association of Lifelong Intake of Barley Diet with Healthy Aging: Changes in Physical and Cognitive Functions and Intestinal Microbiome in Senescence-Accelerated Mouse-Prone 8 (SAMP8). *Nutrients* **2019**, *11*, 1770. [CrossRef] [PubMed]
84. Mozaffarian, D.; Appel, L.J.; Van Horn, L. Components of a Cardioprotective Diet. *Circulation* **2011**, *123*, 2870–2891. [CrossRef]
85. Pour Fard, N.R.; Amirabdollahian, F.; Haghighatdoost, F. Dietary patterns and frailty: A systematic review and meta-analysis. *Nutr. Rev.* **2019**, *77*, 498–513. [CrossRef]
86. Lo, Y.-L.; Hsieh, Y.-T.; Hsu, L.-L.; Chuang, S.-Y.; Chang, H.-Y.; Hsu, C.-C.; Chen, C.-Y.; Pan, W.-H. Dietary Pattern Associated with Frailty: Results from Nutrition and Health Survey in Taiwan. *J. Am. Geriatr. Soc.* **2017**, *65*, 2009–2015. [CrossRef]
87. Trichopoulou, A.; Kouris-Blazos, A.; Wahlqvist, M.L.; Gnardellis, C.; Lagiou, P.; Polychronopoulos, E.; Vassilakou, T.; Lipworth, L.; Trichopoulos, D. Diet and overall survival in elderly people. *BMJ* **1995**, *311*, 1457–1460. [CrossRef] [PubMed]
88. Martinez-Gonzalez, M.A.; Corella, D.; Salas-Salvadó, J.; Ros, E.; Covas, M.I.; Fiol, M.; Wärnberg, J.; Arós, F.; Ruíz-Gutiérrez, V.; Lamuela-Raventos, R.M.; et al. Cohort Profile: Design and methods of the PREDIMED study. *Int. J. Epidemiol.* **2010**, *41*, 377–385. [CrossRef] [PubMed]
89. Kromhout, D.; Menotti, A.; Alberti-Fidanza, A.; Puddu, P.E.; Hollman, P.; Kafatos, A.; Tolonen, H.; Adachi, H.; Jacobs, D.R. Comparative ecologic relationships of saturated fat, sucrose, food groups, and a Mediterranean food pattern score to 50-year coronary heart disease mortality rates among 16 cohorts of the Seven Countries Study. *Eur. J. Clin. Nutr.* **2018**, *72*, 1103–1110. [CrossRef]
90. Zaslavsky, O.; Zelber-Sagi, S.; Shikany, J.M.; Orchard, T.; Wallace, R.; Snetselaar, L.; Tinker, L. Anatomy of the Mediterranean Diet and Mortality Among Older Women with Frailty. *J. Nutr. Gerontol. Geriatr.* **2018**, *37*, 269–281. [CrossRef] [PubMed]
91. TWHI Study. Design of the Women's Health Initiative clinical trial and observational study. *Control. Clin. Trials* **1998**, *19*, 61–109. [CrossRef]
92. Hays, J. The Women's Health Initiative recruit-ment methods and results. *Ann. Epidemiol.* **2003**, *13* (Suppl. S9), S18–S77. [CrossRef]
93. Fried, L.P.; Tangen, C.M.; Walston, J.; Newman, A.B.; Hirsch, C.; Gottdiener, J.; Seeman, T.; Tracy, R.; Kop, W.J.; Burke, G.; et al. Frailty in Older Adults: Evidence for a Phenotype. *J. Gerontol. Ser. A Biol. Sco. Med.Sci.* **2001**, *56*, M146–M157. [CrossRef]
94. Fung, T.T.; Rexrode, K.; Mantzoros, C.S.; Manson, J.E.; Willett, W.C.; Hu, F.B. Mediterranean Diet and Incidence of and Mortality From Coronary Heart Disease and Stroke in Women. *Circulation* **2009**, *119*, 1093–1100. [CrossRef] [PubMed]

95. Campanella, A. The effect of the Mediterranean Diet on lifespan. A treatment-effect survival analysis of a popula-tion-based prospective cohort study in Southern Italy. *Int. J. Epidemiol.* **2021**, *50*, 245–255. [CrossRef]
96. Attili, A.F.; Carulli, N.; Roda, E.; Barbara, B.; Capocaccia, L.; Menotti, A.; Okoliksanyi, L.; Ricci, G.; Festi, D.; Lalloni, L.; et al. Epidemiology of Gallstone Disease in Italy: Prevalence Data of the Multicenter Italian Study on Cholelithiasis (M.I.COL.). *Am. J. Epidemiol.* **1995**, *141*, 158–165. [CrossRef]
97. Cozzolongo, R.; Osella, A.; Elba, S.; Petruzzi, J.; Buongiorno, G.; Giannuzzi, V.; Leone, G.; Bonfiglio, C.; Lanzilotta, E.; Manghisi, O.G.; et al. Epidemiology of HCV Infection in the General Population: A Survey in a Southern Italian Town. *Am. J. Gastroenterol.* **2009**, *104*, 2740–2746. [CrossRef]
98. Buckland, G.; González, C.A.; Agudo, A.; Vilardell, M.; Berenguer, A.; Amiano, P.; Ardanaz, E.; Arriola, L.; Barricarte, A.; Basterretxea, M.; et al. Adherence to the Mediterranean Diet and Risk of Coronary Heart Disease in the Spanish EPIC Cohort Study. *Am. J. Epidemiol.* **2009**, *170*, 1518–1529. [CrossRef]
99. Tosti, V.; Bertozzi, B.; Fontana, L. Health Benefits of the Mediterranean Diet: Metabolic and Molecular Mechanisms. *J. Gerontol. A Biol. Sci. Med. Sci.* **2018**, *73*, 318–326. [CrossRef]
100. Hernaez, A. Increased Consumption of Virgin Olive Oil, Nuts, Legumes, Whole Grains, and Fish Promotes HDL Func-tions in Humans. *Mol. Nutr. Food Res.* **2019**, *63*, e1800847. [CrossRef]
101. van der Kamp, J.W. The HEALTHGRAIN definition of 'whole grain'. *Food Nutr. Res.* **2014**, *58*, 22100. [CrossRef]
102. Maras, J.E.; Newby, P.; Bakun, P.J.; Ferrucci, L.; Tucker, K.L. Whole grain intake: The Baltimore Longitudinal Study of Aging. *J. Food Compos. Anal.* **2009**, *22*, 53–58. [CrossRef]
103. Shock, N. *Normal Human Aging: The Baltimore Longitudinal Study of Aging*; US Government Printing Office: Washington, DC, USA, 1984; NIH Publication No. 84-2450.
104. Sette, S.; D'Addezio, L.; Piccinelli, R.; Hopkins, S.; Le Donne, C.; Ferrari, M.; Mistura, L.; Turrini, A. Intakes of whole grain in an Italian sample of children, adolescents and adults. *Eur. J. Nutr.* **2015**, *56*, 521–533. [CrossRef]
105. Ruggiero, E.; Bonaccio, M.; Di Castelnuovo, A.; Bonanni, A.; Costanzo, S.; Persichillo, M.; Bracone, F.; Cerletti, C.; Donati, M.B.; de Gaetano, G.; et al. Consumption of whole grain food and its determinants in a general Italian population: Results from the INHES study. *Nutr. Metab. Cardiovasc. Dis.* **2019**, *29*, 611–620. [CrossRef] [PubMed]
106. Seal, C.; Brownlee, I. Whole-grain foods and chronic disease: Evidence from epidemiological and intervention studies. *Proc. Nutr. Soc.* **2015**, *74*, 313–319. [CrossRef] [PubMed]
107. Costabile, A.; Klinder, A.; Fava, F.; Napolitano, A.; Fogliano, V.; Leonard, C.; Gibson, G.R.; Tuohy, K. Whole-grain wheat breakfast cereal has a prebiotic effect on the human gut microbiota: A double-blind, placebo-controlled, crossover study. *Br. J. Nutr.* **2007**, *99*, 110–120. [CrossRef] [PubMed]
108. Giacco, R. Effects of the regular consumption of wholemeal wheat foods on cardiovascular risk factors in healthy peo-ple. *Nutr. Metab. Cardiovasc. Dis.* **2010**, *20*, 186–194. [CrossRef] [PubMed]
109. Juntunen, K.S.; Laaksonen, D.; Poutanen, K.S.; Niskanen, L.K.; Mykkänen, H.M. High-fiber rye bread and insulin secretion and sensitivity in healthy postmenopausal women. *Am. J. Clin. Nutr.* **2003**, *77*, 385–391. [CrossRef] [PubMed]
110. Kelly, S.; Hartley, L.; Loveman, E.; Colquitt, J.L.; Jones, H.M.; Al-Khudairy, L.; Clar, C.; Germanò, R.; Lunn, H.R.; Frost, G.; et al. Whole grain cereals for the primary or secondary prevention of cardiovascular disease. *Cochrane Database Syst. Rev.* **2017**, *8*, CD005051. [CrossRef] [PubMed]
111. Kirwan, J.P.; Malin, S.; Scelsi, A.R.; Kullman, E.L.; Navaneethan, S.D.; Pagadala, M.R.; Haus, J.; Filion, J.; Godin, J.-P.; Kochkar, S.; et al. A Whole-Grain Diet Reduces Cardiovascular Risk Factors in Overweight and Obese Adults: A Randomized Controlled Trial. *J. Nutr.* **2016**, *146*, 2244–2251. [CrossRef] [PubMed]
112. Marventano, S. Whole Grain Intake and Glycaemic Control in Healthy Subjects: A Systematic Review and Me-ta-Analysis of Randomized Controlled Trials. *Nutrients* **2017**, *9*, 769. [CrossRef]
113. Canfora, E.; Jocken, J.W.; Blaak, E.E. Short-chain fatty acids in control of body weight and insulin sensitivity. *Nat. Rev. Endocrinol.* **2015**, *11*, 577–591. [CrossRef]
114. Musa-Veloso, K. The effects of whole-grain compared with refined wheat, rice, and rye on the postprandial blood glu-cose response: A systematic review and meta-analysis of randomized controlled trials. *Am. J. Clin. Nutr.* **2018**, *108*, 759–774. [CrossRef]
115. Kirø, C. Higher Whole-Grain Intake Is Associated with Lower Risk of Type 2 Diabetes among Middle-Aged Men and Women: The Danish Diet, Cancer, and Health Cohort. *J. Nutr.* **2018**, *148*, 1434–1444. [CrossRef]
116. Tjønneland, A.; Olsen, A.; Boll, K.; Stripp, C.; Christensen, J.; Engholm, G.; Overvad, K. Study design, exposure variables, and socioeconomic determinants of participation in Diet, Cancer and Health: A population-based prospective cohort study of 57,053 men and women in Denmark. *Scand. J. Public Health* **2007**, *35*, 432–441. [CrossRef]
117. Maki, K.C.; Palacios, O.M.; Koecher, K.; Sawicki, C.M.; Livingston, K.A.; Bell, M.; Cortes, H.N.; McKeown, N.M. The Relationship between Whole Grain Intake and Body Weight: Results of Meta-Analyses of Observational Studies and Randomized Controlled Trials. *Nutrients* **2019**, *11*, 1245. [CrossRef]
118. Ma, X.; Tang, W.-G.; Yang, Y.; Zhang, Q.-L.; Zheng, J.; Xiang, Y.-B. Association between whole grain intake and all-cause mortality: A meta-analysis of cohort studies. *Oncotarget* **2016**, *7*, 61996–62005. [CrossRef] [PubMed]
119. Zong, G. Whole Grain Intake and Mortality From All Causes, Cardiovascular Disease, and Cancer: A Meta-Analysis of Prospective Cohort Studies. *Circulation* **2016**, *133*, 2370–2380. [CrossRef]

120. Wei, H.; Gao, Z.; Liang, R.; Li, Z.; Hao, H.; Liu, X. Whole-grain consumption and the risk of all-cause, CVD and cancer mortality: A meta-analysis of prospective cohort studies. *Br. J. Nutr.* **2016**, *116*, 514–525. [CrossRef]
121. Benisi-Kohansal, S. Whole-Grain Intake and Mortality from All Causes, Cardiovascular Disease, and Cancer: A Sys-tematic Review and Dose-Response Meta-Analysis of Prospective Cohort Studies. *Adv. Nutr.* **2016**, *7*, 1052–1065. [CrossRef] [PubMed]
122. Zhang, B.; Zhao, Q.; Guo, W.; Bao, W.; Wang, X. Association of whole grain intake with all-cause, cardiovascular, and cancer mortality: A systematic review and dose–response meta-analysis from prospective cohort studies. *Eur. J. Clin. Nutr.* **2018**, *72*, 57–65. [CrossRef]
123. Ekmekcioglu, C. Nutrition and longevity—From mechanisms to uncertainties. *Crit. Rev. Food Sci. Nutr.* **2019**, *60*, 3063–3082. [CrossRef]
124. McKeown, N.M.; Livingston, K.; Sawicki, C.M.; Miller, K.B. Evidence mapping to assess the available research on fiber, whole grains, and health. *Nutr. Rev.* **2020**, *78*, 37–42. [CrossRef]
125. Gopinath, B.; Flood, V.M.; Kifley, A.; Louie, J.C.Y.; Mitchell, P. Association Between Carbohydrate Nutrition and Successful Aging Over 10 Years. *J. Gerontol. Ser. A Boil. Sci. Med. Sci.* **2016**, *71*, 1335–1340. [CrossRef] [PubMed]
126. Attebo, K.; Mitchell, P.; Smith, W. Visual Acuity and the Causes of Visual Loss in Australia. *Ophthalmology* **1996**, *103*, 357–364. [CrossRef]
127. Foscolou, A. The Association between Whole Grain Products Consumption and Successful Aging: A Combined Analysis of MEDIS and ATTICA Epidemiological Studies. *Nutrients* **2019**, *11*, 1221. [CrossRef] [PubMed]
128. Panagiotakos, D.B. Ten-year (2002–2012) cardiovascular disease incidence and all-cause mortality, in urban Greek population: The ATTICA Study. *Int. J. Cardiol.* **2015**, *180*, 178–184. [CrossRef]
129. Tyrovolas, S. Successful aging, dietary habits, and health status of elderly individuals: A k-dimensional approach within the multi-national MEDIS study. *Exp. Gerontol.* **2014**, *60*, 57–63. [CrossRef]
130. Fontana, L.; Kennedy, B.; Longo, V.D.; Seals, D.; Melov, S. Medical research: Treat ageing. *Nat. Cell Biol.* **2014**, *511*, 405–407. [CrossRef]
131. Goldman, D.P. Substantial health and economic returns from delayed aging may warrant a new focus for medical research. *Health Aff.* **2013**, *32*, 1698–1705. [CrossRef] [PubMed]
132. Longo, V.D.; Antebi, A.; Bartke, A.; Barzilai, N.; Brown-Borg, H.M.; Caruso, C.; Curiel, T.J.; de Cabo, R.; Franceschi, C.; Gems, D.; et al. Interventions to Slow Aging in Humans: Are We Ready? *Aging Cell* **2015**, *14*, 497–510. [CrossRef] [PubMed]
133. Fontana, L.; Partridge, L. Promoting Health and Longevity through Diet: From Model Organisms to Humans. *Cell* **2015**, *161*, 106–118. [CrossRef] [PubMed]
134. Solon-Biet, S.M.; Mitchell, S.J.; de Cabo, R.; Raubenheimer, D.; Le Couteur, D.; Simpson, S.J. Macronutrients and caloric intake in health and longevity. *J. Endocrinol.* **2015**, *226*, R17–R28. [CrossRef]
135. Weindruch, R.; Sohal, R.S. Caloric Intake and Aging. *N. Engl. J. Med.* **1997**, *337*, 986–994. [CrossRef]
136. Heilbronn, L.K. Effect of 6-month calorie restriction on biomarkers of longevity, metabolic adaptation, and oxidative stress in overweight individuals: A randomized controlled trial. *JAMA* **2006**, *295*, 1539–1548. [CrossRef] [PubMed]
137. Fontana, L.; Partridge, L.; Longo, V.D. Extending Healthy Life Span–From Yeast to Humans. *Science* **2010**, *328*, 321–326. [CrossRef]
138. Heilbronn, L.K. Alternate-day fasting in nonobese subjects: Effects on body weight, body composition, and energy metabolism. *Am. J. Clin. Nutr.* **2005**, *81*, 69–73. [CrossRef]
139. Harvie, M.N.; Pegington, M.; Mattson, M.P.; Frystyk, J.; Dillon, B.; Evans, G.; Cuzick, J.; Jebb, S.; Martin, B.; Cutler, R.G.; et al. The effects of intermittent or continuous energy restriction on weight loss and metabolic disease risk markers: A randomized trial in young overweight women. *Int. J. Obes.* **2010**, *35*, 714–727. [CrossRef] [PubMed]
140. Most, J.; Tosti, V.; Redman, L.M.; Fontana, L. Calorie restriction in humans: An update. *Ageing Res. Rev.* **2017**, *39*, 36–45. [CrossRef] [PubMed]
141. de Cabo, R. Effects of Intermittent Fasting on Health, Aging, and Disease. *N. Engl. J. Med.* **2019**, *381*, 2541–2551. [CrossRef]
142. Stanfel, M.N. The TOR pathway comes of age. *Biochim. Biophys. Acta* **2009**, *1790*, 1067–1074. [CrossRef]
143. Zimmerman, J. Nutritional control of aging. *Exp. Gerontol.* **2003**, *38*, 47–52. [CrossRef]
144. Mair, W.; Morantte, I.; Rodrigues, A.P.C.; Manning, G.; Montminy, M.; Shaw, R.J.; Dillin, A. Lifespan extension induced by AMPK and calcineurin is mediated by CRTC-1 and CREB. *Nat. Cell Biol.* **2011**, *470*, 404–408. [CrossRef] [PubMed]
145. Solon-Biet, S.M.; McMahon, A.C.; Ballard, J.W.O.; Ruohonen, K.; Wu, L.E.; Cogger, V.C.; Warren, A.; Huang, X.; Pichaud, N.; Melvin, R.; et al. The Ratio of Macronutrients, Not Caloric Intake, Dictates Cardiometabolic Health, Aging, and Longevity in Ad Libitum-Fed Mice. *Cell Metab.* **2020**, *31*, 654. [CrossRef]
146. Fontana, L. The science of nutritional modulation of aging. *Ageing Res. Rev.* **2017**, *39*, 1–2. [CrossRef]
147. Simpson, S.J.; Le Couteur, D.G.; James, D.; George, J.; Gunton, J.E.; Solon-Biet, S.; Raubenheimer, D. The Geometric Framework for Nutrition as a tool in precision medicine. *Nutr. Health Aging* **2017**, *4*, 217–226. [CrossRef]
148. Raubenheimer, D.; Simpson, S.J.; Le Couteur, D.; Solon-Biet, S.; Coogan, S.C. Nutritional ecology and the evolution of aging. *Exp. Gerontol.* **2016**, *86*, 50–61. [CrossRef]
149. Lee, K.P.; Simpson, S.J.; Clissold, F.J.; Brooks, R.; Ballard, J.W.O.; Taylor, P.W.; Soran, N.; Raubenheimer, D. Lifespan and reproduction in Drosophila: New insights from nutritional geometry. *Proc. Natl. Acad. Sci. USA* **2008**, *105*, 2498–2503. [CrossRef]
150. Archer, C.R.; Royle, N.; South, S.; Selman, C.; Hunt, J. Nutritional Geometry Provides Food for Thought. *J. Gerontol. Ser. A Boil. Sci. Med. Sci.* **2009**, *64*, 956–959. [CrossRef]

151. Duffield, K.R. Macronutrient intake and simulated infection threat independently affect life history traits of male deco-rated crickets. *Ecol. Evol.* **2020**, *10*, 11766–11778. [CrossRef] [PubMed]
152. Moatt, J.P.; Fyfe, M.A.; Heap, E.; Mitchell, L.J.M.; Moon, F.; Walling, C.A. Reconciling nutritional geometry with classical dietary restriction: Effects of nutrient intake, not calories, on survival and reproduction. *Aging Cell* **2019**, *18*, e12868. [CrossRef] [PubMed]
153. Gibbs, V.K.; Smith, D.L. Nutrition and energetics in rodent longevity research. *Exp. Gerontol.* **2016**, *86*, 90–96. [CrossRef] [PubMed]
154. Senior, A.M.; Solon-Biet, S.M.; Cogger, V.C.; Le Couteur, D.G.; Nakagawa, S.; Raubenheimer, D.; Simpson, S.J. Dietary macronutrient content, age-specific mortality and lifespan. *Proc. R. Soc. B Boil. Sci.* **2019**, *286*, 20190393. [CrossRef] [PubMed]
155. Wali, J.A. Cardio-metabolic consequences of dietary carbohydrates: Reconciling contradictions using nutritional geometry. *Cardiovasc. Res.* **2021**, *117*, 386–401. [CrossRef] [PubMed]
156. Pedersen, A.N.; Kondrup, J.; Børsheim, E. Health effects of protein intake in healthy adults: A systematic literature review. *Food Nutr. Res.* **2013**, *57*, 57. [CrossRef] [PubMed]
157. Lee, D.; Son, H.G.; Jung, Y.; Lee, S.-J.V. The role of dietary carbohydrates in organismal aging. *Cell. Mol. Life Sci.* **2016**, *74*, 1793–1803. [CrossRef]
158. Seidelmann, S.B.; Claggett, B.; Cheng, S.; Henglin, M.; Shah, A.; Steffen, L.M.; Folsom, A.R.; Rimm, E.B.; Willett, W.C.; Solomon, S.D. Dietary carbohydrate intake and mortality: A prospective cohort study and meta-analysis. *Lancet Public Health* **2018**, *3*, e419–e428. [CrossRef]
159. Simpson, S.J.; Le Couteur, D.; Raubenheimer, D.; Solon-Biet, S.; Cooney, G.J.; Cogger, V.C.; Fontana, L. Dietary protein, aging and nutritional geometry. *Ageing Res. Rev.* **2017**, *39*, 78–86. [CrossRef]
160. Le Couteur, D.G. The impact of low-protein high-carbohydrate diets on aging and lifespan. *Cell. Mol. Life Sci.* **2016**, *73*, 1237–1252. [CrossRef] [PubMed]
161. Dehghan, M.; Mente, A.; Zhang, X.; Swaminathan, S.; Li, W.; Mohan, V.; Iqbal, R.; Kumar, R.; Wentzel-Viljoen, E.; Rosengren, A.; et al. Associations of fats and carbohydrate intake with cardiovascular disease and mortality in 18 countries from five continents (PURE): A prospective cohort study. *Lancet* **2017**, *390*, 2050–2062. [CrossRef]
162. Miller, V. Fruit, vegetable, and legume intake, and cardiovascular disease and deaths in 18 countries (PURE): A prospective cohort study. *Lancet* **2017**, *390*, 2037–2049. [CrossRef]
163. Ramsden, C.; Domenichiello, A.F. PURE study challenges the definition of a healthy diet: But key questions remain. *Lancet* **2017**, *390*, 2018–2019. [CrossRef]
164. Wali, J.A.; Milner, A.J.; Luk, A.W.S.; Pulpitel, T.J.; Dodgson, T.; Facey, H.J.W.; Wahl, D.; Kebede, M.A.; Senior, A.M.; Sullivan, M.A.; et al. Impact of dietary carbohydrate type and protein–carbohydrate interaction on metabolic health. *Nat. Metab.* **2021**, *3*, 810–828. [CrossRef] [PubMed]
165. Murray, C.J.L. The state of US health, 1990–2010: Burden of diseases, injuries, and risk factors. *JAMA* **2013**, *310*, 591–608. [CrossRef] [PubMed]
166. Ford, D.W. Association between dietary quality and mortality in older adults: A review of the epidemiological evi-dence. *J. Nutr. Gerontol. Geriatr.* **2013**, *32*, 85–105. [CrossRef]
167. Swaminathan, S.; Dehghan, M.; Raj, J.M.; Thomas, T.; Rangarajan, S.; Jenkins, D.; Mony, P.; Mohan, V.; Lear, S.; Avezum, A.; et al. Associations of cereal grains intake with cardiovascular disease and mortality across 21 countries in Prospective Urban and Rural Epidemiology study: Prospective cohort study. *BMJ* **2021**, *372*, m4948. [CrossRef]
168. Masala, G.; Ceroti, M.; Pala, V.; Krogh, V.; Vineis, P.; Sacerdote, C.; Saieva, C.; Salvini, S.; Sieri, S.; Berrino, F.; et al. A dietary pattern rich in olive oil and raw vegetables is associated with lower mortality in Italian elderly subjects. *Br. J. Nutr.* **2007**, *98*, 406–415. [CrossRef]
169. Carballo-Casla, A.; Ortolá, R.; García-Esquinas, E.; Oliveira, A.; Sotos-Prieto, M.; Lopes, C.; Lopez-Garcia, E.; Rodríguez-Artalejo, F. The Southern European Atlantic Diet and all-cause mortality in older adults. *BMC Med.* **2021**, *19*, 1–11. [CrossRef] [PubMed]
170. Kennedy, E.T. Evidence for nutritional benefits in prolonging wellness. *Am. J. Clin. Nutr.* **2006**, *83*, 410S–414S. [CrossRef]
171. Tessa, J. Physical frailty in older men: Prospective associations with diet quality and patterns. *Age Ageing* **2019**, *48*, 355–360.
172. Le Couteur, D.G. New Horizons: Dietary protein, ageing and the Okinawan ratio. *Age Ageing* **2016**, *45*, 443–447. [CrossRef] [PubMed]
173. Mirzaei, H.; Suarez, J.A.; Longo, V.D. Protein and amino acid restriction, aging and disease: From yeast to humans. *Trends Endocrinol. Metab.* **2014**, *25*, 558–566. [CrossRef]
174. Willcox, D.C.; Willcox, B.J.; Hsueh, W.-C.; Suzuki, M. Genetic determinants of exceptional human longevity: Insights from the Okinawa Centenarian Study. *AGE* **2006**, *28*, 313–332. [CrossRef]
175. Pes, G.M.; Tolu, F.; Dore, M.P.; Sechi, G.P.; Errigo, A.; Canelada, A.; Poulain, M. Male longevity in Sardinia, a review of historical sources supporting a causal link with dietary factors. *Eur. J. Clin. Nutr.* **2014**, *69*, 411–418. [CrossRef]
176. Willcox, B.J.; Willcox, D.C.; Todoriki, H.; Fujiyoshi, A.; Yano, K.; He, Q.; Curb, J.D.; Suzuki, M. Caloric Restriction, the Traditional Okinawan Diet, and Healthy Aging: The Diet of the World's Longest-Lived People and Its Potential Impact on Morbidity and Life Span. *Ann. N. Y. Acad. Sci.* **2007**, *1114*, 434–455. [CrossRef]
177. Maioli, M. Sourdough-leavened bread improves postprandial glucose and insulin plasma levels in subjects with im-paired glucose tolerance. *Acta Diabetol.* **2008**, *45*, 91–96. [CrossRef]
178. Capurso, C.; Bellanti, F.; Buglio, A.L.; Vendemiale, G. The Mediterranean Diet Slows Down the Progression of Aging and Helps to Prevent the Onset of Frailty: A Narrative Review. *Nutrients* **2020**, *12*, 35. [CrossRef] [PubMed]

179. Voelker, R. The Mediterranean Diet's Fight against Frailty. *JAMA* **2018**, *319*, 1971. [CrossRef] [PubMed]
180. Bach-Faig, A.; Berry, E.M.; Lairon, D.; Reguant, J.; Trichopoulou, A.; Dernini, S.; Medina, F.X.; Battino, M.; Belahsen, R.; Miranda, G.; et al. Mediterranean diet pyramid today. Science and cultural updates. *Public Health Nutr.* **2011**, *14*, 2274–2284. [CrossRef]
181. McKeown, T. *The Role of Medicine: Dream, Mirage or Nemesis*; Blackwell: Oxford, UK, 1979.
182. Bunker, J.P. The role of medical care in contributing to health improvements within societies. *Int. J. Epidemiol.* **2001**, *30*, 1260–1263. [CrossRef] [PubMed]
183. Borneo, R.; León, A.E. Whole grain cereals: Functional components and health benefits. *Food Funct.* **2012**, *3*, 110–119. [CrossRef] [PubMed]

MDPI
St. Alban-Anlage 66
4052 Basel
Switzerland
Tel. +41 61 683 77 34
Fax +41 61 302 89 18
www.mdpi.com

Nutrients Editorial Office
E-mail: nutrients@mdpi.com
www.mdpi.com/journal/nutrients

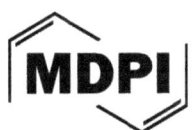

www.ingramcontent.com/pod-product-compliance
Lightning Source LLC
LaVergne TN
LVHW070431100526
838202LV00014B/1577